Advances in Pattern Recognition

For futher volumes:
http://www.springer.com/series/4205

Gabor T. Herman

Fundamentals of Computerized Tomography

Image Reconstruction from Projections

Second Edition

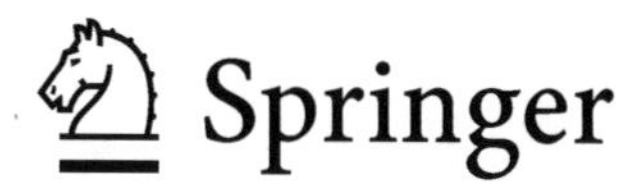

Prof. Gabor T. Herman
City University of New York
Graduate Center
Dept. Computer Science
365 Fifth Avenue
New York NY 10016
USA
gabortherman@yahoo.com

Series editor
Professor Sameer Singh, PhD
Research School of Informatics
Loughborough University
Loughborough, UK

ISSN 1617-7916
ISBN 978-1-4471-2521-1 e-ISBN 978-1-84628-723-7
DOI 10.1007/978-1-84628-723-7
Springer Dordrecht Heidelberg London New York

British Library Cataloguing in Publication Data
A catalogue record for this book is available from the British Library

Printed on acid-free paper

Springer is part of Springer Science+Business Media (www.springer.com)

Preface

Overview and Goals

The problem of image reconstruction from projections has arisen independently in a large number of scientific fields. An important version of the problem in medicine is that of obtaining the density distribution within the human body from multiple x-ray projections. This process is referred to as computerized tomography; it has revolutionized diagnostic radiology over the past three decades. The 1979 Nobel prize in physiology and medicine was awarded to Allan M. Cormack and Godfrey N. Hounsfield for the development of computerized tomography. The 1982 Nobel prize in chemistry was awarded to Aaron Klug, one of the pioneers in the use of reconstruction from electron microscopic projections for the purpose of elucidation of biologically important molecular complexes. The 2003 Nobel prize in physiology and medicine was awarded to Paul C. Lauterbur and Peter Mansfield for their discoveries concerning magnetic resonance imaging, which also included the use of image reconstruction from projections methods.

The author began to work in the field of image reconstruction from projections about 40 years ago. At that time there were only a handful of publications on the topic, published in journals serving diverse fields. Even in 1977, when serious writing of the first edition of this book began, it seemed feasible that the field could be surveyed thoroughly in less than 400 pages. Research progressed faster than the author could write, and by the time the first edition of the book appeared in 1980, it could only be described as an introductory text to what had surely been one of the most explosive and exciting interdisciplinary developments in the history of science.

The first edition has been widely used, as evidenced for example by the over fifteen hundred references to it in the research literature. The revised edition has been prepared so as to maintain the usefulness of the original by bringing its contents in line with the achievements of the last quarter of a century.

This second edition follows closely the structure of the first edition, but it is a painstaking update in the sense that all illustrations and reports on computational experiments and issues are replaced by what is the state of the art at the time of writing the revision. In addition, in those places where progress in the field made the material in the first edition out of date, the currently cutting-edge version completely replaces the old one. Some entirely new topics are introduced; these include the fast calculation of a ray sum for a digitized picture, the task-oriented comparison of reconstruction algorithm performance, blob basis functions and the linogram method for image reconstruction. A few approaches to image reconstruction that were discussed in the first edition but now appear not to have had an influence on the field are not included in the revised edition.

Features

This book is devoted to the fundamentals of this field. Its topic is the **computational and mathematical procedures** underlying the data collection, image reconstruction, and image display in the practice of computerized tomography. It is written from the point of view of the practitioner: points of implementation and application are carefully discussed and illustrated. The major emphasis of the book is on **reconstruction methods**; these are thoroughly surveyed.

After a summary of diverse application areas (from radio astronomy to electron microscopy) the book discusses in some detail the area of x-ray computerized tomography. This is followed by a classification and thorough discussion of reconstruction algorithms and a treatment of the computational problems associated with the display of the results. While all mathematical concepts and claims are carefully stated, they are mostly left unproved in the main body of the work to ensure an easy flow of the presentation. Proofs of the most important of these claims are provided in the final chapter.

Each chapter ends with a section of Notes and References. These are *not* intended to provide a comprehensive history of the topic of the chapter. They always acknowledge the immediate sources on which the chapter is based, sometimes give references to early and current work in the field, but usually do not mention anything between. The References section at the end contains only material that is actually referred to in the book, no attempt has been made to turn it into a complete bibliography of the field.

Target Audiences

The topic of the book is of potential interest in many fields of engineering, science, and medicine. This is well illustrated by the fact that the first edition of the book has been repeatedly cited in such diverse archival publications as *Applied Optics, IEEE Transactions on Image Processing, IEEE Transactions on Medical Imaging, IEEE Transactions on Nuclear Science, International Journal on Imaging Systems and Technology, Journal of the Optical Society of America, Linear Algebra and Its Applications, Measurement Science & Technology, Medical Physics, Nuclear Instruments & Methods in Physics, Optical Engineering, Optics Communications, Physics in Medicine and Biology, Proceedings of the IEEE, Review of Scientific Instruments*, and *Ultramicroscopy*. See also the References of this revised edition: they come from all fields of engineering, science and medicine.

An attempt has been made to carefully introduce all but the most commonly known notions, so that the book should be useful to readers with such diverse backgrounds. Anyone with a degree in an engineering or scientific discipline should have no trouble in following the material presented in the book; the assumed mathematical knowledge is likely be covered in any course that introduces the students to the fundamental concepts of calculus and linear algebra.

Syllabus for an Introductory Course on Image Reconstruction

The book is based on an introductory graduate course that the author has taught during the past thirty years in the Departments of Computer Science at the State University of New York at Buffalo, at the University of Pennsylvania, and at the Graduate Center of the City University of New York. The material has been constantly revised to make it as up-to-date as possible in an introductory text. The following is the presently used syllabus for this course; there is a nearly complete overlap between the syllabus and the contents of the book.

1. DATA COLLECTION. How projection data are obtained in various sciences and medicine, such as electron microscopy, radio astronomy, nuclear medicine, but concentrating on x-ray transmission data. Measurements viewed as line integrals. The nature of noise in experimental measurements: photon noise, scatter, beam hardening, etc.
2. RECONSTRUCTION ALGORITHMS.
   a) Radon transform, the Radon inversion formula, regularization of the singular integral in the Radon inversion formula, numerical evaluation of the regularized integral. Fourier transforms, the projection theorem, convolution, sampling and aliasing, the discrete Fourier transform, and the fast Fourier transform. Filtered backprojection reconstruction methods and Fourier space reconstruction methods, the effect of filtering and interpolation in such methods.

b) Basis functions, the mapping of images into finite-dimensional vectors using series expansion. The reconstruction problem as an optimization problem in finite-dimensional vector spaces, functions to be optimized. Norms, generalized inverses, least squares solutions, maximum entropy solutions, and most likely estimates. Richardson's algorithm and its variants in image reconstruction. Iterative relaxation methods.

c) Comparative evaluation of various reconstruction methods: accuracy under ideal circumstances, noise magnification, computational costs, task-oriented performance, and general applicability.

3. COMPUTER TECHNOLOGY.

   a) Design and maintenance of a large programming system (SNARK09) and database for image reconstruction. The application of SNARK09 in designing, implementing, and evaluating reconstruction algorithms.

   b) Visualization of reconstructed results: surface detection and the display of three-dimensional surfaces.

4. APPLICATIONS. Computerized tomography (CT), x-ray and positron emission scanners, the structure of biological molecules, materials science, anatomical and physiological displays, etc.

Acknowledgments

The author has had the privilege over the last 40 years to work on problems of image reconstruction from projections with a very large number of talented individuals. The list of joint papers in the References gives some indication of this. The preparation for publication of this revised edition was greatly helped by Yair Censor, Ran Davidi, Joanna Klukowska and Stuart Rowland.

Contents

1

Introduction

In this chapter we discuss some of the many different medical, engineering, and scientific areas in which the procedures described in this book are applicable. We also introduce some statistical concepts that are useful for understanding much of the later material.

1.1 Image Reconstruction from Projections

The problem of image reconstruction from projections has repeatedly arisen over the last 50 years in a large number of scientific, medical, and technical fields. The range of applicability is staggering. At one end of the scale, data from electron microscopes are used to reconstruct molecular structures; while at the other end, data from radio telescopes are used to reconstruct maps of radio emission from celestial objects. These seemingly different applications, and many others to be mentioned here, have the same mathematical and computational foundations. It is the purpose of this book to discuss these foundations.

Of all the applications, probably the greatest effect on the world at large has been in the area of diagnostic medicine: *computerized tomography* (CT) has revolutionized radiology. Images of cross sections of the human body are produced from data obtained by measuring the attenuation of x-rays along a large number of lines through the cross section. Most of this book uses CT as the framework within which the problems and solutions are presented. We therefore say very little about it in this section, but survey some of the numerous other applications.

We start with a simple artificial problem to demonstrate the underlying ideas. While the solution to this problem is of no known practical usefulness, the problem is very similar to a practical problem in astrophysics (to be mentioned in the following), and shares its basic structure with other applications of image reconstruction from projections.

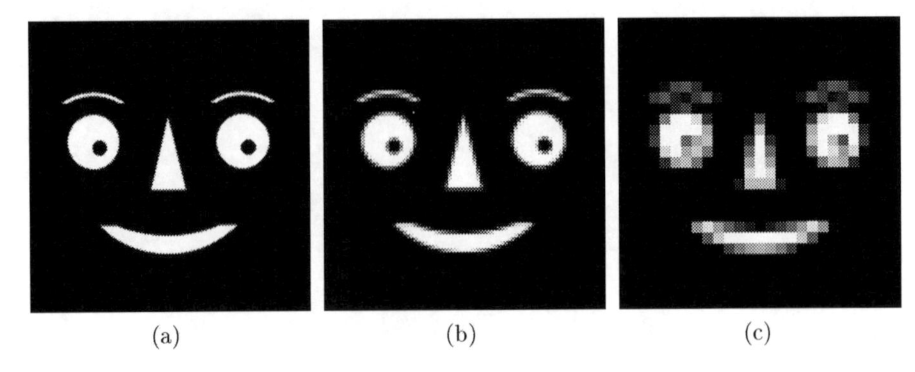

(a) (b) (c)

Fig. 1.1: Three different digitizations of the same picture: (a) is a 243×243 digitization, (b) is an 81×81 digitization, and (c) is a 27×27 digitization.

Suppose that we have a rectangular area containing some sources of light. A simple example is a television screen displaying a still picture. Suppose that we also have a "detector" that can measure the *total* intensity of light in the picture. That, of course, would not help us to record the details in the picture. One way of getting at the details is to make a "collimator," by cutting a small square hole into a sheet of nontransparent material. If we put the collimator in front of the picture, the detector measures only the light emanating from the small region behind the square hole. By moving the hole in discrete steps across the picture and measuring the intensity each time, we can build up an image of the picture. The image is made up of small square regions whose brightness is proportional to the average intensity in the original picture in the corresponding region. We can move the collimator so that the small square regions are abutting and cover the whole picture. In such a case, the resulting image (referred to as a *digitization* of the picture later in this book) resembles the picture, provided only that the collimator's hole is small enough. This is illustrated in Fig. 1.1.

Suppose now that we lack the capability of cutting a small square hole into our opaque sheet. It may then appear that we can no longer produce an image of our picture. However, image reconstruction from projections comes to our rescue. We now illustrate the processes of "projection taking" and "reconstruction" on our simple problem.

The process of projection taking in this case consists of moving the opaque sheet across the picture in small discrete steps in a fixed direction. After each move, we use our detector to measure the total intensity of light in the uncovered part of the picture. Subtraction of the measured value of the total intensity at any time instance from the measured value of the total intensity at the next time instance provides us with the total intensity of light in each of a set of parallel abutting thin strips of known location (see Fig. 1.2). We can now repeat this process with the opaque sheet moving in a different direction. This way we get the total intensity of light in each of another set of

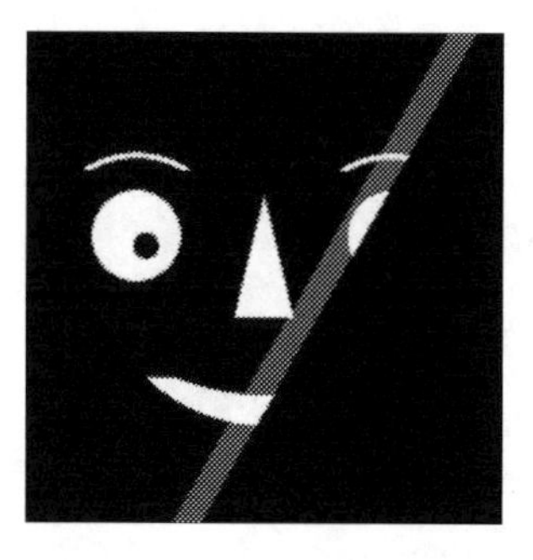

Fig. 1.2: The process of projection taking. The line integral of the brightness along the central line of a strip (shown half-illuminated) is estimated by dividing the total brightness in the strip by the width of the strip.

parallel abutting thin strips of known location. We estimate the *line integral* of the brightness along the central lines of these strips, by dividing the total brightness in the strip by the width of the strip. Doing this repeatedly (say 90 times, rotating the orientation of the opaque sheet by 2° each time), we obtain many such sets of measurements. Each set of estimated line integrals is often called a *projection*, but in this book we preferentially use the word *view*, since "projection" is also used for a number of other things. The collection of all the estimated line integrals is referred to as the *projection data*.

The process of *reconstruction* produces an image of the picture from projection data of the picture. How this is done is the main topic of this book. In Fig. 1.3 we compare the 81×81 digitization of a picture with an 81×81 reconstruction from 90 views with 121 estimated line integrals in each.

This example illustrates the informal definition given in the following paragraph. While not all that comes under the heading "image reconstruction from projections" is covered by this informal definition (for example, in Chapter 13

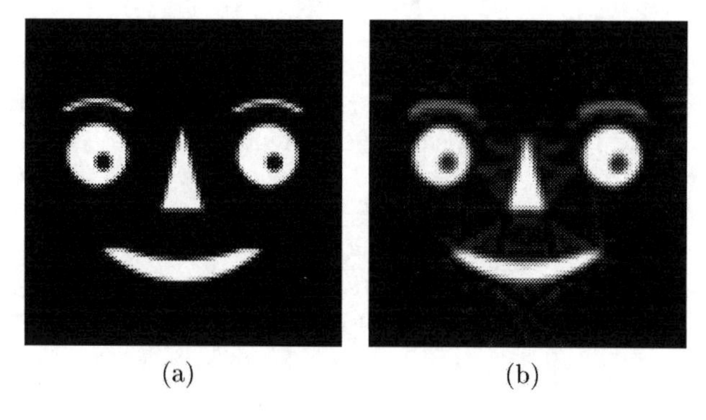

Fig. 1.3: The 81×81 digitization of a picture (a) compared to an 81×81 reconstructions from 90 views with 121 measurements in each view (b).

we discuss truly three-dimensional reconstruction), it is adequate for describing our attitude toward image reconstruction throughout most of this book.

Image reconstruction from projections is the process of producing an image of a two-dimensional distribution (usually of some physical property) from estimates of its line integrals along a finite number of lines of known locations.

We now turn to some real-life applications. The order in which we take these is according to the size of the object to be reconstructed. The reader is warned that the following is by no means an exhaustive survey of all the application areas of image reconstruction from projections.

Actually, our simple artificial problem has a close analog in *astrophysics*. There are instruments for measuring the brightness distribution of radio sources in the sky that are of too low resolution to provide astrophysicists with the information they seek. However, if the moon moves across the portion of the sky that is of interest, it acts in an analogous fashion to the opaque sheet of our artificial example. The directions of the paths of the moon across the sky vary, providing us with a number of views, which in this field are referred to as profiles obtained from *lunar occultation* observations. From such observations the two-dimensional brightness distribution of radio sources can be reconstructed. Among the other applications of image reconstruction we mention its use for discovering the x-ray structure of supernova remnants and the electron-density distribution in the solar corona. In the latter case, display techniques allow us to make movies of the dynamic changes in the solar corona as would be observed from above the north pole of the sun's rotation, a view that cannot possibly be observed from earth! Coming down to earth, we note that there are numerous applications, such as applying tomographic methods to geodesy and to volcanology. However, we concentrate on the application in which image reconstruction from projections is probably applied more frequently than in any other, namely diagnostic medicine.

X-ray *transmission computerized tomography* (CT) is discussed in some detail in the succeeding chapters. Here we just indicate its nature using a few illustrations. Figure 1.4(a) shows a photograph of an x-ray CT scanner and Fig. 1.4(b) shows an engineering drawing of an apparatus for data collection in x-ray CT. The tube contains a single x-ray source, the detector unit contains an array of x-ray detectors. Suppose for the moment that the x-ray Tube and Collimator on the one side and the Data Acquisition/Detector Unit on the other side are stationary, and the patient on the table is moved between them at a steady rate. By shooting a fan beam of x-rays through the patient at frequent regular intervals and detecting them on the other side, we can build up a two-dimensional x-ray projection of the patient that is very similar in appearance to the image that is traditionally captured on an x-ray film. Such a projection is shown in Fig. 1.5(a). The brightness at a point is indicative of the total attenuation of the x-rays from the source to the detector. This mode of operation is *not* CT, it is just an alternative way of taking x-ray images. In the CT mode, the patient is kept stationary, but the tube and the detector unit rotate (together) around the patient. The fan beam of x-rays from the

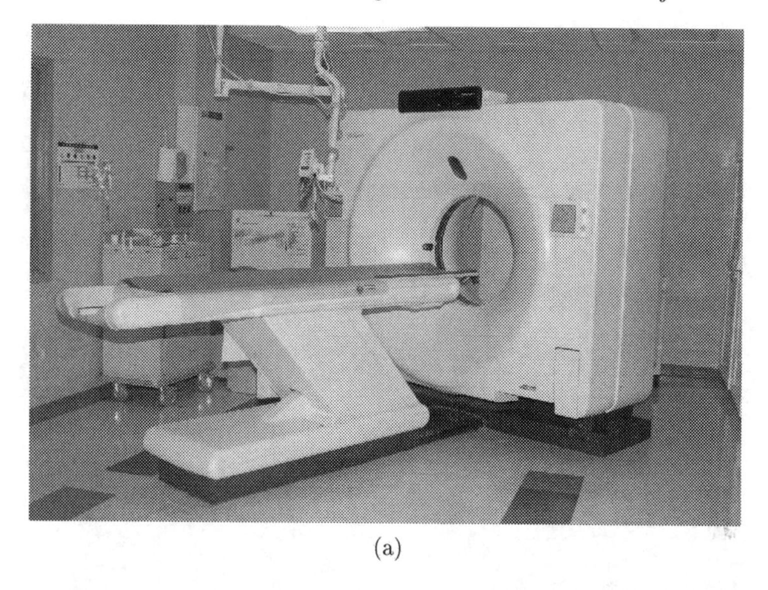

(a)

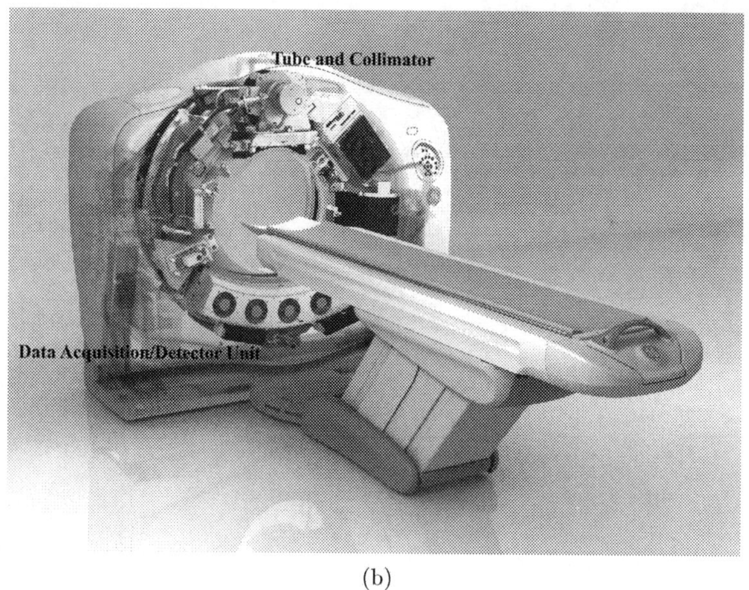

(b)

Fig. 1.4: (a) A CT scanner of the LightSpeed Series of GE Healthcare. (Illustration provided by C. Yee of Jacobi Medical Center.) (b) Engineering rendering of a CT scanner released in 2008. (Photo provided by GE Healthcare.)

source to the detector determines a slice in the patient's body. The location of such a slice is shown by the horizontal line in Fig. 1.5(a). Data are collected for a number of fixed positions of the source and detector; these are referred

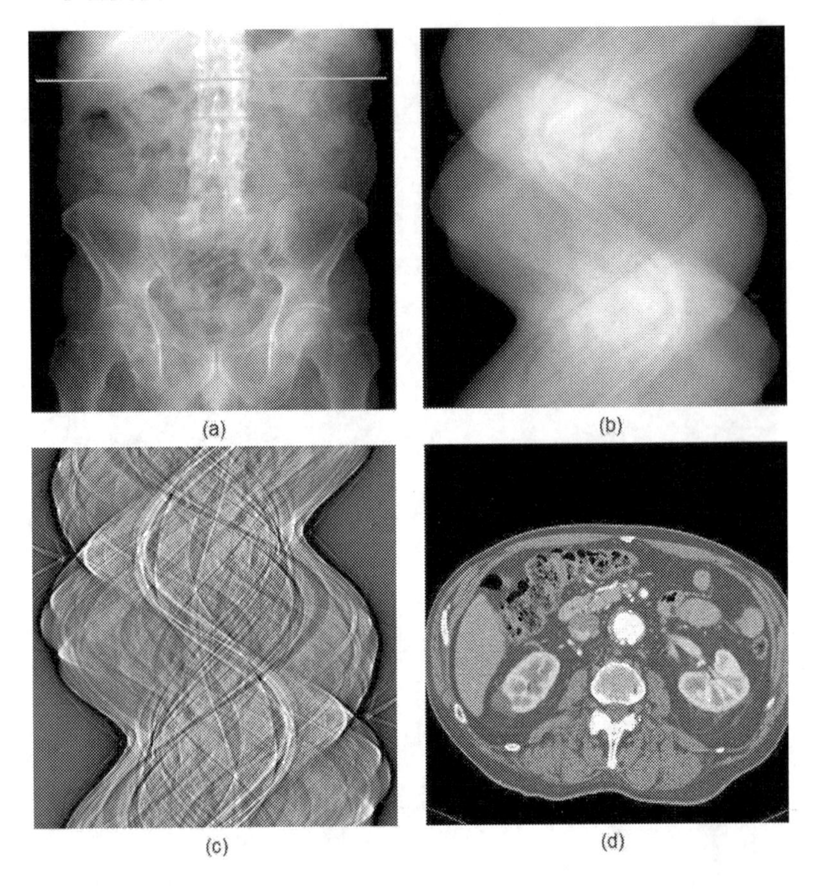

Fig. 1.5: (a) A digitally rendered (x-ray) radiograph with a horizontal line marking the location of the cross section for which the following images were obtained. (b) Sinogram of the projection data. (c) Sinogram of the convolved projection data. (d) A reconstruction from the projection data. (All images were obtained using a Siemens Sensation CT scanner by R. Fahrig and J. Starman at Stanford University.)

to as *views*. For each view, we have a reading by each of the detectors. All the detector readings for all the views can be represented as a *sinogram*, shown in Fig. 1.5(b). The intensities in the sinogram are proportional to the line integrals of the x-ray attenuation coefficient between the corresponding source and detector positions. From these line integrals, a two-dimensional image of the x-ray attenuation coefficient distribution in the slice of the body can be produced by the techniques of image reconstruction. Such an image is shown in Fig. 1.5(d). Inasmuch as different tissues have different x-ray attenuation coefficients, boundaries of organs can be delineated and healthy tissue can be distinguished from tumors. In this way CT produces cross-sectional slices of the human body without surgical intervention. (The picture in Fig. 1.5(c) is a sinogram of the "convolved projection data," which is to be defined in (10.12).)

In addition to providing an excellent tool for diagnosis, the images produced by CT can be used for the planning of radiation therapy, in which beams of penetrating radiation are directed at malignancies in the body with the aim of destroying them. The goal is to deliver a sufficiently high dose to target volumes, such as tumor cells, but to avoid depositing a harmfully high dose to organs at risk. Modern devices use multileaf collimators that allow the treatment planner to control the intensity of radiation within relatively thin beams; this is referred to as *intensity modulated radiation therapy* (IMRT), see Fig. 1.6. The mathematical problem of IMRT can be considered to be

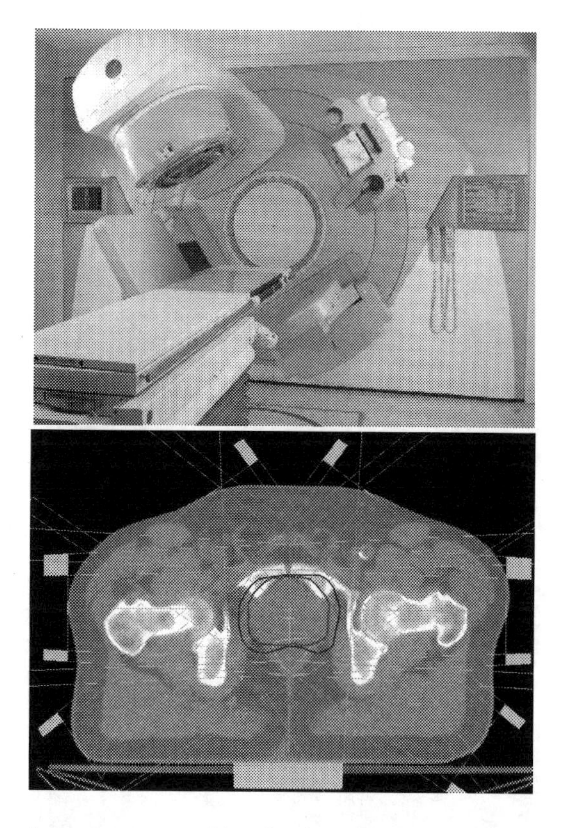

Fig. 1.6: Top: A treatment machine for intensity modulated radiation therapy (Elekta Synergy^{TM}) with multileaf collimator and a CT device for online image guided radiation therapy. (Illustration provided by Elekta, Inc.) Bottom: A CT slice of a cancer patient. Six beam angles are used and the treatment is planned so that the 75.6 Gy isodose line (in black) covers the target volume (in gray), but it bends so as to avoid the greater part of the rectum (outlined in white just below the center of the image). (Illustration provided by Y. Xiao of Thomas Jefferson University.)

"dual" to that of CT: in CT we try to recover the distribution of the x-ray attenuation in the body from measurements of total attenuation within thin beams of x-rays, in IMRT we are given information regarding the desired dose distribution in the body and we need to calculate the radiation intensity that needs to be sent into the body along thin beams in order to achieve such a dose distribution. Some of the mathematical techniques discussed later are applicable to both problems.

Another method of extreme usefulness in diagnostic medicine is *magnetic resonance imaging* (MRI). When an object is placed in a magnetic field gradient, the frequencies of magnetic resonance signals from its nuclei and unpaired electrons depend upon the value of the local applied magnetic field, as well as upon those molecular interactions usually studied by magnetic res-

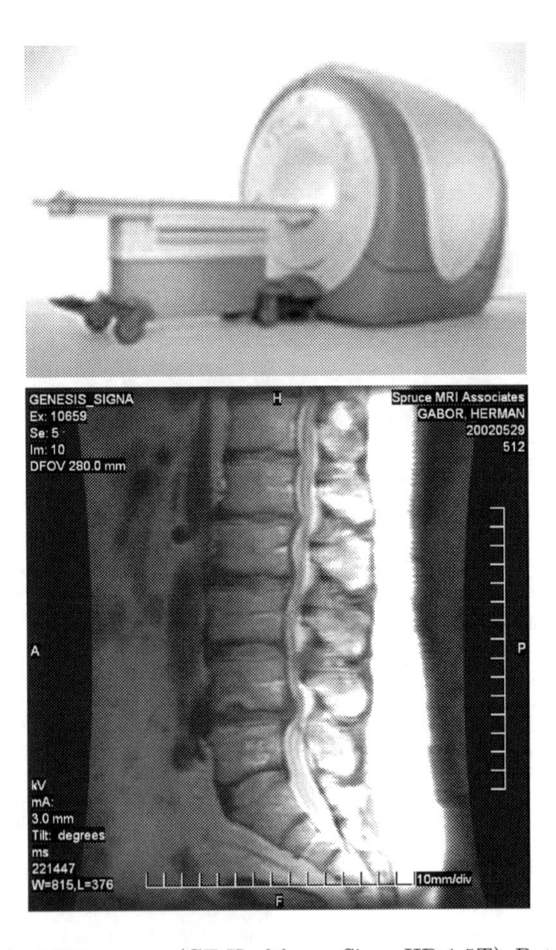

Fig. 1.7: Top: An MRI scanner (GE Healthcare Signa HD 1.5T). Bottom: A sagittal slice through the spine of the author obtained by such a scanner. Note the bulging disc pressing on the spinal nerve; this required surgical intervention.

onance methods. The integrated signal from the intersection of a surface of constant magnetic field with a three-dimensional object is one point on a one-dimensional projection of a three-dimensional signal. In a uniform linear field gradient, a plot of such signals against frequency is a one-dimensional projection, in a direction perpendicular to the gradient axis, of the total signal intensity. If the direction of the field gradient is varied other projections may be produced, and a two- or three-dimensional image may be reconstructed. However, such a "projection imaging" approach is not frequently used in practice: MRI usually relies on collecting data regarding the Fourier transform of the object to be imaged and then inverting this Fourier transform. (The associated mathematics is discussed below in Sections 8.4 and 9.1.) An MRI scanner and its output are illustrated in Fig. 1.7.

Emission computerized tomography has as its major emphasis the quantitative determination of the moment-to-moment changes in the chemistry and flow physiology of injected or inhaled compounds labeled with radioactive atoms. In this case the distribution to be reconstructed is the distribution of radioactivity in the body cross section, and the measurements are used to estimate the total activity along lines of known locations. Figure 1.8 illustrates

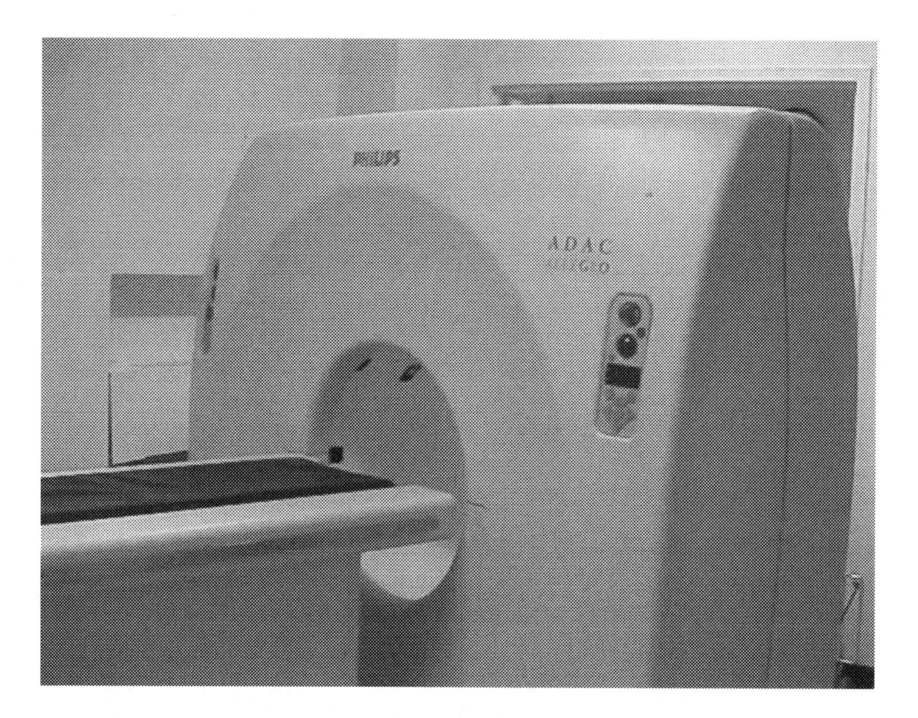

Fig. 1.8: A PET scanner that has 17,864 scintillation crystals to collect its data. Whole-body imaging is performed by acquiring seven to eight data sets (of approximately three-minutes duration each) with bed motion between acquisitions. (Illustration provided by J. Karp of the University of Pennsylvania.)

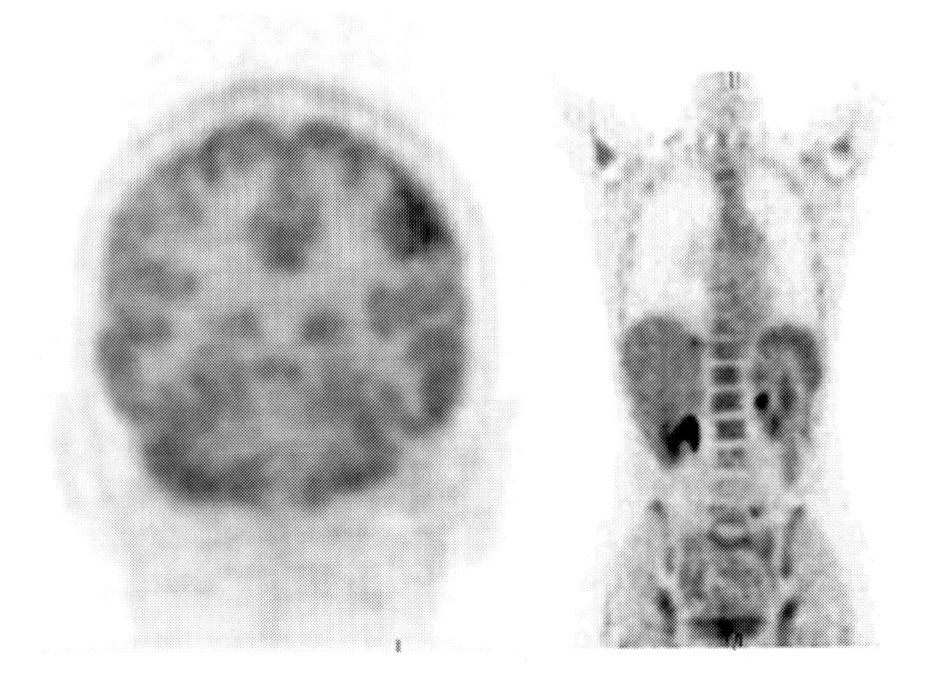

Fig. 1.9: Coronal sections of reconstructions of patients who have been injected with fluoro-deoxy-glucose (FDG) tagged with a radioactive isotope whose decay generates positrons that annihilate and produce pairs of gamma rays to be detected by the crystals to identify a line that contains the location of the annihilation. From the total activity along a large number of such lines the distribution of the annihilation frequency, and hence of the FDG, can be reconstructed. Left: Brain scan of an epilepsy patient; see the increased FDG uptake (dark) at about two o-clock, indicating the seizure focus site. Right: Whole-body scan of a patient with melanoma; see the increased FDG uptake in a small spot near the top, anterior part of the liver, indicating a lesion. (Images were obtained by the Philips Allegro scanner shown in Fig. 1.8 and were provided by J. Karp of the University of Pennsylvania.)

a device, a so-called *positron emission tomography* (PET) scanner, for doing this and Fig. 1.9 shows two clinical images produced by this device. As explained in the caption of that figure, the device allows us to image how the compound (in this case FDG) distributes itself in the body; if the compound uptake is increased in lesions, then the images can be used for locating such lesions.

Both x-ray CT and emission computerized tomography use potentially harmful ionizing radiation for their data collection, but this is not the case for MRI. Another modality of data collection with no demonstrated adverse effect on the patient is *ultrasound*.

In Fig. 1.10, we show a photograph of an apparatus used to collect ultrasonic data regarding the female breast. From these data one obtains three

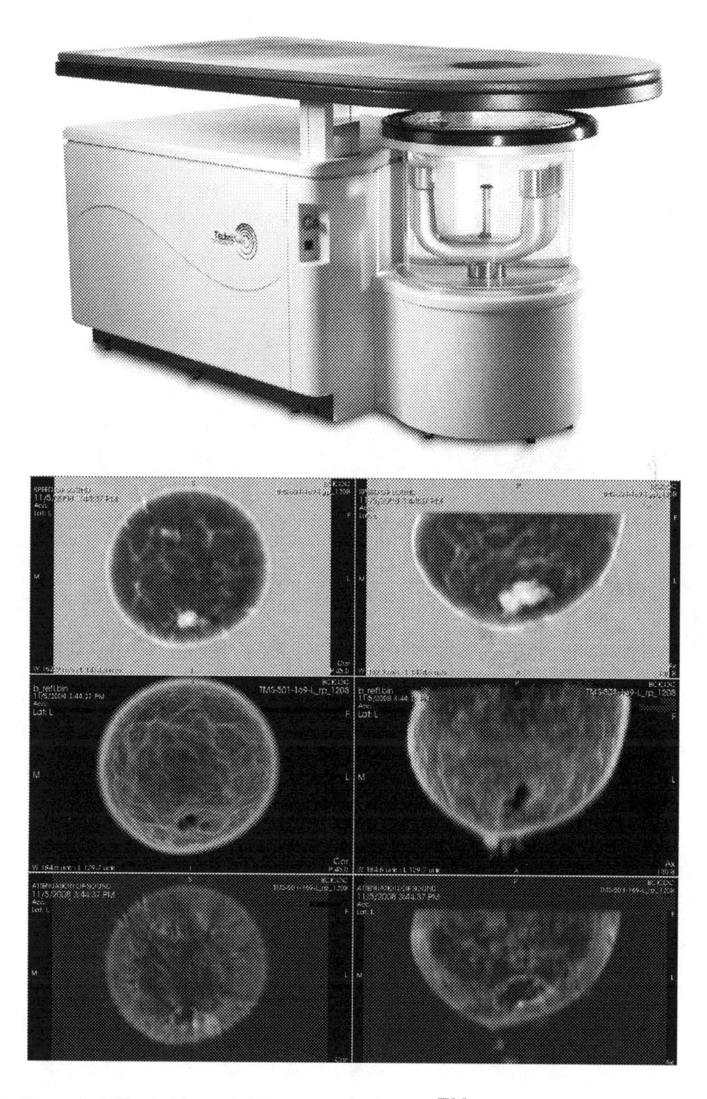

Fig. 1.10: Top: A Whole Breast Ultrasound (WBU^{TM}) scanner (TechniScan Medical Systems) used for collecting data to reconstruct breast images. Bottom: A screenshot of the speed of sound (top), reflection (middle) and the attenuation of sound (bottom) of a complex cyst, shown in coronal (left column) and axial (right) correlated slices. (Illustrations provided by TechniScan Medical Systems.)

separate but correlated reconstructions, providing different tissue characteristics. The three reconstructions looked at together give a great deal of information about the nature of the tumors (if any) present. The figure also shows a screenshot on the scanner's viewer of the coronal slices (left column) and axial slices (right column) in the three 3D reconstructions.

Another method for tomographic imaging the body uses light. We give an illustration of such *optical tomography* in Fig. 1.11.

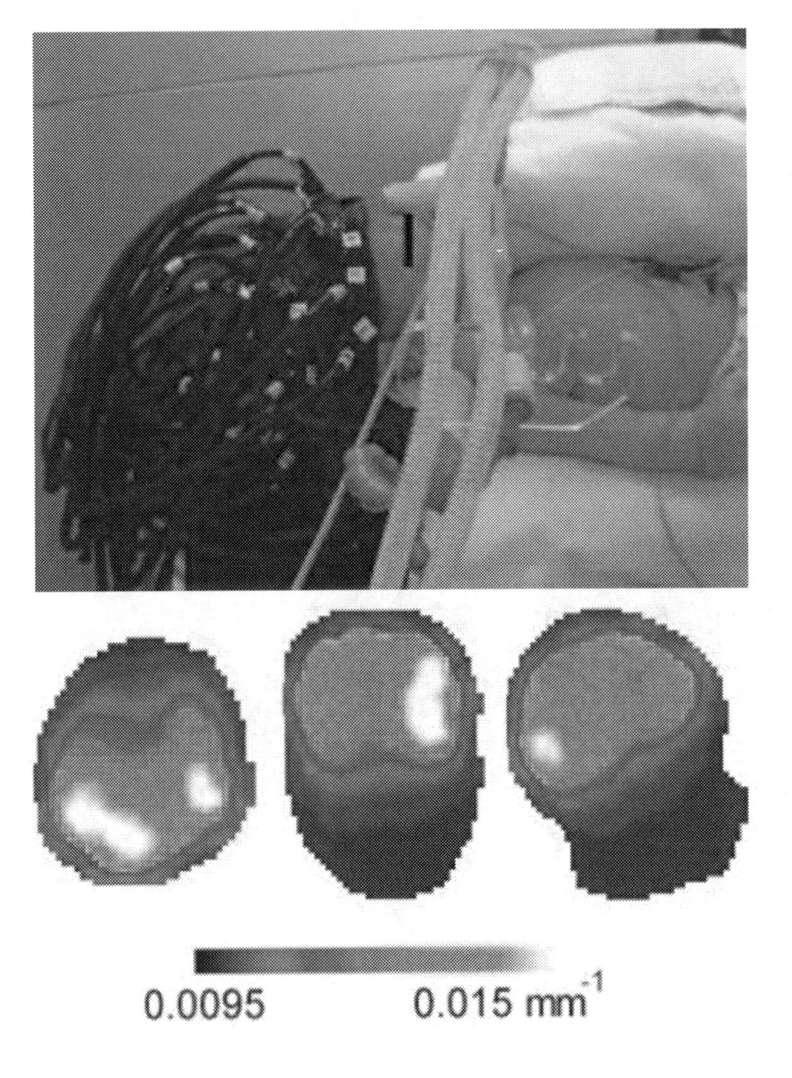

Fig. 1.11: Optical tomography. Top: A four-day old infant is being optically imaged using 29 source-detector pairs around her head. Bottom: Slices across the reconstructed 3D images of differences in light absorption at the the wavelength of 815 nm, caused by differences in blood distribution. Sequences of such images can be used to assess physiological functioning. (Illustration provided by S. Arridge of the University College London.)

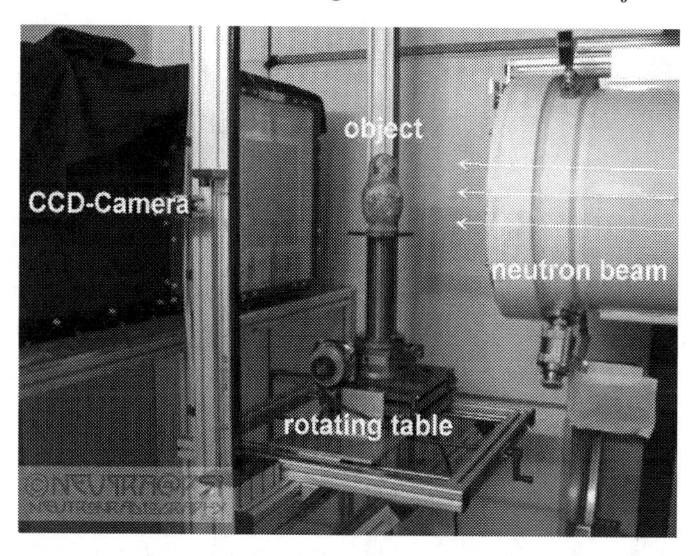

Fig. 1.12: Apparatus for neutron tomography data collection. (Illustration provided by the Neutron Imaging and Activation Group, Paul Scherrer Institute, Switzerland, http://neutra.web.psi.ch.)

Getting away from medicine, we note that image reconstruction from projections has been found useful in *nondestructive testing*. For example, a collection of transmission beam neutron radiographs can be used for the reconstruction (and hence inspection) of such objects as turbine blades and even whole engines. Such metallic objects would not be well penetrated by x-rays. Figure 1.12 shows a setup for collecting the necessary data. A typical neutron radiograph collected by such a device is shown in Fig. 1.13, together with two slices through the 3D reconstruction from multiple such radiographs.

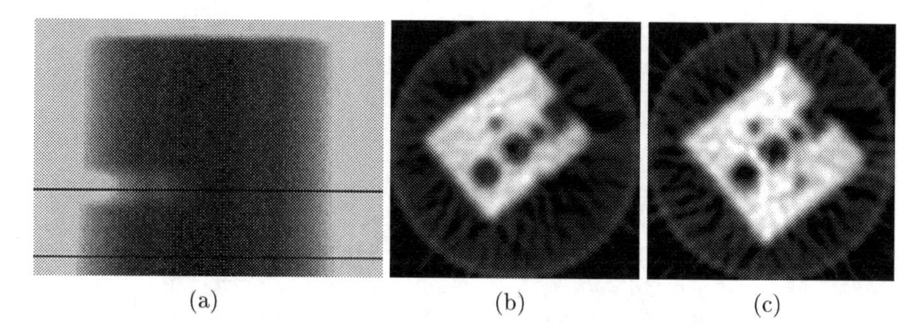

Fig. 1.13: (a) A neutron radiograph with the location of two cross sections indicated. (b) and (c) Reconstructions of the indicated cross sections. (Illustration provided L. Ruskó of the University of Szeged, Hungary.)

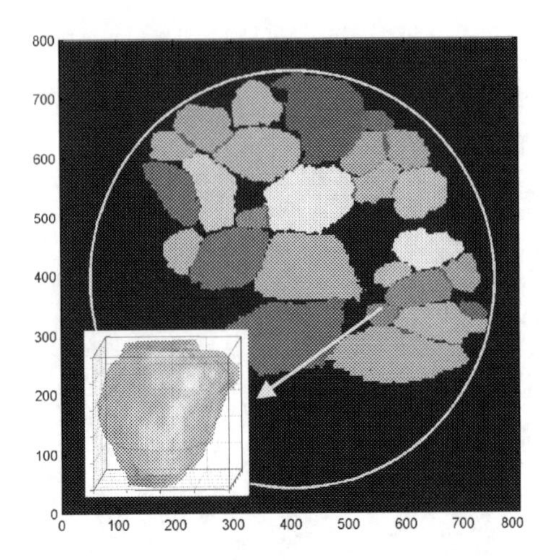

Fig. 1.14: Grains in a polycrystal. Multiple grains in a cross section are shown, a single one of them is displayed three-dimensionally. (Illustration provided by H.F. Poulsen of the Risø National Laboratory, Denmark.)

An emerging application of image reconstruction from projections is in *materials science*. In nature most materials such as rocks, ice, sand, and soil appear as aggregates comprised of a set of small crystals. Similarly, modern society is built on applications of metals, ceramics and other hard materials, which are also polycrystalline. An example of a *polycrystal* is shown in Fig. 1.14. The individual crystals are known as *grains*. Each grain is characterized by its position and shape as well as by the *orientation* of the 3D *crystalline lattice* (the discrete lattice of atom positions). The latter property is known as the *grain orientation*. The physical, chemical and mechanical properties of the material are to a large extent governed by the geometrical features of this 3D complex.

Three-dimensional x-ray diffraction (3DXRD) is one way to collect data for recovering the distribution and orientation of grains; see Fig. 1.15. The method is based on reconstruction using x-rays with a setup similar to that of CT. The vital difference is that in CT the absorption of the incident beam through the sample is probed, while in 3DXRD the diffracted beam is probed as it diverges from the sample on the exit side. The *diffraction pattern* on the detector typically is composed of a set of distinct *diffraction spots*. Acquiring images at a set of rotation angles, each grain gives rise to 5 to 30 spots, with positions and intensity distributions determined by the local orientation of the crystalline lattice. From such data it is possible to reconstruct not only the geometry of the grains, but also the variation of the orientations within the grains. Since orientations need three variables to specify them, an interesting aspect of such reconstructions is that what is reconstructed is an image of a distribution of three-dimensional vectors; see Fig. 1.16.

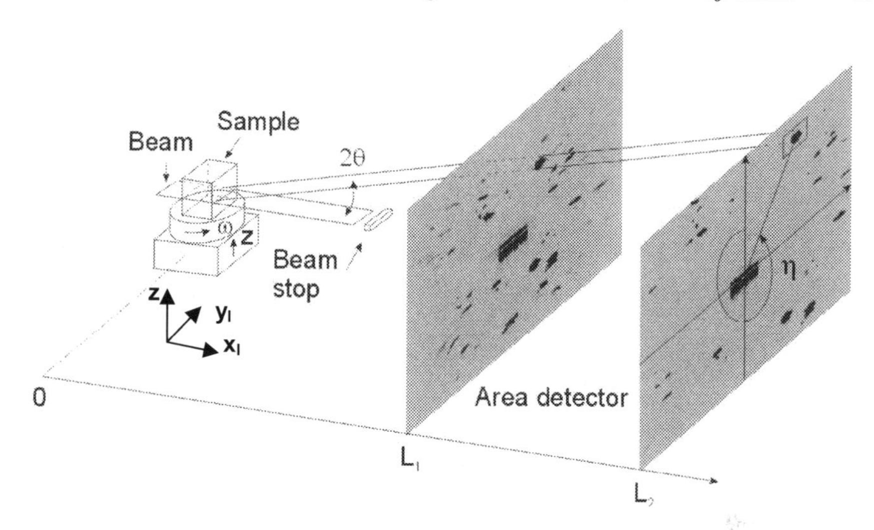

Fig. 1.15: The 3DXRD data collection geometry. Detectors are positioned perpendicular to the beam at various distances. (Illustration provided by H.F. Poulsen of the Risø National Laboratory, Denmark.)

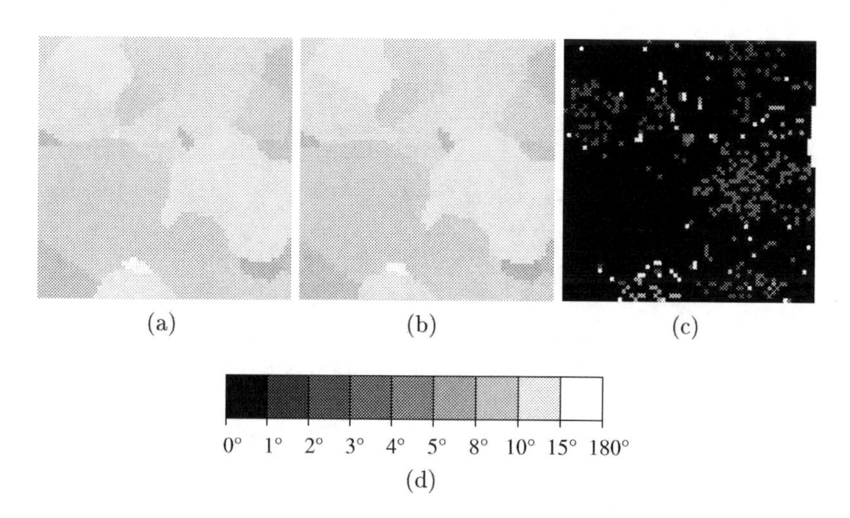

Fig. 1.16: (a) A test pattern of polycrystal orientations (obtained by electron microscopy). (b) A reconstruction from simulated noisy diffraction data. (c) Differences between the test and the reconstructed orientation distributions. (d) Gray scale indicating the angles in the difference map. Note that at nearly everywhere the difference angle is less than 15° and in the large majority of cases it is less than 1°.

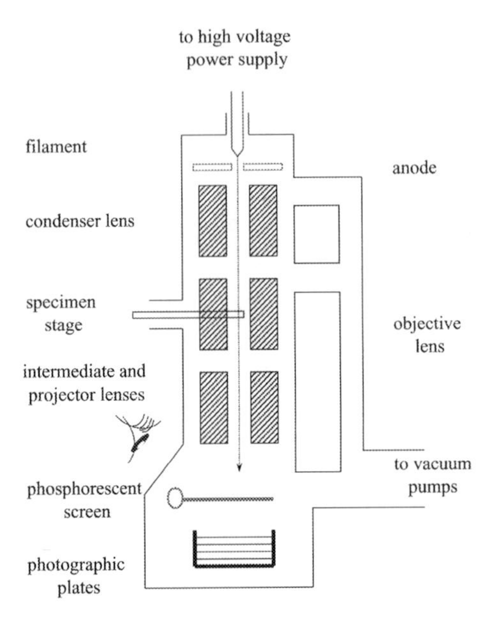

Fig. 1.17: Schematic drawing of a transmission electron microscope. (Illustration provided by C. San Martín of the Centro Nacional de Biotecnología, Spain.)

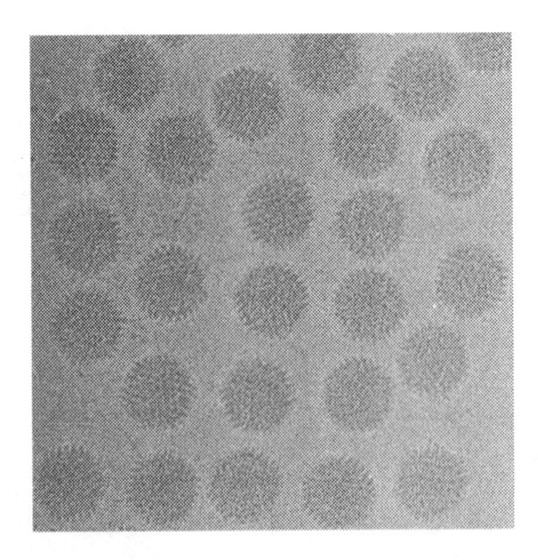

Fig. 1.18: Part of an electron micrograph containing projections of multiple copies of the human adenovirus type 5. (Illustration provided by C. San Martín of the Centro Nacional de Biotecnología, Spain.)

Three-dimensional reconstruction of nano-scale objects (such as biological macromolecules) can be accomplished using data recorded with a transmission *electron microscope* (see Fig. 1.17) that produces *electron micrographs*, such as the one illustrated in Fig. 1.18, in which the grayness at each point is indicative of a line integral of a physical property of the object being imaged. From multiple electron micrographs one can recover the structure of the biological object that is being imaged; see Fig. 1.19.

This completes our survey of some of the applications of image reconstruction from projections. Except for some further discussion of x-ray CT, the rest of this book is devoted to the theory, rather than applications, of image reconstruction.

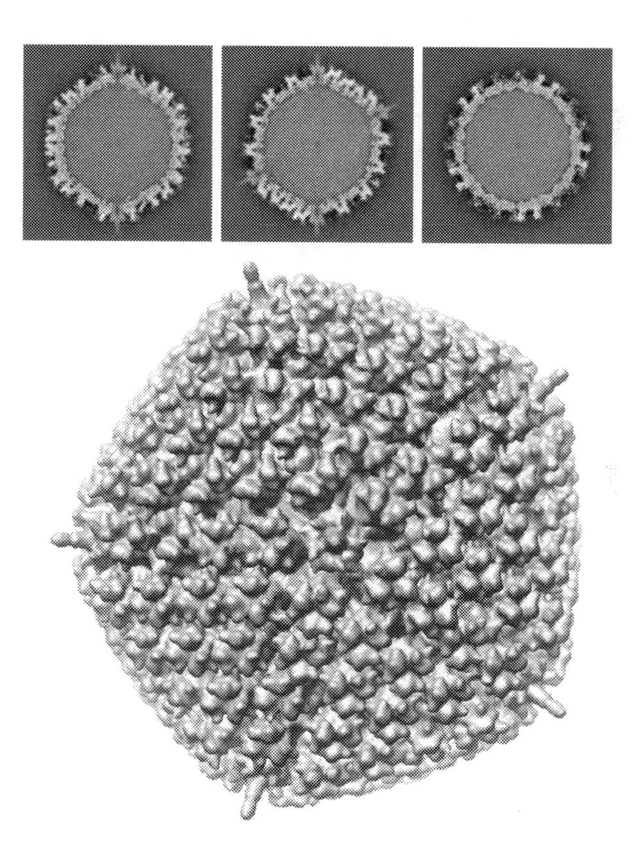

Fig. 1.19: Top: Reconstructed values, from electron microscopic data such as in Fig. 1.18, of the human adenovirus type 5 in three mutually orthogonal slices through the center of the reconstruction. Bottom: Computer graphic display of the surface of the virus based on the three-dimensional reconstruction. (Illustration provided by C. San Martín of the Centro Nacional de Biotecnología, Spain.)

1.2 Probability and Random Variables

In order to discuss the processes involved in CT we need to know some of the basic concepts of probability theory. That is the purpose of this section. The reader may wish to skim it at first reading and return to it at times when the notions introduced here are actually used.

As an example, consider the situation depicted in Fig. 1.20. There is a slab of material and the line L goes through it. If an x-ray photon enters the slab along the line L through its top face, it will continue to travel along the line L until it is absorbed or scattered. Some photons will be neither absorbed nor scattered before exiting through the bottom face. We shall say such photons are *transmitted* through the slab. The point is that for any individual x-ray photon we cannot be certain whether or not it will be transmitted. All we can say is that, for any fixed energy $\bar{e}$, there is a fixed *probability* ρ that a photon at that energy that enters the slab is transmitted. We call ρ the *transmittance* at energy $\bar{e}$ of the slab along line L, and we define it as follows. The definition is typical of how the "probability" of something happening is defined.

To define ρ we carry out a "thought experiment." Such an experiment could be physically carried out if we had at our disposal an infinite amount of time and instruments with unlimited precision. We shoot photons at energy $\bar{e}$ one by one through the slab along the line L, and we test whether they are transmitted. Let $t_1(n)$ denote the number of photons transmitted out of the first n in this experiment. (The subscript 1 refers to the fact that this is the first such thought experiment, in the following we discuss a whole series of them.) Then ρ is defined as the limit of $t_1(n)/n$ as n tends to infinity:

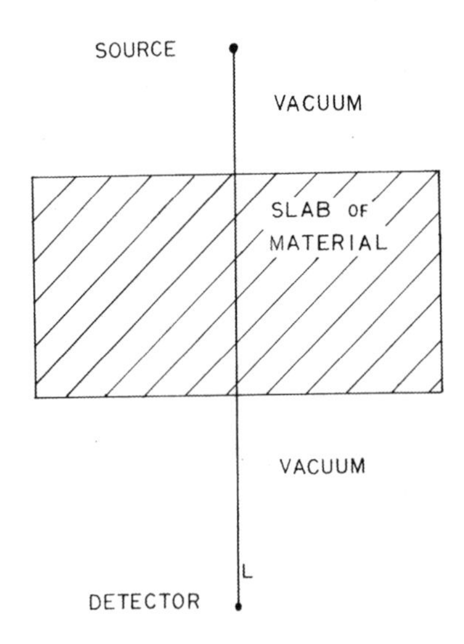

Fig. 1.20: Definition of transmittance.

$$\rho = \lim_{n \to \infty} (t_1(n)/n) . \tag{1.1}$$

That is, the transmittance ρ is a number such that given a positive real number ε, however small, there will always be an integer n_0, such that the difference between ρ and $t_1(n)/n$ is less than ε for all n greater than n_0.

Note that it is not a priori obvious that $t_1(n)/n$ has a limit as n tends to infinity. The claim that it does is based on physical experiments that approximate the thought experiment just described. Note also that it is assumed that the same value of ρ will be provided if the experiment is carried out again. More precisely, let the same thought experiment be carried out the second time, and let $t_2(n)$ denote the number of photons transmitted out of the first n in the second experiment. Then $\rho = \lim_{n \to \infty} (t_2(n)/n)$.

Even though the values of ρ defined by the limits of the two identical thought experiments are the same, it does not mean that we can assume that $t_1(n) = t_2(n)$, for any fixed n. Both $t_1(n)$ and $t_2(n)$ may assume any integer value between zero (no photons are transmitted) and n (all photons are transmitted). However, some of these values are more likely than others. It is reasonable to inquire as to what is the probability $p_{n,\rho}(m)$ that m photons out of n get transmitted.

To define $p_{n,\rho}(m)$, we carry out the previously described thought experiment repeatedly up to the point when n photons have entered the slab. Let $t_i(n)$ denote the number of transmitted photons in the ith thought experiment. Let $s(N)$ denote the number of times $t_i(n) = m$, for $1 \leq i \leq N$. Then

$$p_{n,\rho}(m) = \lim_{N \to \infty} (s(N)/N) . \tag{1.2}$$

Note that $p_{n,\rho}(m) = 0$ if m is negative or if m is greater than n. Since $p_{n,\rho}(m)$ is supposed to be the probability of m photons being transmitted out of n, this is reassuring. Also it is easy to see, by comparing the thought experiments used to define ρ and $p_{n,\rho}(m)$, that $p_{1,\rho}(1) = \rho$. It is somewhat more difficult to show that, in general for $0 \leq m \leq n$,

$$p_{n,\rho}(m) = \frac{n!}{m!(n-m)!} \rho^m (1-\rho)^{n-m} , \tag{1.3}$$

where, as usual, $m!$ denotes $m \times (m-1) \times (m-2) \times \cdots \times 2 \times 1$, with $0!$ defined to be one. Equation (1.3) is referred to as the *binomial probability law*. The values of $p_{30,0.7}(m)$, for $0 \leq m \leq 30$, are plotted in Fig. 1.21.

More generally, if S_X is a finite or a countably infinite set (such as the set all integers) of all possible outcomes of an experiment, then S_X together with the probability $p_X(x)$ of the outcome for each x in S_X is referred to as the *discrete random variable* X. Mathematically, we must have that $p_X(x) \geq 0$ for all x in S_X, and that the sum of the $p_X(x)$ over S_X is 1. In this book, we only allow experiments whose outcome is a number, or possibly a column vector of numbers. For example, for a fixed n, the set of all integers m together with the probability $p_{n,\rho}(m)$ is the *binomial random variable* with parameters n and ρ.

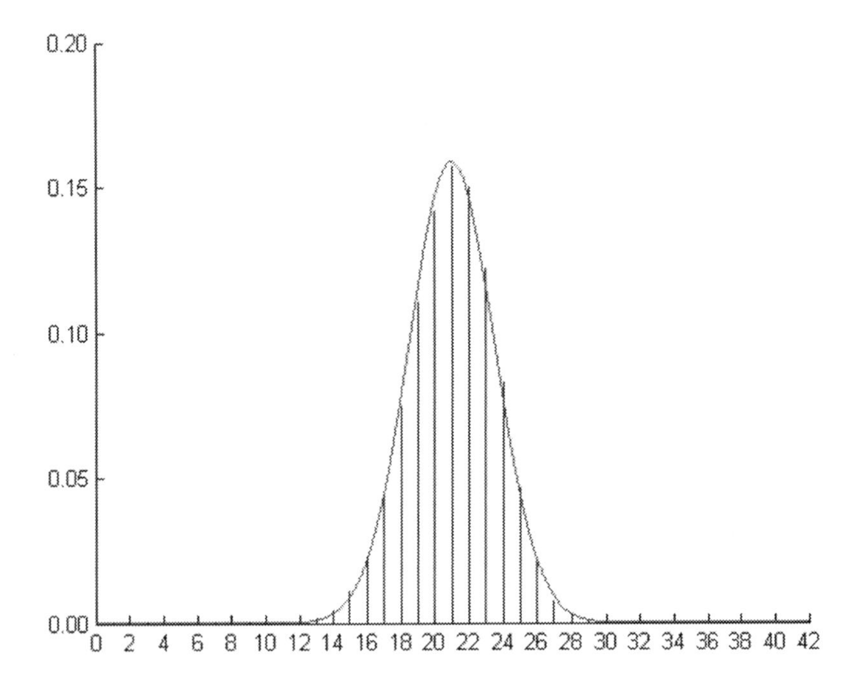

Fig. 1.21: Plot of the binomial probability function $p_{30,0.7}$, see (1.3), with values indicated by the vertical lines and of the Gaussian probability density function, see (1.10), with $\mu_X = 21$ and $V_X = 6.3$, shown as a continuous curve.

We call the outcome of a single experiment a *sample* of the random variable. For example, the value of $t_i(n)$, for a fixed i, in the thought experiment above is a sample of the binomial random variable with parameters n and ρ.

In summary, the number of photons that may be transmitted when n photons enter the slab is a discrete random variable. The actual number of photons transmitted in a single experiment with n photons entering the slab is a sample of the random variable. Later on we will see other examples of discrete random variables. A particularly important one for our purposes is associated with the number of photons emitted by an x-ray source in the direction of a detector during a unit period of time.

Two important properties of a discrete random variable X are its *mean* μ_X and its *variance* V_X, defined by

$$\mu_X = \sum_{x \in S_X} x p_X(x), \tag{1.4}$$

$$V_X = \sum_{x \in S_X} (x - \mu_X)^2 p_X(x). \tag{1.5}$$

Note that the averaged outcome of a very large number of experiments will approximate the mean. Also, the variance will be approximated by taking the average of the squares of the distances of the samples from the mean. Thus, the variance is a measure of the spread of the possible outcomes around the mean. For the binomial random variable with parameters n and ρ, the mean is $n\rho$ and the variance is $n\rho(1-\rho)$. The *standard deviation* σ_X of the random variable X is defined to be the nonnegative square root of its variance.

We introduce one more notion for the special case when all elements of S_X are real numbers. Let a denote either $-\infty$ or a real number and let b denote either a real number or ∞, such that $a < b$. Then we define

$$P_X(a,b] = \sum_{\substack{x \in S_X \\ a < x \leq b}} p_X(x). \tag{1.6}$$

Thus, $P_X(a,b]$ denotes the probability that a sample of the discrete random variable X is in the interval $(a,b]$.

We now discuss the notion of a *continuous random variable* X for the special case when the associated set S_X of possible outcomes is the set of all real numbers. In this case we use a *probability density function* p_X that maps S_X into the range $[0,1]$ (the closed interval of real numbers from 0 to 1) in such a way that the probability that a sample of X is in the interval $(a,b]$ is

$$P_X(a,b] = \int_a^b p_X(x)dx. \tag{1.7}$$

Note that this implies in particular that the integral of the $p_X(x)$ over S_X is 1. The *mean*, *variance* and *standard deviation* of such a continuous random variable X are defined by

$$\mu_X = \int_{-\infty}^{\infty} x p_X(x)dx, \tag{1.8}$$

$$V_X = \int_{-\infty}^{\infty} (x-\mu_X)^2 p_X(x)dx \tag{1.9}$$

and $\sigma_X = \sqrt{V_X}$.

The most important family of continuous random variables are the *Gaussian* (also called *normal*) *random variables* X that have the property that, for all real numbers x,

$$p_X(x) = \frac{1}{\sqrt{2\pi V_X}} \exp\left(-\frac{(x-\mu_X)^2}{2V_X}\right). \tag{1.10}$$

As usual, $\exp(x)$ denotes the value of the mathematical constant e raised to the power x. Such a probability density function can be seen in Fig. 1.21.

All Gaussian random variables "look the same" in the following well-defined sense. Let $(c, d]$ be an interval such that $-\infty \leq c < d \leq \infty$. Suppose that X and Y are Gaussian random variables. Then $P_X(\mu_X + c\sigma_X, \mu_X + d\sigma_X] = P_Y(\mu_Y + c\sigma_Y, \mu_Y + d\sigma_Y]$. In particular, they all look the same as the *standard Gaussian random variable* N, which is the Gaussian random variable with $\mu_N = 0$ and $V_N = 1$. This has the practically useful consequence that if we have a method (a table or a program) that allows us to calculate $P_N(c, d]$ for any interval $(c, d]$, then we can calculate $P_X(a, b]$ for any Gaussian random variable X and any interval $(a, b]$, since $P_X(a, b] = P_N\left(\frac{a-\mu_X}{\sigma_X}, \frac{b-\mu_X}{\sigma_X}\right]$. In particular, $P_N(-1, 1] > 0.67$, which implies that a sample of any random Gaussian variable will lie within one standard deviation of its mean in more than two cases out of three. We also know that $P_N(-2, 2] > 0.95$ and $P_N(-3, 3] > 0.995$. We can make use of these facts to estimate μ_X of a Gaussian random variable from a sample or samples. In more than 95 cases out of a 100, a sample will be within two standard deviations of μ_X. If we had a way of estimating the standard deviation (and we often do), then having observed a single sample we can say that we are 95% *confident* that the mean lies between two numbers, which are the sample plus/minus twice the standard deviation. Similarly, we can say that we are 99.5% confident that the mean lies between the sample plus/minus three standard deviations.

The reason for the importance of the Gaussian random variables is twofold. First, many random variables that occur in practice (in particular in things related to CT) can be closely approximated by some Gaussian random variable. We illustrate this in Fig. 1.21, where we plot the probabilities of the binomial random variable with $n = 30$ and $\rho = 0.7$ and the probability density function of the Gaussian random variable with the same mean (i.e., $n\rho = 21$) and the same variance (i.e., $n\rho(1 - \rho) = 6.3$). Second, even if we start with a random variable X that is not at all similar to any Gaussian random variable, if we average a sufficient number (typically, thirty or more) of samples of X, then the random variable that corresponds to this average of samples will be very similar to a Gaussian random variable.

A mathematically precise statement of this is called the *central limit theorem*, it can be stated as follows. Let X be any random variable, discrete or continuous, with S_X consisting of real numbers and $V_X > 0$. For a fixed positive integer n, consider the following process for obtaining samples z of a random variable Z_n: pick n independent samples using X, sum them together, subtract $n\mu_X$, and divide by $\sqrt{nV_X}$. Then it will be the case that, for any interval $(a, b]$,

$$\lim_{n \to \infty} P_{Z_n}(a, b] = P_N(a, b]. \tag{1.11}$$

In words, the central limit theorem says that by taking the sum of a sufficiently large number of independent samples of any random variable X, then normalizing the sum by subtraction of $n\mu_X$ and by division by $\sqrt{n}\sigma_X$, we get something that is indistinguishable from the standard Gaussian random variable!

A good example is provided if we start with the discrete random variable X for which $S_X = \{0, 1\}$ and p_X is set to $p_{1,0.7}$; i.e., $p_X(0) = 0.3$ and $p_X(1) = 0.7$. Let Y be the discrete random variable that is obtained by adding 30 random samples of X; then S_Y is the set of integers between 0 and 30 and p_Y is $p_{30,0.7}$ (recall the definition of the binomial random variables). The Z_{30} of (1.11) is obtained by taking a sample of Y, subtracting from it 21 and dividing the result by $\sqrt{6.3}$, which is just slightly larger than 2.5. If we now consider the interval (1,3], we see that $S_{Z_{30}}$ has five elements in this interval, the ones that correspond to 24, 25, 26, 27, and 28 in S_Y. So $P_{Z_{30}}(1,3] = \sum_{m=24}^{28} p_{30,7}(m)$, which is approximately 0.159. Comparing this with $P_N(1,3]$, which is approximately 0.157, we see that for the interval $(1,3]$ the right-hand side of (1.11) is well approximated by its left-hand side already at the value $n = 30$. Except for the shift and the scaling that is used in the central limit theorem, the relationship between the two sides of (1.11) at $n = 30$ is demonstrated in Fig. 1.21. In fact, the discussion here indicates that, for every ρ strictly between 0 and 1, the binomial random variable determined by $p_{n,\rho}$ will be similar to a Gaussian random variable, provided that the n is chosen large enough.

In the definition of Z_n we used the expression *independent samples.* This means exactly what the language implies: when we pick one of the n samples we totally ignore the values that have been picked prior to that, we just pick a random sample from X. One might be tempted to describe the random variable whose samples are the sums of n independent samples of X by using the notation nX. But that notation is usually used for something quite different: assuming again that all elements of S_X are real numbers and that n is a positive integer, nX denotes the random variable for which $S_{nX} = \{nx \mid x \in S_X\}$, that is the set of all numbers nx for which x is in S_X, and $p_{nX}(nX) = p_X(X)$. It is easy to see that $\mu_{nX} = n\mu_X$ and $\sigma_{nX} = n\sigma_X$. On the other hand, it is a consequence of a soon-to-be-stated fact that, although the mean of the sum of n independent samples of X is also $n\mu_X$, the standard deviation of the sum is not $n\sigma_X$ but $\sqrt{n}\sigma_X$. Taking the average (rather than the sum) of n independent samples of X, we get a random variable whose mean is μ_X and whose standard deviation is $\sigma_X/\sqrt{n}$. Furthermore, according to the central limit theorem, this random variable becomes indistinguishable, as n increases, from the Gaussian random variable of mean μ_X and standard deviation $\sigma_X/\sqrt{n}$. Thus, if it is our desire to estimate μ_X accurately, we can do this by averaging n independent samples of X for some large n, since (using a previously introduced terminology) we can be 99.5% confident that μ_X lies between the calculated average plus/minus $3\sigma_X/\sqrt{n}$, which can be made arbitrarily small by choosing n large enough.

One can think of the random variable nX introduced in the previous paragraph as the value of a *function on random variables* when that function is applied to X. Similarly, if X is a discrete random variable with elements of S_X positive numbers, then $\ln(X)$ is a random variable such that $S_{\ln(X)}$ consists of the natural logarithms of elements of S_X and, for x in S_X, $p_{\ln(X)} \ln(x) = p_X(x)$.

Given any two continuous random variables X and Y over the real numbers, their sum $X+Y$ is a continuous random variable such that S_{X+Y} is also the set of real numbers and, for any real number z,

$$p_{X+Y}(z) = \int_{-\infty}^{\infty} p_X(x) p_Y(z-x) dx. \tag{1.12}$$

(A similar definition can be given for discrete random variables using a sum instead of the integral.) This corresponds to the process of sampling by picking a random sample x of X, then independently picking a random sample y of Y, and then producing the sample z by adding x and y. It is not difficult to prove that $\mu_{X+Y} = \mu_X + \mu_Y$ and $V_{X+Y} = V_X + V_Y$. We note that it is essential for these to be true that X and Y are sampled independently (statisticians would do this more formally, using the concept of *independent random variables*); as we have seen above, if we in fact chose Y to be the same random variable as X and always pick from S_Y what we have picked from S_X, then we would get the random variable $2X$, with $V_{2X} = 4V_X$. (We note by the way that the integral in (1.12) is the *convolution* of the functions p_X and p_Y; convolutions play an essential role in some methods for image reconstruction from projections and will be discussed further later on, especially in Chapter 8.) This concept of sum generalizes to any number of random variables: we sample $X_1 + \ldots + X_n$ by independently picking a sample of each of $X_1, \ldots, X_n$ and adding them together. It is a standard result in probability theory that

$$\mu_{X_1+\cdots+X_n} = \mu_{X_1} + \cdots + \mu_{X_n} \tag{1.13}$$

(this is true even if $X_1, \ldots, X_n$ are not independent) and

$$V_{X_1+\cdots+X_n} = V_{X_1} + \cdots + V_{X_n}. \tag{1.14}$$

In CT we frequently have to work with the ratios of two random variables. For example, in Section 2.5, we use A to denote the number of photons counted during an actual measurement and C to denote the number of photons counted during a calibration measurement, and then we take the ratio of these numbers. To put this into the context of the current discussion, let A and C be two random variables such that both S_A and S_C consist of the set of positive integers. Then A/C is the random variable for which $S_{A/C}$ is the set of positive rational numbers and, for any positive rational number q,

$$p_{A/C}(q) = \sum_{\substack{a,c \text{ positive integers} \\ (a/c)=q}} p_A(a) p_C(c). \tag{1.15}$$

Further concepts of probability theory will be introduced as and when they are needed.

Notes and References

An early book devoted mainly to the applications of image reconstruction from projections is [113]. That book contains survey articles on using image reconstruction to solve problems of finding the internal structure of the solar corona, the radio brightness of a portion of the sky, the distribution of radionuclides indicating the physiological functioning of the human body, and the dynamic behavior of the beating heart of a patient. Early applications of image reconstruction from projections to medicine were reported in [229], which includes articles on x-ray, proton, ultrasound, and emission computerized tomography. Another collection of articles that gives a rather mathematical approach to the field is [143] and a more recent book with a similar attitude is [211]. A relatively recent development is "discrete tomography" that also has interesting applications [125]; for a recent example see [278], which discusses this approach in geotomography. A recent book that concentrates on applications in various aspects of materials research, but covers quite a few topics in the process, is [18].

For a description of using lunar occultation observations for the reconstruction of two-dimensional brightness distribution of radio sources, see [257]. For a general tutorial of image reconstruction in radio astronomy, see [27]. For the reconstruction of the x-ray structure of a supernova remnant, see [204]. A survey on the reconstruction of the three-dimensional solar corona is given in [3], for a more recent article on the topic see [85]. For the use of tomography in geodesy see [149] and for its use in volcanology see [9, 172].

The first report in the open literature on an apparatus demonstrating the potential of reconstructive tomography in medicine was [213]. The procedure used for doing reconstruction in that paper is essentially the same as the backprojection method (to be discussed in Chapter 7). A more accurate method was proposed by A.M. Cormack in a paper [57] that also demonstrated the potential usefulness of reconstruction from x-ray projections in diagnostic medicine. The first commercially available x-ray CT scanner was designed by G.N. Hounsfield [145, 146]; it was used for scanning the head only. CT body scanning was introduced in [171]. The 1979 Nobel prize in physiology and medicine was awarded to G.N. Hounsfield and A.M. Cormack for their pioneering contributions to the development of computerized tomography. A book covering the technological state of the art for CT is [155].

Two books that cover the state of the art (up to 2004) in IMRT are [215, 268]. Two articles that discuss how the series expansion methods that were previously applied in image reconstruction from projections (and are presented in some detail below) can also be applied to IMRT are [42, 43]. A related development is intensity modulated proton therapy (IMPT); for a recent overview see [243]. It is also possible to do computerized tomography with protons, which has the potential of improving IMPT [240].

A brief early article (with a long bibliography) on medical magnetic resonance imaging was written by P.C. Lauterbur [170]. The 2003 Nobel prize in physiology and medicine was awarded to P.C. Lauterbur and P. Mansfield for their discoveries concerning MRI. The original approach of Lauterbur was using reconstruction from projections; while nowadays most work is based on a different approach using Fourier transforms, there are some interesting developments that use projection imaging [152]. A book that discusses the technology of MRI, as well as some of its important applications to diagnostic medicine, is [13]; watch out for the soon-to-appear fourth edition! A review article on an important recent development in the field of MRI is [169].

A pioneering report on medical emission computerized tomography is [164] and an early survey of the topic is given by [35]. For more recent developments regarding PET, both basic science and clinical applications, see [17, 230, 263]. Clinical evaluation of the type of algorithms that can be used to produce reconstructions from the data collected by a PET scanner, such as the one shown in Fig. 1.8, to produce images, such as shown in Fig. 1.9, is reported in [53].

An early work on the topic of reconstructing the spatial distribution of acoustic absorption within tissue from acoustic projections is [101]. Two recent papers that are very relevant to Fig. 1.10 are [151, 269]. Note the 33-year spread between these publications! A thorough basic treatment of inverse problems for acoustic, electromagnetic and elastic wave scattering is [168]. Reconstruction from data collected by light (i.e., optical tomography) is a more recent development. A recent review of the topic is [91] and a very recent article is [162]. The methodology behind our Fig. 1.11 is discussed in [14]. The recent development of using reconstruction from data obtained by T-rays (alternatively called terahertz radiation) is discussed in [270].

The background material to our illustration of tomographic nondestructive testing (Figs. 1.12 and 1.13) can be obtained from [20, 173]. Other recent examples from the field of nondestructive testing are [96, 228]. For a general description of 3DXRD methodology, see [221]. For the specific algorithm used to obtain the reconstruction shown in Fig. 1.16, see [2, 233]. Recent developments combine diffraction data with attenuation data [150], use phase contrast tomography [207] or Friedel pairs [189], and image crystal growth [251].

The pioneering paper proposing the use of reconstruction from electron microscopic projections for the purpose of elucidation of biologically important molecular complexes was published by D.J. DeRosier and A. Klug [65]; the 1982 Nobel prize in chemistry was awarded to A. Klug for such work. Another example of an early paper on such techniques is [246]. The methods used in producing Fig. 1.19 are described in [238]; see also [236]. Two recent books that cover this field comprehensively are [83, 84]. A more recent paper that elucidates the tendency toward reconstruction from projections of larger cellular structures is [258]. Software tools for reconstruction from electron microscopic projections are described in the recent papers [239, 248].

Further details on probability and random variables can be found in [217], which provides additional material and the original references in this area. Two books written for users of statistics, rather than statisticians, are [1, 205].

2

An Overview of the Process of CT

In this chapter we describe, in the most general terms, the whole process of x-ray computerized tomography. Our intention is to give a brief overview. Hence, some terms with which the reader may not be familiar are introduced without proper definition. We ask the reader's indulgence; such terms will be carefully defined in subsequent chapters.

2.1 What Are We Trying to Do?

The aim of CT is to obtain information regarding the nature of material occupying exact positions inside the body. Generally speaking, the process as it is discussed in most of this book is as follows. A CT scanner is used to produce for a specified cross section of the body a sinogram, such as the one illustrated in Fig. 1.5(b). From this sinogram, we need to produce a two-dimensional image of the x-ray attenuation coefficient distribution in the cross section, as illustrated in Fig. 1.5(d).

In addition, the reconstruction of a series of parallel cross sections enables us to discover and display the precise shape of selected organs, as illustrated in Fig. 2.1. Such displays are obtained by further computer processing of the reconstructed cross sections (see Chapter 14).

2.2 Traditional Tomography

Prior to the introduction of CT, sectional imaging was done using various modes of (not computerized) *tomography*. We now describe a mode of tomography (*linear tomography*), illustrated in Fig. 2.2.

If we are interested in a cross section C of a patient, we can obtain a fairly good estimate by the following tomographic method. We place a photographic plate P parallel to the cross section C on one side of the patient, and an x-ray source on the other side. By moving the x-ray source at a fixed speed parallel

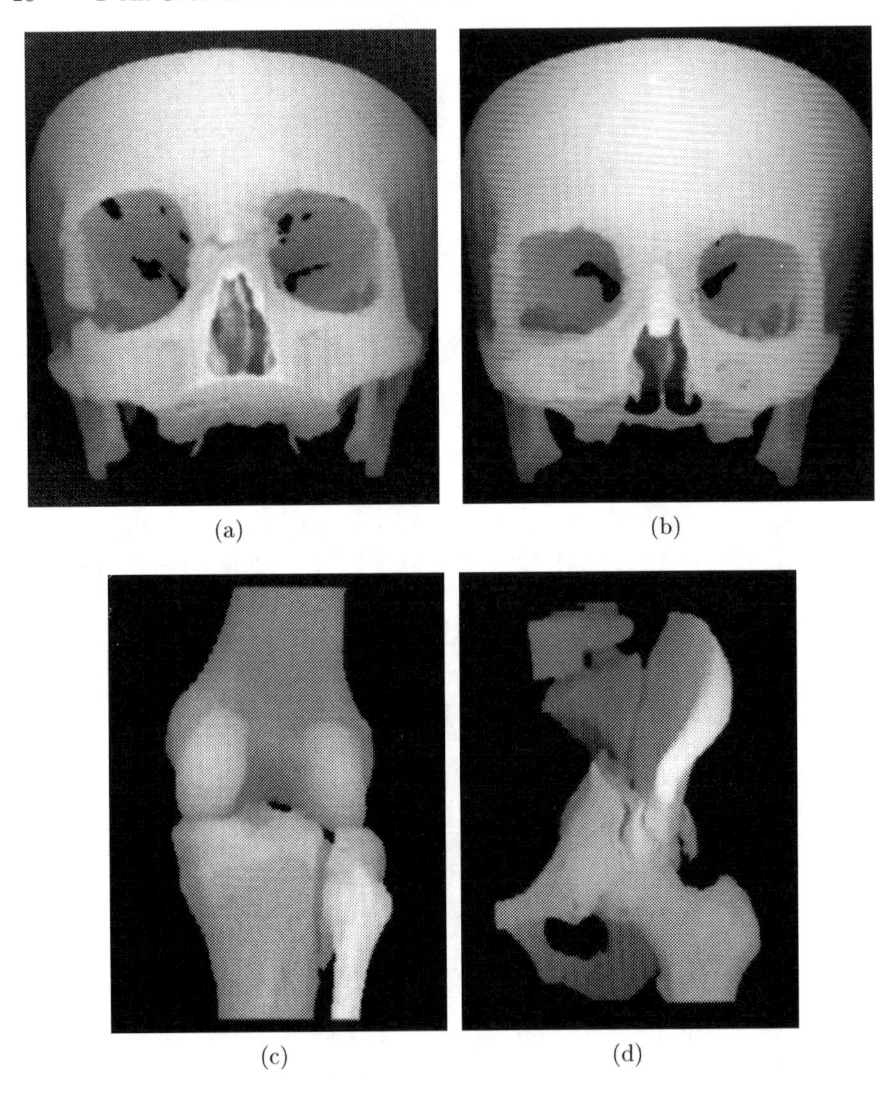

Fig. 2.1: Three-dimensional displays of bone structures of patients produced during 1986–8 by software developed in the author's research group at the University of Pennsylvania for the General Electric Company. (a) Facial bones of an accident victim prior to operation. (b) The same patient at the time of a one-year postoperative follow-up. (c) A tibial fracture. (d) A pelvic fracture.

to C in one direction, and moving P at an appropriate speed in the opposite direction, we can ensure that a point in C always projects onto the same point in P, but a point in the patient above or below C is projected onto different points in P. Thus on the photographic plate the section C will stand out, while the rest of the body will be blurred out.

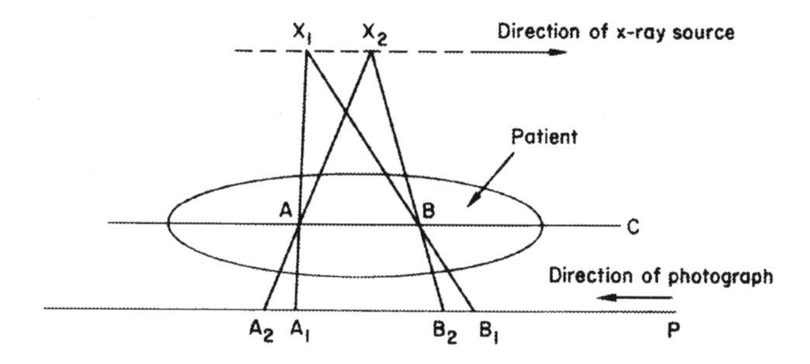

Fig. 2.2: Linear tomography. C: patient cross section; A and B: two points in the cross section C; X_1 and X_2: positions of the x-ray source at times t_1 and t_2; P: the photographic plate; A_1 and A_2: positions of a fixed point on P at times t_1 and t_2; B_1 and B_2: positions of another fixed point on P at times t_1 and t_2. (Reproduced from [100], with permission from Elsevier.)

More closely related to CT is *transaxial tomography*. An example of this is shown in Fig. 2.3. The patient sits in a special rotating chair in an upright position. The x-ray film lies flat on a rotating horizontal table beside the patient. The table is positioned a little below the desired focal plane. X-rays are directed obliquely through the patient and onto the film. The x-ray tube remains stationary throughout the exposure. The patient and film both rotate in the same direction and at the same velocity. Only those points actually in the focal plane remain in sharp focus throughout a rotation. Points above and below the focal plane are blurred. The section thickness is determined by the angle between the x-ray tube and film. The more obliquely the central ray is directed toward the film the thinner is the tomographic section.

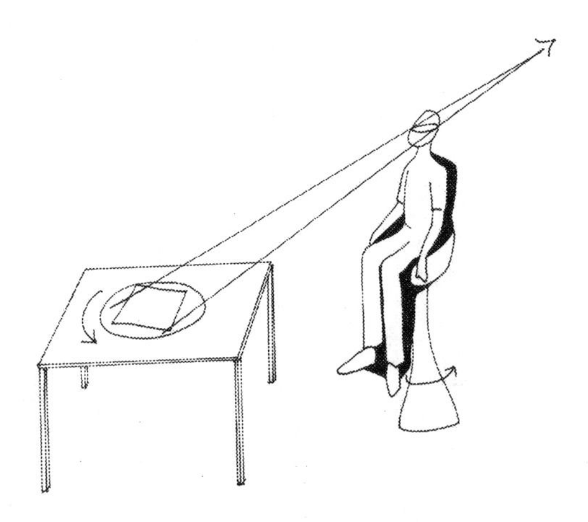

Fig. 2.3: Transaxial tomography.

In traditional forms of tomography, objects that are out of the focal plane are visible in the image, although in a blurred form. In CT, the images of cross sections are not influenced by the objects outside those sections. For this reason, the images produced by CT are much sharper, and hence generally of greater clinical utility. We will therefore forgo further discussion of traditional tomography and concentrate only on CT.

2.3 Data Collection for CT

A typical method by which data are collected for transverse section imaging in CT is indicated in Fig. 2.4. A large number of measurements are taken. Each of these measurements is related to an x-ray source position combined with an x-ray detector position. Both the source and the detector lie in the plane of the section to be imaged. For each combination of source and detector positions, two physical measurements are taken: a *calibration measurement* and an *actual measurement*. We now explain what these measurements are for a single fixed source and detector position combination.

During the calibration measurement, the object whose cross section we hope to image is not in the path of the x-ray beam from the source to the

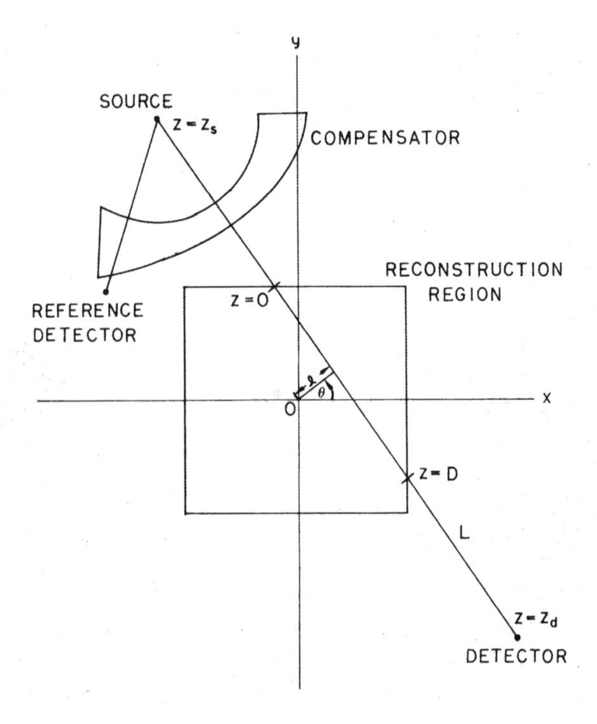

Fig. 2.4: Data collection for CT.

detector. In fact, it is assumed that the part of the beam that intersects the so-called *reconstruction region* (see Fig. 2.4) traverses through a homogeneous *reference material* such as air or water. The calibration measurement tells us how many out of a large but fixed number of photons that leave the source are counted by the detector. A *reference detector* serves the purpose of compensating for fluctuations in the strength of the x-ray source. Compensation can be done by dividing the number of photons counted by the detector by the number of photons counted by the reference detector. During the actual measurement, the object of interest is inserted into the reconstruction region, (partially) replacing the reference material. It is an important restriction that the object of interest does *not* occupy any point outside the reconstruction region. On the other hand, we allow the possibility of additional objects occupying fixed positions outside the reconstruction region during both the calibration and the actual measurement. An example of this is the object marked *compensator* in Fig. 2.4. (It compensates for the thinness of a transverse section of human body near the edges. This makes the number of photons reaching the detector at different positions more uniform and so reduces the range of photon counts that a detector needs to handle.) The actual measurement is defined in the same way as the calibration measurement, except that the cross section to be imaged is now in position. It influences the photon count by the detector, but not the photon count by the reference detector.

In summary, the size of the actual measurement as compared to the size of the calibration measurement depends on the photon absorbing and scattering properties of the object to be reconstructed as compared to those properties of a reference material.

We obtain a calibration measurement and an actual measurement for each of many source and detector position combinations. From these two sets of numbers we wish to produce a third set, namely, the set of CT numbers for the cross section of the object under investigation. These numbers, when coded into grayscale images, give the type of pictures that we see in Fig. 1.5(d). In the next section we discuss the physical interpretation of these numbers and images.

2.4 Voxels, Pixels, and CT Numbers

In a vacuum all x-ray photons that leave a source in the direction of a detector will reach the detector. When a material is placed between the source and the detector, some of the photons that leave the source in the direction of the detector will be removed from the beam (absorbed or scattered). The probability that a photon gets removed depends on the energy of the photon and on the material between the source and the detector.

The *linear attenuation coefficient* $\mu_{\bar{e}}^{t}$ of a tissue t at energy $\bar{e}$ is defined as follows. Let ρ be the probability that a photon of energy $\bar{e}$, which enters a uniform slab of the tissue t of unit thickness, on a line L perpendicular to the face of the slab, will not be absorbed or scattered in the slab (i.e., ρ is the transmittance at energy $\bar{e}$ of the slab along the line L, see Section 1.2 and especially Fig. 1.20). We define

$$\mu_{\bar{e}}^{t} = -\ln \rho, \tag{2.1}$$

where ln denotes the natural logarithm. Note that the size of the linear attenuation coefficient is dependent on the unit of length used. As is justified in Section 15.1, the linear attenuation coefficient is measured in units of inverse length. For example, the linear attenuation of water at 73 keV is 0.19 cm^{-1}.

In what follows we shall be working with the *relative linear attenuation* at energy $\bar{e}$. At any point of space, we define the relative linear attenuation to be $\mu_{\bar{e}}^{t} - \mu_{\bar{e}}^{a}$, where t is the tissue occupying the point of space during the actual measurement and a is the material occupying the point during the calibration measurement. Since we assume that the exterior of the reconstruction region is the same during the two sets of measurements, the relative linear attenuation is zero for all points outside the reconstruction region for all energies. Note also that for all points inside the reconstruction region $\mu_{\bar{e}}^{a}$ is the same, since the reference material is supposed to be homogeneous during the calibration measurement.

Now suppose that we are interested in a cross-sectional slice of the human body that is, say, 3 mm thick. We can subdivide this slice into small 3 mm long blocks with equal, square-shaped cross sections. These blocks are usually referred to as *volume elements*, or *voxels*, for short. Roughly speaking, a *CT number* is proportional to the average relative linear attenuation in a voxel. Since the relative linear attenuation itself is energy dependent, this definition needs further clarification, which is given in the next section. Typically, the background material is assumed to have the linear attenuation of water (thus the CT number of water is zero), and the scale of CT numbers is adjusted so that the CT number of air is approximately -1000.

Suppose, for example, that the reconstruction region in Fig. 2.4 is a square $41.6 \times 41.6\ \text{cm}^2$, and we wish to use voxels that are $3 \times 0.65 \times 0.65\ \text{mm}^3$. Then there is a 640×640 array of such voxels that exactly fills the reconstruction region, providing us with a 640×640 array of CT numbers. In displaying the cross section, we display the CT numbers. In this case, we want to display a 640×640 array of small squares, with the uniform grayness in each one being proportional to the CT number of the voxel in the appropriate position. These small squares are referred to as *picture elements*, or *pixels*, for short.

2.5 The Problem of Polychromaticity

When an x-ray beam passes through the body, its attenuation at any point depends on the material at that point and on the energy distribution (*spectrum*) of the beam. In CT the spectrum is made up from many energy levels (*polychromatic*) and it changes (*hardens*) as the beam passes through the object. Thus, the attenuation at a point may vary with the direction of the beam passing through it. If we had a spectrum of only one energy level (*monochromatic*), this would not be the case. Each point would have a uniquely assigned attenuation coefficient, and reconstruction of the distribution of these coefficients would be a well-defined aim of computerized tomography.

We would like the following statement to be true: "The CT number assigned to a voxel is a property of the tissue occupying the voxel and does not depend on the location of the voxel in the slice." This is obviously desirable for diagnostic purposes. Also, as we shall see in the following, the truth of the statement is assumed in the development of mathematical procedures for calculating CT numbers.

A suitable definition for CT numbers is one in which a CT number is a multiple of the average relative linear attenuation of a voxel at a specified energy $\bar{e}$, to which we refer as the *effective energy.* Suppose now that we have a monochromatic x-ray source with photon energy $\bar{e}$. For a fixed position of the source and detector pair, let C_m be the calibration measurement (the count of the number of photons that get from the source to the detector without the object to be reconstructed being between them, divided by the count of the reference detector), and let A_m be the actual measurement (the count of the number of photons that get from the source to the detector with the object of interest in place, divided by the count of the reference detector). We define the *monochromatic ray sum*, m, for this beam by

$$m = -\ln\left(A_m/C_m\right), \tag{2.2}$$

and we refer to the set of ms for all source and detector pair positions as the *monochromatic projection data.* Based on the physical and mathematical facts to be discussed, we know that the relative linear attenuation inside the slice at the effective energy $\bar{e}$ can be accurately estimated from the monochromatic projection data.

In practice, the x-ray beam is polychromatic. Let C_p and A_p denote the calibration and actual measurement, respectively, for a particular source–detector pair position with the polychromatic x-ray beam. We define the *polychromatic ray sum, p,* for this x-ray beam by

$$p = -\ln\left(A_p/C_p\right), \tag{2.3}$$

and we refer to the set of ps for all source and detector pair positions as the *polychromatic projection data.*

Our problem is the following. For any source and detector position we can obtain p, but the reconstruction procedure requires m. The question naturally arises: Does p uniquely determine m? Unfortunately, except in unrealistically restrictive cases, the answer is "no."

A more pragmatic question is: Given p, can we approximate m well enough so that it leads to diagnostically useful CT numbers? There the answer appears to be "yes," as is illustrated in the following chapters.

2.6 Reconstruction Algorithms

We now briefly discuss the major topic of this book: the method for obtaining CT numbers from the monochromatic projection data. In practice, we apply this method using corrected polychromatic projection data in place of the (usually unavailable) monochromatic projection data.

Since we wish to implement our method on a computer, we need precise instructions on how the CT numbers are to be obtained from the monochromatic projection data. A finite sequence of unambiguous instructions that tell us how to get, step by step, from some given input to the desired output is an *algorithm*. Instructions that a physician writes up for unskilled laboratory assistants on what tests to perform next on a sample, based on the outcome of previous tests, should (and usually do) form an algorithm. The instructions provided by the Internal Revenue Service on how to fill out a tax return should also form an algorithm; the fact that they do not gives rise to the honorable profession of tax accountancy.

Basically the same procedure would have to be described differently depending on at whom the description is aimed. A computing machine needs a very detailed description (a computer program) in order to perform the same calculations that a mathematician would perform from just a few brief formulas.

In order to design an algorithm for obtaining CT numbers from monochromatic projection data, we first replace the problem by a simplified mathematical idealization of it. This has the same standing as the classical assumption one makes in calculating the earth's orbit; namely, that all the mass of the earth is concentrated in a single point at its center. While the assumption is blatantly false, as long as it leads to correct calculations, there is every reason to use it: it makes the theory and the resulting calculations tractable. There is very little we could do in calculating the earth's orbit if we had to know the location of every fly before such a calculation could be carried out.

The simplifying assumptions we make in setting up the theory for reconstruction algorithms are: (1) slices are infinitely thin; (2) for any particular source and detector pair position, all x-ray photons travel in the same straight line (which lies in the infinitely thin slice). A consequence of the first assumption is that the distinction between voxels and pixels disappears. Indeed, since the slice is infinitely thin, it can be thought of as a picture whose grayness at any point (x, y) is proportional to the relative linear attenuation $\mu_{\bar{e}}(x, y)$ at that point. This is the reason why the theory behind reconstruction algorithms is often referred to as "image reconstruction from projections."

Let L be the straight line that is the path of all the x-ray photons for a particular source–detector pair and let m be the corresponding monochromatic ray sum. Based on our definition of a linear attenuation coefficient, it is proved in Section 15.2 that

$$m \simeq \int_0^D \mu_{\bar{e}}(x, y)\, dz. \tag{2.4}$$

In this formula, $\simeq$ denotes "approximately equal," z is the distance of the point (x, y) on the line L, and the integration limits 0 and D are clear from Fig. 2.4.

Since $\mu_{\bar{e}}(x,y) = 0$ for points (x,y) outside the reconstruction region, $\int_0^D \mu_{\bar{e}}(x,y)$ is the integral of $\mu_{\bar{e}}(x,y)$ along the line L. Thus our problem is to calculate the values of $\mu_{\bar{e}}(x,y)$ from estimates of its integrals along a number of lines, namely from the monochromatic projection data.

In some sense this problem was solved in 1917 by Radon. Let ℓ denote the distance of the line L from the origin, let θ denote the angle made with the x axis by the perpendicular drawn from the origin to L (see Fig. 2.4), and let $m(\ell,\theta)$ denote the integral of $\mu_{\bar{e}}(x,y)$ along the line L. Radon proved (see Section 15.3) that

$$\mu_{\bar{e}}(x,y) = -\frac{1}{2\pi^2} \lim_{\varepsilon \to 0} \int_{\varepsilon}^{\infty} \frac{1}{q} \int_0^{2\pi} m_1(x\cos\theta + y\sin\theta + q, \theta)\, d\theta\, dq, \qquad (2.5)$$

where $m_1(\ell,\theta)$ denotes the partial derivative of $m(\ell,\theta)$ with respect to ℓ. While the exact details of this formula are likely to be obscure to a non-mathematician, its implication should be clear: the distribution of the relative linear attenuations in an infinitely thin slice is uniquely determined by the set of *all* its line integrals.

This seems to indicate that the reconstruction problem has been solved since 1917. However, there are some practical difficulties in applying to CT this mathematical solution to the idealized problem:

(a) Radon's formula determines a picture from all its line integrals. In CT we have only a finite set of measurements. Even if these were *exactly* the projections along a number of straight lines, a finite number of them would not be enough to determine the picture uniquely, or even accurately. Based on the finiteness of the data alone one can easily produce objects for which the reconstructions will be very inaccurate (see Section 15.4).

(b) The measurements in computed tomography can only be used to estimate the line integrals. Inaccuracies in these estimates are due to the width of the x-ray beam, scatter, hardening of the beam, photon statistics, detector inaccuracies, etc. Radon's inversion formula is sensitive to these inaccuracies.

(c) Radon gave a mathematical formula; we need an *efficient* algorithm to evaluate it. This is not necessarily trivial to obtain. There has been a very great deal of activity to find algorithms that are fast when implemented on a computer and yet produce acceptable reconstructions in spite of the finite and inaccurate nature of the data. Much of this book is devoted to this topic.

Notes and References

The mathematical and computational procedures underlying CT as described in this chapter are summarized in Fig. 2.5. Much of this material is based on [111]. A more up-to-date coverage of CT can be found in [155].

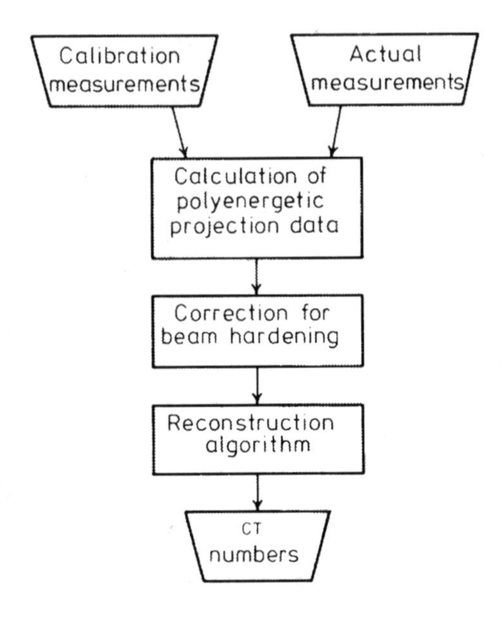

Fig. 2.5: Outline of the mathematical and computational procedures underlying CT. (Reproduced from [111]. Copyright by the Institute of Physics.)

The three-dimensional displays in Fig. 2.1 were produced by the software 3D98 [261], which was probably the first software system for 3D display and analysis that was integrated into a commercial CT scanner (namely the GE CT/T 9800).

The discussion of traditional tomography is based on [100]; see also [253]. These papers contain further early references. A more recent sample reference is [159] and a survey of relatively modern developments is given in [68].

The physics of x-ray generation and interaction with matter is discussed in books on radiological physics such as [54].

For a more detailed discussion on the nature of algorithms in general see, e.g., the relevant entries in [226]. A relatively recent book that discusses reconstruction-related algorithms is [211].

The Radon transform was introduced in [225]; that paper contains a derivation of the inversion formula (2.5).

3

Physical Problems Associated with Data Collection in CT

The main topic of this book is a discussion of the algorithms by which the distribution of the relative linear attenuation at an effective energy $\bar{e}$, namely $\mu_{\bar{e}}(x,y)$, is calculated from estimates of its line integrals along a finite number of lines. The measurements in CT are taken in order to estimate these line integrals. In this chapter we discuss the physical limitations and problems that arise in estimating the line integrals from the calibration and actual measurements. Except for the problems of photon statistics and beam hardening, our discussion will be limited to a summary of the problems with some indications on how their effects may be reduced. We also discuss the different scanner configurations that are used in computerized tomography. In Chapter 5 we illustrate the effects on the quality of the reconstruction of the different sources of error in the data collection.

3.1 Photon Statistics

A very basic limitation to the accuracy of measurements taken in CT is the statistical nature of the process of x-ray photon production, photon interaction with matter, and photon detection. We discuss these processes one by one.

Consider the experiment in which we count the actual number of photons emitted in a unit period of time in the direction of a detector by a stable x-ray source that emits on average λ photons in a unit period of time in the direction of the detector. Such an experiment gives rise to a discrete random variable, which we denote by Y_λ (see Section 1.2). The set S_{Y_λ} of the possible outcomes of the experiment consists of the nonnegative integers (the photon counts). In this book we accept without further discussion the physical result that

$$p_{Y_\lambda}(y) = \frac{\lambda^y \exp(-\lambda)}{y!}. \tag{3.1}$$

In Fig. 3.1 we show the values of $p_{Y_\lambda}(y)$ for $y = 0, \ldots, 50$ when (a) $\lambda = 5$ and (b) $\lambda = 25$.

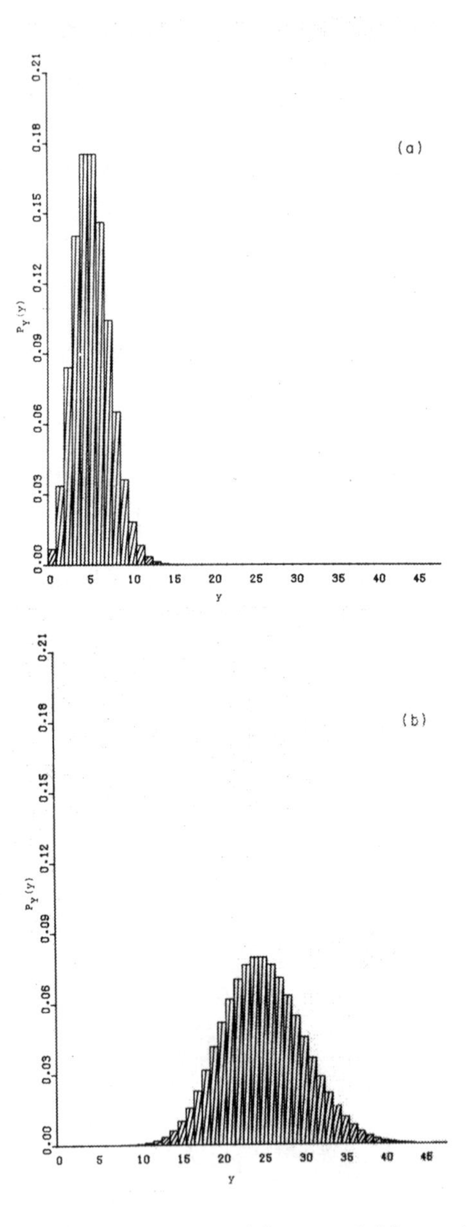

Fig. 3.1: Plots of the functions (a) p_{Y_5} and (b) $p_{Y_{25}}$ in (3.1).

Equation (3.1) is referred to as the *Poisson probability law*, and a discrete random variable Y_λ satisfying it is called the *Poisson random variable* with parameter λ. We note three important properties of this random variable:

(i) its mean is λ,

(ii) its variance is λ,
(iii) it is very similar to the Gaussian random variable X with mean λ and variance λ, as defined by (1.10), provided that λ is large (greater than 100), in the sense that, for any interval $(a, b]$ such that $b - a$ is a positive integer, $P_{Y_\lambda}(a, b] \simeq P_X(a, b]$.

This has important practical implications. Suppose, for example, that we are interested in estimating λ, the average number of photons emitted per unit time by a stable x-ray source in the direction of a detector. If we have a way of counting all the photons reaching the detector, we may estimate λ by the count of the number of photons during a particular period of unit time (i.e., by a sample of the random variable). If the true value of λ is 10,000, then there is at most a 1 in 20 chance that we make an error 200 (two standard deviations) or more using this approach. (Recall from Section 1.2 that we are 95% confident that the mean of a Gaussian random variable is within two standard deviations of a random sample from it.) Alternatively, we may count the number of photons for 100 units of time, and divide the count by 100 to give us an estimate of λ. The total number of photons during this longer period is on average 1,000,000, and in 19 cases out of 20, the actual count will be between 998,000 and 1,002,000. So in 19 cases out of 20, the estimate of λ will be between 9,980 and 10,020; i.e., the error is 20 or less. By increasing the time period used for counting photons by a factor of 100 we have reduced the size of the likely error in our estimate by a factor of 10. We observe a similar phenomenon in the following when we discuss how the accuracy of the calibration and actual measurements in CT is dependent on the total number of x-ray photons used.

Now we look at the statistical nature of the interactions of x-ray photons with matter. Suppose that a photon leaves the source in direction of the detector along a line L (see Fig. 2.4). Then there is a fixed probability ρ that the photon will get as far as the detector without being absorbed or scattered. This probability depends on the energy of the photon and the material intersected by the line L between the source and the detector. We call ρ the *transmittance* along L of the material between the source and the detector at that particular energy. If everything between the source and the detector remains stationary for a period of time and during this time 10,000 photons of the same energy leave the source in direction of the detector along the line L, then the number of photons reaching the detector will be approximately, but almost never exactly, $10{,}000\rho$. The rest of the photons will be absorbed or scattered.

A photon that reaches the detector is not necessarily counted. For each energy, there is a fixed probability that a photon that reaches the detector is counted by the detector. We call σ the *efficiency* of the detector at that particular energy. Continuing with the case discussed in the previous paragraph, the number of photons out of the original 10,000 that will not be absorbed or scattered and will be counted is approximately, but almost never exactly, $10{,}000\rho\sigma$. The following important statement is proved in Section 15.5.

Let λ denote the average of the number of photons at energy $\bar{e}$ that are emitted in one unit of time by a stable x-ray source along a line L in the direction of a detector. Let ρ denote the transmittance along L of the material between the source and detector at energy $\bar{e}$. Let σ denote the efficiency of the detector at energy $\bar{e}$. Then the number of photons that

(i) are at energy $\bar{e}$,
(ii) reach the detector without having been absorbed or scattered, and
(iii) are counted by the detector in one unit of time,

is a sample of the Poisson random variable with parameter $\lambda\rho\sigma$.

We are now in position to discuss what is being measured during the data collection phase of CT, as described in Section 2.3. For this discussion we assume that the x-ray beam is monochromatic, the x-ray source and detectors are negligible in size (hence all photons from the source to the detector travel in the same straight line), and that a photon that has been absorbed or scattered along this line never reaches the detector. In subsequent sections we talk about the errors introduced by the physical unattainability of these assumptions.

Let us look at the exact nature of the process involved in getting the C_m and the A_m of (2.2). Suppose that a monochromatic x-ray source of energy $\bar{e}$ is such that the fraction of emitted photons that leave in the direction of the reference detector is ϕ_r, and the fraction of emitted photons that leave in the direction of the actual detector is ϕ_d (see Fig. 2.4). Suppose further that the averages of the total number of photons emitted during the periods of the calibration and actual measurements are λ_c and λ_a, respectively. Let ρ_r be the transmittance at energy $\bar{e}$ of the material between the source and the reference detector, and let ρ_c and ρ_a be the transmittance at energy $\bar{e}$ of the material between the source and the actual detector during the calibration and the actual measurement, respectively. Let σ_r, respectively σ_d, be the efficiency at energy $\bar{e}$ of the reference detector, respectively of the detector.

Consider now how we get a value of C_m. The actual number of photons emitted is a sample y_c from Y_{λ_c}. The actual number of photons counted by the reference detector is a sample c_r from the binomial distribution with parameters y_c and $\phi_r\rho_r\sigma_r$ and the actual number of photons counted by the actual detector is a sample c_a from the binomial distribution with parameters y_c and $\phi_d\rho_c\sigma_d$. To avoid divisions by zero and (later on) having to take the logarithm of zero, in the unlikely case that either c_r or c_a is 0, we set its value to 1. Finally, we define $C_m = c_a/c_r$. This is quite a complicated sampling process, especially since c_r and c_a are related to each other by the fact that the binomial distributions from which they are picked have the parameter y_c in common, but this parameter itself changes from sample to sample.

Ignoring the full complexity of the statistics for the moment, let us argue based just on means. The means of the binomial distributions with parameters

y_c and $\phi_r\rho_r\sigma_r$ and with parameters y_c and $\phi_d\rho_c\sigma_d$ are $y_c\phi_r\rho_r\sigma_r$ and $y_c\phi_d\rho_c\sigma_d$, respectively. Hence, it is reasonable to claim that

$$C_m \simeq \phi_d\rho_c\sigma_d/\phi_r\rho_r\sigma_r. \tag{3.2}$$

By a completely analogous argument for the actual measurement process, we obtain that

$$A_m \simeq \phi_d\rho_a\sigma_d/\phi_r\rho_r\sigma_r. \tag{3.3}$$

Combining (3.2) and (3.3) with (2.2), we get that

$$m \simeq -\ln\left(\rho_a/\rho_c\right). \tag{3.4}$$

In Section 15.2 we show that

$$-\ln\frac{\rho_a}{\rho_c} = \int_0^D \mu_{\bar{e}}(x,y)\,dz. \tag{3.5}$$

This is why the monochromatic ray sum m can be used as an estimator to $\int_0^D \mu_{\bar{e}}(x,y)\,dz$ in an algorithm that calculates $\mu_{\bar{e}}(x,y)$ at individual points from the line integrals of $\mu_{\bar{e}}(x,y)$ (see Section 2.6).

The important question is: How accurate an estimator is m of $-\ln(\rho_a/\rho_c)$? As illustrated in Section 15.5, in a realistic CT situation, it can be assumed that m is a sample of a random variable M such that

$$\left|\mu_M + \ln\left(\rho_a/\rho_c\right)\right| < S, \tag{3.6}$$

and

$$V_M \simeq S, \tag{3.7}$$

where

$$S = \left(\phi_d\lambda_a\rho_a\sigma_d\right)^{-1} + \left(\phi_r\lambda_a\rho_r\sigma_r\right)^{-1} + \left(\phi_d\lambda_c\rho_c\sigma_d\right)^{-1} + \left(\phi_r\lambda_c\rho_r\sigma_r\right)^{-1}. \tag{3.8}$$

If we can make this quantity S very small, then we ensure accurate estimation of $-\ln\left(\rho_a/\rho_c\right)$ by m.

Note that one way of making S very small is to make the number of photons leaving the source (λ_c and λ_a) large. Except for the problem of possibly saturating the counting capability of the detectors there is no difficulty in making λ_c very large, and thereby making the last two terms in S negligibly small. In such a case we see that S becomes inversely proportional to λ_a. Unfortunately, one cannot make the number of photons leaving the source during the actual measurement arbitrarily large, since this would result in an unacceptable radiation dose to the patient and may slow the process of projection taking so that errors due to motion become important (see the following). Note, however, that by ensuring that ϕ_r is much larger than ϕ_d and that the transmittance ρ_r between the source and the reference detector is relatively large (near 1), it is possible that we can also make the second term (3.8) negligibly small. This leaves us with

$$S \simeq 1/\phi_d \lambda_a \rho_a \sigma_d, \tag{3.9}$$

which shows in particular that the error in our estimation of $-\ln(\rho_a/\rho_c)$ depends on the transmittance ρ_a during the actual measurement; lesser transmittance results in greater error.

As can be seen from the preceding, a certain amount of error in the measurements due to the statistical nature of the processes of x-ray photon production, photon interaction with matter, and photon detection is unavoidable. The properties of the error, considered as a random variable, are understood. As we shall see, some reconstruction algorithms attempt to make use of these properties. Since the errors in the measurements affect the outcome of the reconstruction process, it is important to understand both the nature of these errors and the way in which the results produced by a given reconstruction algorithm are influenced by such errors.

3.2 Beam Hardening

The x-ray beam used in CT is polychromatic, consisting of photons at different energies. Because the attenuation at a fixed point is generally greater for photons of lower energy, the energy distribution spectrum of the x-ray beam changes (hardens) as it passes through the object. X-ray beams reaching a particular point inside the body from different directions are likely to have different spectra (having passed through different materials before reaching the point in question) and thus will be attenuated differently at that point. This makes it difficult to assign a single value to the attenuation coefficient at a point in the body.

A possible solution to this difficulty is to assign to the point the attenuation coefficient of photons at a particular energy (what we referred to as the effective energy). If we used monochromatic x-ray beams consisting of photons only at that single energy, beams from different directions would be attenuated in the same way at a fixed point. Reconstruction of such attenuation coefficients is a well-defined aim of computed tomography.

In this section we discuss mathematical formulas that describe the nature of polychromatic ray sums and methods that may be used to find the corresponding monochromatic ray sums. It is shown in Section 15.6 that the polychromatic ray sum p approximates an integral of the form

$$p \simeq -\ln \int_0^E \tau_e \exp\left(-\int_0^D \left(\mu_e(z) - \mu_e^a\right) dz\right) de. \tag{3.10}$$

We now give a detailed explanation of the meaning of the symbols in (3.10).

It is assumed that the source emits a polychromatic x-ray beam with photons at energies between 0 and E. We use τ_e to denote the value at energy e of the probability density function of the continuous random variable that describes the statistical distribution of the energies of the photons counted during the calibration measurement. Here we have adopted the somewhat nonstandard notation of using τ_e to denote the value of a function of energy at the energy e. We refer to this probability density function as the *detected spectrum during the calibration measurement*.

The symbols D and z have the same meaning as in the last chapter (see Fig. 2.4) and $\mu_e(z)$ is a function of two variables (the energy e and the distance z), whose value is the linear attenuation coefficient at energy e at the point z on the line L during the actual measurement. On the other hand, μ_e^a is a function of one variable only (the energy e), whose value is the linear attenuation of the reference material a at energy e. Thus, $\int_0^D (\mu_e(z) - \mu_e^a)\, dz$ is the integral of the relative linear attenuation at energy e along the line L. Note, in particular, that the polychromatic ray sum depends only on the relative linear attenuations (at all energies between 0 and E) and on the detected spectrum during the calibration measurement. Rewriting (2.4) in this notation we get

$$m \simeq \int_0^D \left(\mu_{\bar{e}}(z) - \mu_{\bar{e}}^a\right) dz. \tag{3.11}$$

Recall now that CT numbers represent relative linear attenuations at the effective energy $\bar{e}$; and that they are to be obtained from estimates of the monochromatic projection data, which are themselves calculated from the experimentally obtained polychromatic projection data. The method of estimating the monochromatic projection data from the polychromatic projection data is the topic of the rest of this section.

We start with a theoretical discussion of a special situation. Suppose that during the actual measurement there are only two types of material, a and b, in the reconstruction region (a is the reference material). Consider a fixed source–detector pair, and assume that the total length of the parts of the line L that go through material b is B. From (3.10) and (3.11) we get

$$p \simeq -\ln \int_0^E \tau_e \exp\left(-B\left(\mu_e^b - \mu_e^a\right)\right) de \tag{3.12}$$

and

$$m \simeq B\left(\mu_{\bar{e}}^b - \mu_{\bar{e}}^a\right). \tag{3.13}$$

Combining (3.12) and (3.13) we get

$$p \simeq -\ln \int_0^E \tau_e \exp\left(-\frac{\mu_e^b - \mu_e^a}{\mu_{\bar{e}}^b - \mu_{\bar{e}}^a} m\right) de. \tag{3.14}$$

The important thing to observe in (3.14) is that, provided either $\mu_e^b > \mu_e^a$ for all energies between 0 and E or $\mu_e^b < \mu_e^a$ for all energies between 0 and E, its right-hand side is a monotonic function of m. (Note that τ_e is positive for all e.) Hence, given any value of p, there is only one value of m that makes the two sides of (3.14) equal. In practice we can use the plot of the right-hand side of (3.14) to correct for beam hardening; we simply find the value of m for which the value of the right-hand side is the experimentally obtained polychromatic ray sum p.

Equation (3.14) was obtained under the rather restrictive assumption that there are only two different types of material in the reconstruction region. If the organ we are looking at is a head inserted into a water bag, this assumption is not too badly violated, since the contents of the head are bone and material whose x-ray attenuation properties are not too dissimilar to water. Thus (3.14) may be used for correcting for beam hardening in such a situation, but in general it is not as good as some other methods to be discussed in the following.

While the precise method based on (3.14) must be considered to be unreliable because of the too restrictive nature of the underlying assumptions, the general approach suggested by it is very attractive: specify a function q of the polychromatic ray sum p such that if we use $q(p)$ as our estimate of the monochromatic ray sum m, then we get reasonably good reconstructions of the relative linear attenuations at the effective energy $\bar{e}$.

Natural candidates for such a function are *polynomials*, i.e., functions of the form

$$q(p) = a_n p^n + a_{n-1} p^{n-1} + \cdots + a_1 p + a_0, \tag{3.15}$$

where n (the order of the polynomial) is a fixed integer and $a_0, \ldots, a_n$ are fixed coefficients that need to be determined so that $q(p)$ provides an acceptable estimate of m for our purpose. There are two computational advantages of polynomial approximations to others (for example, approximation by combination of exponentials): the coefficients are easy to calculate and, once they are calculated, (3.15) is easy to evaluate, especially since a low value of n (less than 5) usually suffices (see Section 5.6).

In certain cases there is no single function q such that replacement of m by $q(p)$ in (2.5) would lead to acceptable reconstructions. One is then forced to use either multiple correcting functions specific to the source–detector pair positions or an iterative correction procedure, where the correcting function q for the next iteration is based on a reconstruction during the previous iteration (see Section 5.6).

3.3 Other Sources of Error

If we wish to base our reconstruction algorithm on (2.5), then we have to know the values of $m(l, \theta)$ (the line integral of $\mu_{\bar{e}}(x, y)$ along L, see Fig. 2.4) for certain l and θ (i.e., for certain lines L). Photon statistics and beam hardening are two reasons why physical measurements can provide us only with approximations of $m(l, \theta)$. In this section we briefly discuss further reasons.

One source of error is that both the x-ray source (more precisely the focal spot of the x-ray source) and the detector have a certain size, and thus the

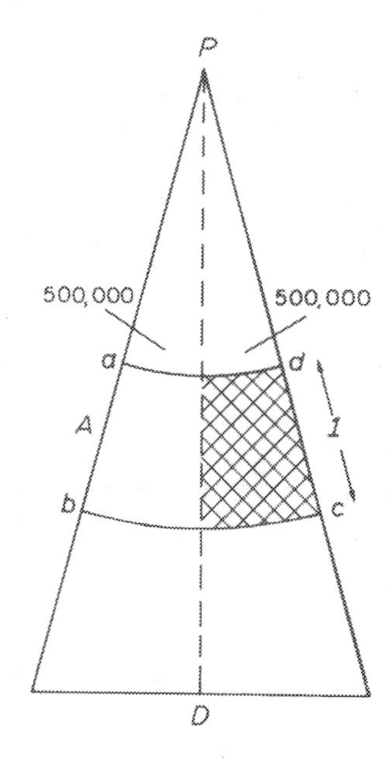

Fig. 3.2: Illustration of the partial volume effect.

photons that are counted do not all travel along the same line, but rather they travel along one of a bundle of lines forming a rather complicated shape.

One consequence of the non-negligible size of the focal spot and detector is the so-called *partial volume effect*, which we now explain on a simple two-dimensional example. Suppose we have a point monochromatic x-ray source P and a line segment detector D; see Fig. 3.2. Suppose that the linear attenuation coefficient (see Section 2.4) is everywhere zero except in that half of the area A that is cross-hatched in Fig. 3.2, where its value is two. It is assumed that the length of intersection with A of any line from P to D is unity. Suppose also that the reference material has linear attenuation coefficient zero (vacuum) and that the number of photons read by the reference detector during both calibration and actual measurement is 1000. Hence the number of photons that leave the source in direction of the detector is about the same during calibration and actual measurement. Suppose this number is 1,000,000. Thus the calibration measurement is $C_m \simeq 1000$. Breaking the x-ray beam into two equal halves as shown in Fig. 3.2 we see that approximately 500,000 photons will enter both halves of A. In the left half, where the linear attenuation coefficient is zero and hence transmittance is one, all 500,000 photons reach the detector. In the right half, where the linear attenuation is two, and hence transmittance is $e^{-2} \simeq 0.135$, the number of photons that reach the detector is about 68,000. Hence the total number of detected photons is about 568,000 and the actual measurement is $A_m \simeq 568$. Using (2.2) we get $m \simeq 0.566$. This is an estimate, see (2.4), of the average of the line integral of the relative linear attenuation between the source and points on the detector. However, it is easy to see that the true value of this average is 1.0. The reason for this rather large error (43.4%) in the estimation of the average is that the beam is only partially blocked by attenuating material and the processes of taking exponentials and logarithms give a disproportionately great importance to the unblocked portion of the beam.

In principle, one can reduce the size of the source and the detector by putting lead shielding with long narrow pinholes in front of both of them, but this would have two undesirable consequences. One is that the error due to photon statistics would considerably increase, because the value of ϕ_d in (3.9) would become very small. The second consequence arises when we search for possibly small features in large organs (such as tumors in the lung) by taking cross-sectional slices. If the physical slices are thin, we have to use many slices to ensure that we do not miss what we are looking for. This results in longer time to be spent by the computer that provides the reconstructions and possibly by the radiologist who needs to examine them.

We have just given one example of a phenomenon that is rather common in CT: methods that can be used to combat error due to one physical phenomenon result in increasing the error due to another one. A further example of this is the way one handles *motion artifacts*.

It is an underlying assumption in CT that the $m(l, \theta)$, which we try to measure, are integrals along different lines of the same function $\mu_{\bar{e}}(x, y)$. However, this assumption is violated if some of these lines L go through a moving organ, such as the lung or the heart, and if the actual measurements are taken at different times for different lines, since the function $\mu_{\bar{e}}(x, y)$ changes as the organ moves. One way of combating this is to use multiple arrays of detectors and possibly even multiple sources (more about this in the next section), so that all the measurements can be taken within a small period of time during which organ motion is insignificant. However, this results in an increase of error due to detection of *scattered* photons, a phenomenon that we now discuss.

Note that in Section 3.1 we have assumed that the detector counts a photon only if it has left the source in the direction of the detector and has reached the detector without having been absorbed or scattered. If there is a single source and a single detector, this is a reasonable assumption, since a scattered photon can reach the detector only if it has been scattered in a direction very nearly the same as its original direction or if it has been multiply scattered away from and then back towards the detector. These events are sufficiently unlikely, so that the error due to scatter in a single source single detector case is rather small. However, if we have an array of detectors, a photon scattered out of its path towards one detector may very well reach another detector and be counted by it. Since the ratio of scattered photons to unscattered photons that reach a detector is dependent on the object to be reconstructed (and in a rather complicated way), the error introduced by scatter cannot be completely removed from the measurements prior to reconstruction. Collimation, which absorbs photons coming towards a detector from directions other than the source, can reduce the number of scattered photons that are counted by the detector.

Finally, we discuss some errors that are due to the device used for collecting the data not functioning exactly as intended.

It is important that the source and the detectors do not change their behavior between the calibration measurement and the actual measurement. For example, in our derivation in Section 3.1 we have assumed that the efficiency σ_d, of the detector is the same during the calibration and the actual measurement. Change in detector efficiency would make (3.4) invalid.

Detector efficiency is assumed to be independent of the number of photons the detector has to count. This may be difficult to achieve in practice, since detectors can be saturated by too many photons getting to them. One way of combating this is by insertion of a compensator (see Fig. 2.4) that ensures that even along lines that either miss or hardly touch the object to be reconstructed, the total attenuation is significant enough for the detector not to get saturated. Alternatively, one can achieve this by using water as the reference material into which one inserts the object to be reconstructed during the actual measurement. One reason for preferring the former of these two methods is that it requires less radiation dose to achieve the same photon statistics. (This is because in the latter option photons that have already transited through the patient's body may get absorbed and so not reach the detector.)

Mechanical stability is also of importance; the lines along which data are collected should be the same lines that the algorithms assume as the lines of data collection.

There are other possible sources of errors in data collection, but their discussion is beyond the scope of this book.

3.4 Scanning Modes

Figure 3.3 shows five classical designs that had been used by devices for data collection in CT. While various variants of these scanning modes existed, we restrict our attention to these five basic modes. We discuss some of the advantages and disadvantages of each from the point of view of their proneness to the errors we have discussed in the previous section. This will be followed by a discussion of the scanning mode that is considered state-of-the-art for commercial scanners at the time of writing this revised edition.

In the first scanning mode, see Fig. 3.3(a), there is a single x-ray source and a single detector. There are two motions involved. First, both the detector and the source are moved in parallel in a direction perpendicular to the line connecting the source to the detector. During this time projection data are collected for one set of parallel lines. Second, the apparatus is rotated by a

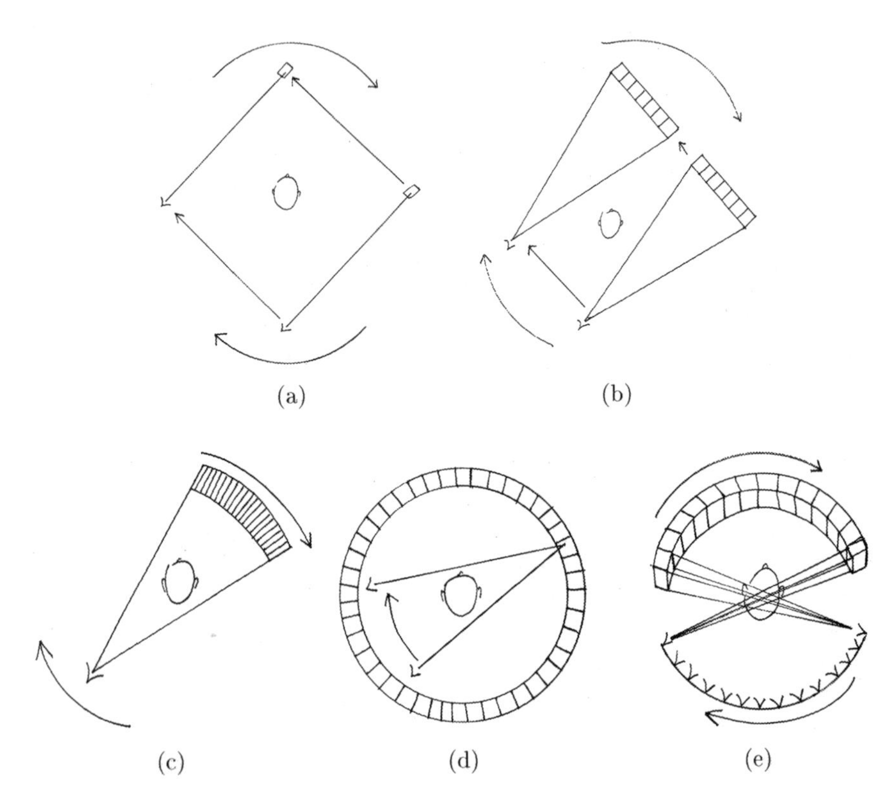

Fig. 3.3: Classical scanning modes in CT. (a) Pencil beam "incremental" scanner (single source, single detector, translate-rotate). (b) Fan beam "incremental" scanner (single source, multiple detector, translate-rotate). (c) Fan beam "spinning" scanner (single source, multiple detector, rotate only). (d) Fan beam "spinning" scanner (single rotating source, stationary ring of detectors). (e) Cone beam "cylindrical" scanner (multiple source, multiple-planar detector).

small amount (e.g., 1°). By repetition of these two motions, data are collected for a number (e.g., 180) of sets of parallel lines.

There are a number of attractive features of this method of data collection. There is very little noise due to scatter. The detector can be calibrated at the beginning of each of the parallel scans, since we can ensure that the first line of a scan misses the reconstruction region. The source–detector combination can be moved in small steps, ensuring that enough data are collected for reconstruction. (There will be more about this in later chapters.) An undesirable feature of this method of data collection is the time it takes; typically several minutes. Such a scanning mode is inappropriate for imaging organs that cannot stay stationary for more than a few seconds, such as the lung.

The second scanning mode in Fig. 3.3(b) was introduced to speed up the data collection process without losing most of the desirable features of the first scanning mode. Instead of one detector, an array of detectors is used (e.g., 30). As the source and detector array move in parallel, data are collected for several sets of parallel lines. When the apparatus is rotated, the rotation can be by a much larger angle than in the first scanning mode (e.g., 10°), and yet the total number of sets of parallel lines is usually increased. Such scanners can collect all their data in slightly over 10 seconds, an acceptable breath holding period for most patients. Apart from increase in cost, the only obvious disadvantage of this scanning mode over the first one is the increased effect of scatter.

The third scanning mode in Fig. 3.3(c) involves only one motion. A single x-ray source is faced by a large enough array of detectors so that the angle subtended by the detector array at the source encloses the whole reconstruction region. The source and detector-array combination rotates around the patient. The data are collected for a large number of sets of lines (typically of the order of 500 sets with about the same number of lines in each); the lines in each set diverge from the source position to the detectors in the array. All data for one set are collected simultaneously. The complete data collection can be achieved in a matter of seconds (typically five or less). One potential problem with this arrangement is that calibration has to be done before the patient is inserted for possibly a whole series of scans, since in all positions of the apparatus the line between the source and the central detectors goes through the patient. Very stable detectors seem to have overcome this difficulty. Also, the detectors have to be narrow so that sufficient amount of data are collected for the reconstruction. This method of data collection was standard for commercial CT scanners for about twenty years from the late 1970s.

An alternative fast method of data collection, with only one motion, is the fourth scanning mode in Fig. 3.3(d). A stationary array of detectors has the x-ray source move inside it in a circle. The line from one of the detectors to the source forms a diverging set of lines as the source moves. Calibration of the detector for this set of lines is possible while the line from the detector to the source is outside the reconstruction region. The number of detectors has to be large compared with the previous scanning mode, unless one is willing to have radiation that goes through the body but ends up between detectors. The latter is undesirable, since the body is subjected to potentially harmful radiation that does not contribute diagnostic information. Also, it is more difficult to reduce scatter by collimation than in the previous scanning mode since the direction from detector to source changes as the source moves.

None of these scanning modes is appropriate for precise imaging of a rapidly moving organ such as the heart. Not only is the speed of data collection far too slow (the heart goes through a whole cycle in about one second), but also it is difficult to achieve a slice-to-slice coherence if the data are collected at different times for each cross-sectional slice. The fifth scanning mode, Fig. 3.3(e), was designed to overcome these difficulties. An array of x-ray sources (e.g., 28) is arranged in a semicircle. They can be electronically switched on and off. They project the body onto a curved fluorescent screen, so that when an x-ray source is switched on a large part of the body (say the whole thorax) is imaged simultaneously, providing us with projection data for a cone beam of lines diverging from the source. It is possible to complete the data collection in as little as one-hundredth of a second, removing any possibility of organ motion interfering with the reconstruction process. Note that this method of data collection is essentially different from the other four, inasmuch as a series of two-dimensional projections of a three-dimensional object is collected rather than a series of one-dimensional projections of a two-dimensional object. While this arrangement solves the problems that motivated its introduction, it has its own special difficulties. For example, the number of views that can be taken is severely limited both by the cost and the size of the x-ray tubes, and the error due to scatter is unavoidably much more significant than in the previous scanning modes. It is also very expensive, especially if the whole sources–detectors combination needs to be rotated around the patient for high spatial resolution in the reconstructions. For such reasons, this scanning mode has not made it into clinical practice.

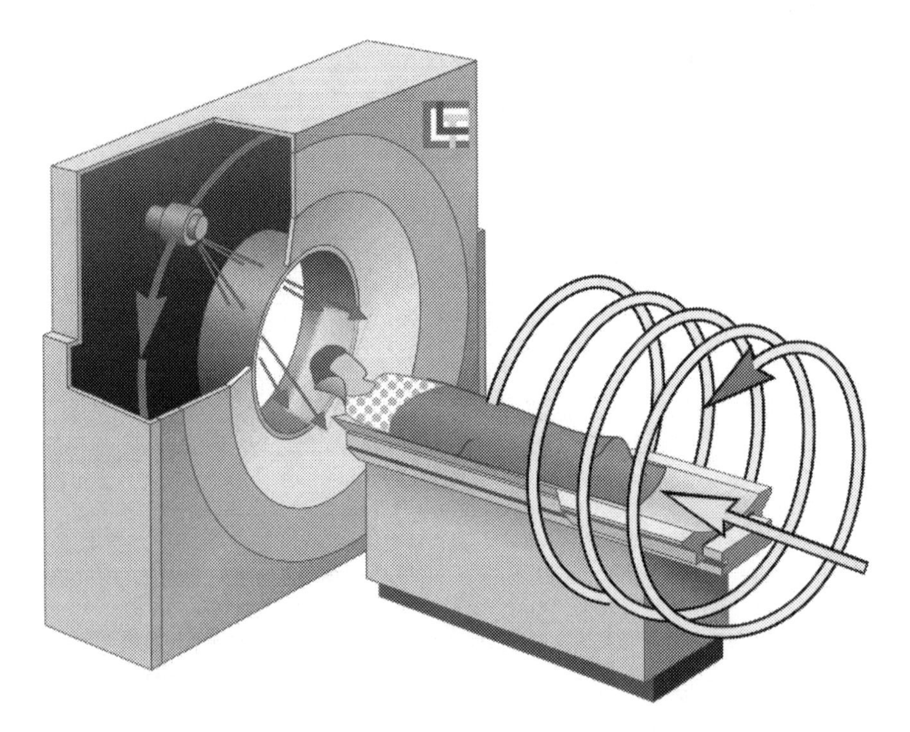

Fig. 3.4: Helical (also known as spiral) CT. (Illustration provided by G. Wang of the Virginia Polytechnic Institute & State University.)

Helical CT (also referred to as *spiral CT*) first started around 1990 and has become standard for medical diagnostic x-ray CT. Typically such a system is single source and multiple detectors (which were initially in a single one-dimensional array as in Fig. 3.3(c), but then were replaced by detectors in a two-dimensional array similar to the detectors in Fig. 3.3(e)); the innovation over the previously mentioned scanning modes is the presence of an independent motion: while the source–detectors rotate around the patient, the table on which the patient lies is continuously moved between them (typically orthogonally to the plane of rotation), see Fig. 3.4. Thus, the trajectory of the source relative to the patient is a helix (hence the name "helical CT"). Helical CT (especially in its cone-beam mode) allows rapid imaging as compared with the previous commercially-viable approaches, which has potentially many advantages. One example is when we wish to image a long blood vessel that is made visible to x-rays by the injection of some contrast material: helical CT may very well allow us to image the whole vessel before the contrast from a single injection washes out and this may not be possible by the slower scanning modes. Since our mathematical and algorithmic development in this book is mainly devoted to the reconstruction of two-dimensional slices from one-dimensional projections (as in Figs. 2.4 and 3.3(c)), we do not get into further discussion of helical CT here. We return to the topic in Chapter 13, where we illustrate the data collection for a dynamically changing object using helical CT and an algorithm for reconstructing the object from such data. We point out that the CT scanners illustrated in Fig. 1.4 are in fact modern helical CT scanners, but at the level of detail of that figure they could just as well be used as illustrations for the older fan beam spinning scanners whose nature is indicated in Fig. 3.3(c).

There are many existing and possible variants of these scanning modes, and many more advantages and disadvantages to each than we have space to mention. However, the configurations discussed here include all the basic arrangements that we need to consider when discussing reconstruction algorithms.

Notes and References

Justification for using the Poisson probability law to describe photon generation can be found in standard books, such as [77]. More detailed discussion of the nature of Poisson random variables is also a standard topic; see, e.g., [217]. A recent paper discussing the noise properties of sinograms in x-ray CT is [267].

The material on beam hardening is based on [111], which gives many early references. An example of an iterative beam-hardening correction procedure is given in [153]. A comparative study is reported in [141]. Examples of recent developments on beam-hardening correction (from the nondestructive testing literature) are [163, 264]. We return to this topic in Section 5.6. It was pointed out in [192] that general-purpose beam-hardening correction methods may, under some circumstances, result in a so-called pseudo-enhancement, which may result in an incorrect diagnosis. This clinically important issue was subsequently addressed in a number of papers; a recent example is [209]. An alternative to correcting for beam hardening is to attempt to make use of the nature of the x-ray spectrum. An early example of such an approach was proposed in [7, 191]. For a much more recent approach see [222].

The shape of the x-ray beam in CT, and what one might do about the errors introduced by it, is discussed in [26]. A discussion of the partial volume is given in [95]. The nature of scatter and correction for it is dealt with in [252]; see also [78].

The first commercially available CT scanner was manufactured by EMI Ltd; see [146]. This scanner was of the type shown in Fig. 3.3(a). A scanner of the type shown in Fig. 3.3(c) is reported on in [70]; see also [218]. A scanner of the type shown in Fig. 3.3(e) is the dynamic spatial reconstructor (DSR) reported on in [232] and its use for imaging physiological functions was detailed in [231]. A table of the physical characteristics of the early commercial scanners is given by [32]. Our classification of classical scanning modes is based on that provided in [271].

A recent article on helical (spiral) CT is [266], it gives a good survey of this very important development. A book that also deals with this topic is [155]. Two early papers are [58, 156]. Sample papers that report on recent technological and application developments of helical CT are [279] and [87], respectively.

In this chapter, as indeed in the whole of this book, we have concentrated on x-ray CT. Data collection in other applications of image reconstruction from projections will have their own physical problems; for a recent example see [22] that discuses a model of noise in low-dose electron microscopy.

4

Computer Simulation of Data Collection in CT

While the aim of CT is the reconstruction of real objects from their actual x-ray projections, the theoretical development of CT owes a lot to reconstruction of mathematically described objects (*phantoms*) from computer simulated projection data. The basic reason for this is that computer simulation enables us to investigate individually various phenomena that cannot be separated physically. For example, x-ray data always contain noise due to both photon statistics and scatter, but simulation can indicate the specific separate effects of noise and scatter.

As can be seen from the previous chapter, a software package capable of realistic simulation of data collection using various scanning modes has to be fairly complex. Nevertheless, a number of such packages have been written. In producing many of the figures for this book we have made repeated use of one of them, called SNARK09. (The name originates from the Lewis Carroll nonsense poem entitled "The Hunting of the Snark.") SNARK09 provides a uniform framework for implementing reconstruction algorithms and for evaluating their performance. All two-dimensional reconstruction algorithms discussed in this book, as well as a number of others, are incorporated in it. In this chapter we discuss the way SNARK09 creates test data for reconstruction algorithms.

4.1 Pictures and Digitization

It is useful at this stage to make precise a number of concepts we need in the rest of this chapter and elsewhere in the book.

When we talk about a *picture*, we assume that it has two components:

(i) the *picture region,* which is a square whose center is at the origin of the coordinate system;
(ii) a *picture function* of two variables whose value is zero outside the picture region.

Sometimes, when this leads to no confusion, we call the function in (ii) the "picture." However, identical functions may give rise to different pictures if the picture regions are different. We often refer to the value of the picture at the point (x, y) as the *density* at (x, y).

An n-element *grid* subdivides the picture region into n^2 equal squares. Each of these smaller squares is called a *pixel* (short for *picture element*).

An $n \times n$ *digitized picture* is one whose value in the interior of any pixel of an n-element grid is uniform. The $n \times n$ *digitization* of a picture is an $n \times n$ digitized picture such that the integral of the original picture over any pixel of an n-element grid is equal to the integral of the digitization over the same pixel (see Fig. 1.1). In CT, the picture region is the reconstruction region and the density of the picture at the point (x, y) is the relative linear attenuation at the effective energy of the tissue at the point (x, y).

4.2 Creation of a Phantom

We now describe how a test phantom is created in SNARK09. A test phantom is nothing but a picture on which we wish to test reconstruction algorithms or data collection methods.

The phantom is put together by superimposing a number of *elemental objects*, placed at desired positions, at desired orientations and of desired size and density. The density of the elemental objects may be negative. The density of the picture at any point is then defined as the sum of the densities associated with all the elemental objects within which the point lies. To obtain an estimate of the density within a pixel, the user specifies a number K, which has the effect that the density within a pixel is determined by averaging the values of the density at $K \times K$ uniformly-spaced points within the pixel. Thus, the density assigned to a pixel can be expressed by the sum

$$\frac{1}{K^2} \sum_{k=1}^{K^2} \sum_{j=1}^{J} \delta_{k,j} d_j, \tag{4.1}$$

where J is the number of elemental objects in the phantom, d_j is the density of the jth elemental object. $\delta_{k,j} = 1$ if the kth of the $K \times K$ points in the pixel is in the jth elemental object, and $\delta_{k,j} = 0$ otherwise. Note that the digitized picture produced by this method is only an approximation to the digitization of the phantom.

An elemental object in SNARK09 may be a rectangle, an ellipse, an isosceles triangle, or a segment or a sector of a circle. The location of an elemental object is described by five variables CX, CY, U, V, and ANG. For each type of elemental object the explanation of these variables is given by Fig. 4.1. The boundary of an elemental object is considered to be part of the object.

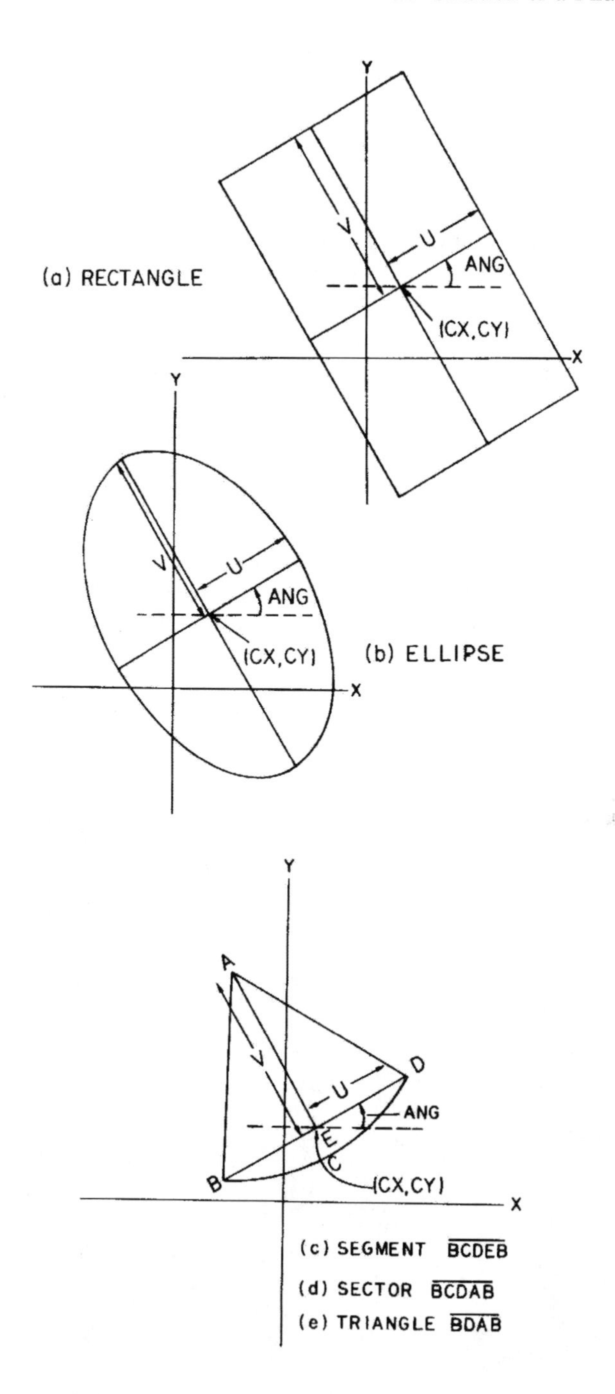

Fig. 4.1: Elemental objects. In SNARK09, an elemental object consists of both the boundary and the interior of a rectangle, or an ellipse, or a triangle, or a segment or a sector of a circle, respectively.

4.3 A Piecewise-Homogeneous Head Phantom

A most important application to date of image reconstruction from projections has been in the area of diagnostic radiology. A region of the body for which such procedures have been widely and successfully used is the head. For this reason, all ideas and methods introduced in this book are demonstrated on a typical cross section of the human head, containing tumors, a blood clot, ventricles and, of course, the skull enclosing the brain.

Our primary purpose is to introduce methods of image reconstruction from projections and to illustrate how they perform under various circumstances. Since we wish to control precisely the circumstances and to compare the results of the reconstructions with a known original, rather than using an actual cross section of a human head, we use a mathematically defined head phantom. In this and in the next section we describe how we arrived at the head phantoms that will be used repeatedly throughout the book.

We studied a cross section of a human head that was reconstructed by CT (see Fig. 4.2). Based on this cross section we described a skull enclosing the brain with ventricles, two tumors, and a hematoma (blood clot) using five ellipses, eight segments of circles, and two triangles. The tumors were placed so that they are vertically above the blood clot in the display. This facilitates reporting on our results as will be seen later on. The positioning of these ellipses, segments, and triangles is shown in Fig. 4.3.

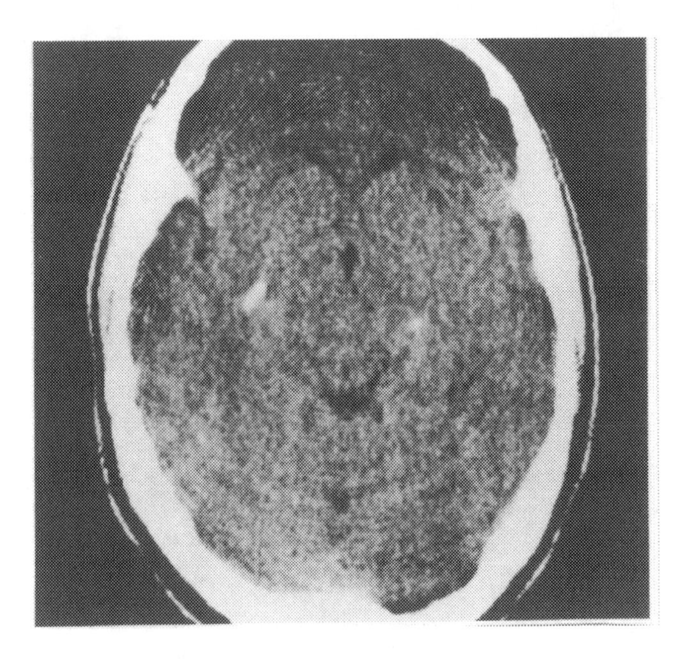

Fig. 4.2: Central part of an x-ray CT reconstruction of a cross section of the head of a patient. This served as the basis for our piecewise-homogeneous head phantom.

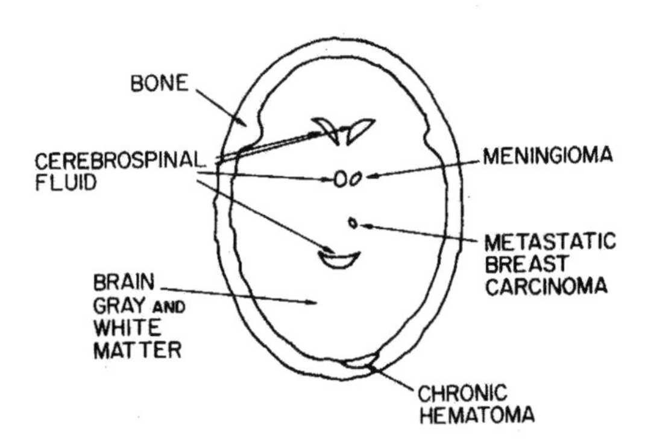

Fig. 4.3: Outlines of the elemental objects that make up the piecewise-homogeneous head phantom, with tissue type indicated for each object.

We assume that the reference material is air whose linear attenuation coefficient can be taken to be zero for all energies. Hence the density of the phantom at a point (x, y) is the linear attenuation coefficient at some fixed energy of the tissue at (x, y). Table 4.1 gives the linear attenuation coefficients of the various tissues in our head phantom at different energies. Table 4.2 gives a precise mathematical description of the location and densities of the elemental objects in Fig. 4.3, assuming 60 keV photons.

We used SNARK09 to obtain the density in each of 243 $\times$ 243 pixels of size 0.0752 cm with $K = 11$. The resulting array of numbers is represented in Fig. 4.4. The nature of this display deserves careful discussion. The densities given to the elemental objects were such that the resulting values are the linear attenuation coefficients at 60 keV of the appropriate tissue types measured in cm^{-1}. Thus the values range between zero (background, can be thought of as air) and 0.416 (bone of the skull). However, the interesting part of the picture is the interior of the skull. The values there range from 0.207 (cerebrospinal fluid) to 0.216 (metastatic breast tumor). The small differences between tissues inside the skull would not be noticeable if we used black to

Table 4.1: Linear attenuation coefficients (in cm^{-1}) as a function of photon energy for tissues that occur in the piecewise-homogeneous head phantom.

energy (keV)	bone	brain (gray and white matter)	metastatic breast carcinoma	meningioma	chronic hematoma	cerebro-spinal fluid
41	0.999	0.265	0.284	0.269	0.266	0.260
52	0.595	0.226	0.237	0.227	0.228	0.222
60	0.416	0.210	0.216	0.213	0.212	0.207
84	0.265	0.183	0.186	0.187	0.184	0.181
100	0.208	0.174	0.175	0.176	0.175	0.171

Table 4.2: Specifications of the elemental objects used to produce Fig. 4.4. The densities are: bone in air (Object 1), brain in bone (Object 2), cerebrospinal fluid in brain (Objects 3, 8, 10 and 12), carcinoma in brain (Object 4), meningioma in brain (Object 5), hematoma in bone (Object 6), bone in hematoma (Object 7), brain in cerebrospinal fluid (Objects 9, 11 and 13) and bone in brain (Objects 14 and 15). The word *density* here refers to differences of linear attenuation coefficients measured in cm^{-1} at 60 keV; in the polychromatic case, similar densities need to be specified for all energies in the x-ray spectrum.

No.	type	CX	CY	U	V	ANG	density
1	ellipse	0.000	0.000	8.625	6.4687	90.00	0.416
2	ellipse	0.000	0.000	7.875	5.7187	90.00	-0.206
3	ellipse	0.000	1.500	0.375	0.3000	90.00	-0.003
4	ellipse	0.675	-0.750	0.225	0.1500	140.00	0.006
5	ellipse	0.750	1.500	0.375	0.2250	50.00	0.003
6	segment	1.375	-7.500	1.100	0.6250	19.20	-0.204
7	segment	1.375	-7.500	1.100	4.3200	19.21	0.204
8	segment	0.000	-2.250	1.125	0.3750	0.00	-0.003
9	segment	0.000	-2.250	1.125	3.0000	0.00	0.003
10	segment	-1.000	3.750	1.000	0.5000	135.00	-0.003
11	segment	-1.000	3.750	1.000	3.0000	135.00	0.003
12	segment	1.000	3.750	1.000	0.5000	225.00	-0.003
13	segment	-1.000	3.750	1.000	3.0000	225.00	0.003
14	triangle	5.025	3.750	1.125	0.5000	110.75	0.206
15	triangle	-5.025	3.750	1.125	0.9000	-110.75	0.206

display zero, white to display 0.5 and corresponding grayness for values in between. In order to see clearly the features in the interior of the skull, we use zero (black) to represent the value 0.204 (or anything less) and 255 (white) to

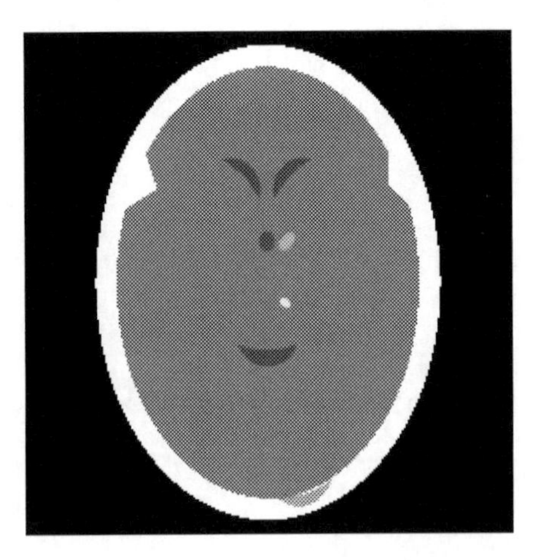

Fig. 4.4: A piecewise-homogeneous head phantom.

represent the value 0.21675 (or anything more). This way the small change in density by 0.001 corresponds to a change of twenty in display grayness, which is visible. We used this method to produce Fig. 4.4 and the **displays of all the reconstructions of the head phantoms** used as illustrations in this book.

4.4 Head Phantom with a Large Tumor and Local Inhomogeneities

In Fig. 4.5(a) we show an actual brain cross section. The left half of the image shows a malignant tumor that has a highly textured appearance. In order to simulate the occurrence of a similarly textured object in our phantom we need to use many additional elemental objects. This was done by adding to the list of elemental objects (Table 4.2) that produced Fig. 4.4 a much longer list of elemental objects, each coinciding exactly with a pixel; this resulted in the phantom shown in Fig. 4.5(b). Because of the medical relevance of imaging brains with such tumors, for the rest of this book we use the head phantom with this tumor added to it. (Due to our display method, it seems that there is a large range of values in the tumor. However, this is an illusion: the range of values in the tumor is less than 7% of the range of values in the picture that is displayed in Fig. 4.4. Another way of saying this is that the range of the difference between the pictures represented by Figs. 4.4 and 4.5(b), is less than 7% of the range within either of those pictures.)

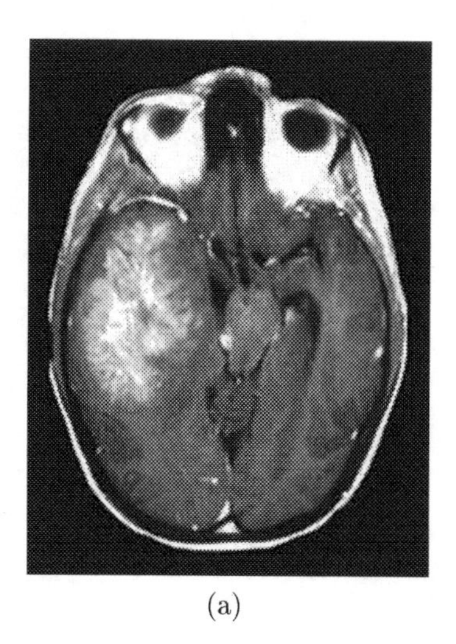

(a)

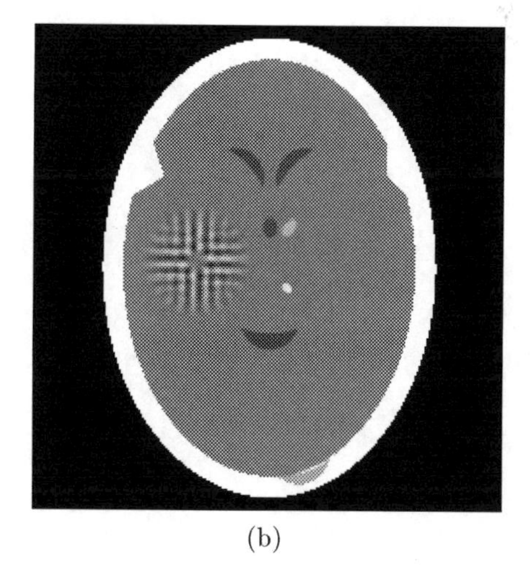

(b)

Fig. 4.5: (a) An actual brain cross section with a tumor. (Image is reproduced, with permission, from the Roswell Park Cancer Institute website.) (b) The head phantom of Fig. 4.4 with a "large tumor" added to it.

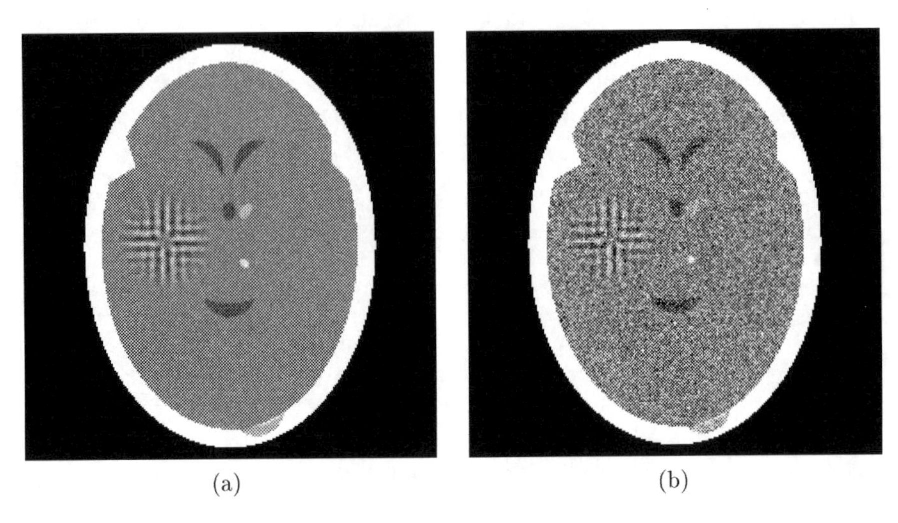

Fig. 4.6: Head phantoms with local inhomogeneities. (a) $\sigma_X = 0.0025$. (b) $\sigma_X = 0.01$.

One problem with the phantoms as defined so far is that a brain is far from being homogeneous: it has gray matter, white matter, blood vessels and capillaries carrying oxygenated blood to and deoxygenated blood from the brain, etc. This is even more so for bone, whose strength to a large extent is derived from its structural properties (it is more like the Eiffel tower than a monolith of solid stone). There are methods that can obtain remarkably accurate reconstruction of piecewise homogeneous objects, but their performance may not be medically efficacious when applied to CT data from real objects with local inhomogeneities. So as not to fall into the trap of drawing too optimistic conclusions from experiments using piecewise homogeneous objects, we superimposed on our head phantom a random local variation that is obtained by picking, for each pixel and for each energy level, a sample from the Gaussian random variable X with mean $\mu_X = 1$ and a variance V_X that reflects the level of local inhomogeneity present in our object (see (1.10)) and then multiplying the previously estimated linear attenuation coefficient at that energy level with that sample. In Fig. 4.6 we show the results of this for 60 keV for two different values of $\sigma_X = \sqrt{V_X}$. The value that we use for the phantoms in the rest of this book is $\sigma_X = 0.0025$, shown in Fig. 4.6(a).

4.5 Creation of the Ray Sums

The simulation of the data collection in SNARK09 is based on (2.3):

$$p = -\ln\left(A_p/C_p\right). \tag{4.2}$$

We first discuss how the calibration measurement C_p is calculated. It is given by

$$C_p = C_0/C_r, \tag{4.3}$$

where C_0 is the number of photons counted by the detector under consideration and C_r is the number of photons counted during the same period by a reference detector. As discussed in Section 3.1, both C_0 and C_r are samples of Poisson random variables, which can be approximated by Gaussian random variables if their means are large. In SNARK09 it is assumed that C_0 and C_r are samples of the same Gaussian random variable (with a user-provided mean), and so the expected value of C_p is one. In fact, if the user of the programming system requests the simulation of the physically unattainable case of no error due to photon statistics, the value of C_p is taken to be exactly one. Otherwise, a random number generator is used to produce C_0 and C_r.

A subtle point is that, except in the case of the fifth scanning mode (Fig. 3.3(e)), C_p is not to be calculated separately for each source–detector pair. This is because of the way calibration is done in the different scanning modes (see Section 3.4). In the first two scanning modes (Figs. 3.3(a) and (b)), C_p is the same for all source–detector pair positions that are used to obtain data for one set of parallel lines. Similarly, in the fourth scanning mode (Fig. 3.3(d)), C_p is the same for all lines that diverge from the same detector as the source moves. The situation with the third scanning mode is essentially different: C_p is the same for all lines that connect the source to a particular detector as the apparatus moves. All these lines are tangential to the same circle, and this may cause a ringlike feature to appear in the reconstruction if an error has been made during the calibration measurement. (This artifact can be observed in Fig. 4.2, which was produced by an early CT scanner.)

We now turn to how the actual measurement A_p is calculated. It is given by

$$A_p = A_0/A_r, \tag{4.4}$$

where A_0 is the number of photons counted by the detector under consideration and A_r is the number of photons counted by the reference detector. Again A_r is taken to be a sample of a Poisson random variable with a user-provided mean, say λ. The calculation of A_0 is more complex since it is during this calculation that SNARK09 introduces polychromaticity, the shape of the x-ray beam, and scatter.

In order to understand this clearly, we have to go back to the way we create a phantom (Section 4.2). The phantom is put together from a number of elemental objects each with an associated density. Since the phantom represents the distribution of relative linear attenuation at a fixed energy, we need only one density associated with each elemental object. If we want to represent the relative linear attenuation at a different energy, we need to use different densities for the elemental objects. In order to describe the interaction of a polychromatic x-ray beam with the phantom, densities for all energies in the beam need to be given.

SNARK09 solves this problem as follows. It assumes that the x-ray spectrum is discrete; i.e., it consists of a mixture of photons that are of one of a finite number of different energies. For each energy the user has to specify the percentage of photons at that energy (based on the detected spectrum during the calibration measurement, see Section 3.2) and the density at that energy of all the elemental objects. (In general, the user also needs to specify the absorption properties of the reference material at the different energies, but since in our example the reference material is air we do not dwell on the details of this point.)

Since the density (in our case: relative linear attenuation at a fixed energy) at a point is the sum of the densities of all the elemental objects within which the point lies, the integral of the density along a line L is the sum over all elemental objects of the products of the length of intersection of L with the elemental object and the density in the elemental object.

Assume for now that we have a point source, a point detector, with a line L between them, and no scatter. Then (3.10), when combined with (4.2) and (4.4), yields

$$A_0 \simeq \lambda \int_0^E \tau_e \exp\left(-\int_0^D \left(\mu_e(z) - \mu_e^a\right) dz\right) de, \tag{4.5}$$

where we have made use of the assumptions that the expected values of C_p and A_r are 1 and λ, respectively. In SNARK09, the expression on the right-hand side of (4.5) is evaluated as follows.

Let I be the number of discrete energy levels and J be the number of elemental objects. Let $d_{j,i}$ be the density of the jth elemental object at energy level i, let ℓ_j be the length of intersection of the line L with the jth elemental object (ℓ_j may be 0), and let t_i be the probability that a photon counted during the calibration measurement is at energy level i (these probabilities are user specified). Then A_0 is taken to be a sample of a Poisson random variable with mean

$$\lambda \sum_{i=1}^{I} t_i \exp\left(-\sum_{j=1}^{J} \ell_j d_{j,i}\right). \tag{4.6}$$

If the user wishes to simulate the physically unattainable case of no photon statistics, SNARK09 sets A_0 equal to the value provided by (4.6). To simulate the shape of the x-ray beam, SNARK09 calculates A_0 as the weighted average of the values of (4.6) for a number of different lines between the source and the detector.

To simulate scatter, SNARK09 replaces the value A_0 for a detector position by a weighted average of the values of A_0 for that detector position and the neighboring detector positions. The scatter contribution of a detector position to another one is assumed to depend only on the distance between the two detector positions. Mathematically, we express this by saying that the values A_0 with scatter taken into consideration are obtained by *convolution* of the values of A_0 without scatter and a fixed *scatter function*. (The notion of convolution, which is essential for some of the reconstruction algorithms, is explained in Section 8.1.) This model for the scattering process is a very much simplified version of what really happens; scatter simulated by SNARK09 resembles true physical scatter only in its gross characteristics.

In the next chapter we give examples of how SNARK09 simulates the different processes just described and of the effects of these processes on the quality of the reconstruction.

4.6 Fast Calculation of a Ray Sum for a Digitized Picture

As long as the number J of elemental objects composing a phantom is not particularly large, evaluating a formula such as the one that occurs in (4.6) is not computationally demanding: for each line, we loop through all the elemental objects j, and using the location and shape of the elemental object we calculate the length ℓ_j of the intersection of that line with that elemental object. However, the situation changes essentially by the introduction of local inhomogeneities. Mathematically, the introduction of local inhomogeneities can be thought of as just the introduction of extra elemental objects, one per pixel, with densities assigned to them that represent the calculated inhomogeneities at those pixels in the phantom, as described at the end of Section 4.4. However, the number of pixels tends to be large (in our head phantom it is 59,049) and to loop through all of them for each line would result in a considerable computational burden.

Fortunately, there is an alternative. Using an approach often referred to as a *digital difference analyzer* (*DDA*, for short), one can rapidly obtain, for each line, the location of all the pixels intersected by that line and the lengths of those intersections. Then the inner sum in (4.6) can be rapidly evaluated using only those pixels that are intersected by the line. Since typically only a small fraction of pixels is intersected by any line, this results in a very significant computational speedup. The same idea can be, and is, used in the implementation of the so-called series expansion reconstruction algorithms, discussed later in Section 6.3 and, in more detail, in Chapters 11 and 12.

The idea of a DDA for locating for a line L the pixels that are intersected by L and the lengths of the intersections is described in Fig. 4.7. Let us denote, as in Fig. 2.4, by θ the angle that L makes with the y (vertical) axis. We make two nonessential assumptions to simplify the presentation of the idea behind the DDA; it is easy to work out how the details of our presentation need to be changed if these nonessential assumptions are not satisfied. The assumptions are that $0 \leq \tan\theta < 1$ and that the point b where L "first" intersects the picture region lies on the top horizontal edge.

Given geometrical information about the location of the line, we can easily calculate the coordinates of the point b. We denote the length of a side of a

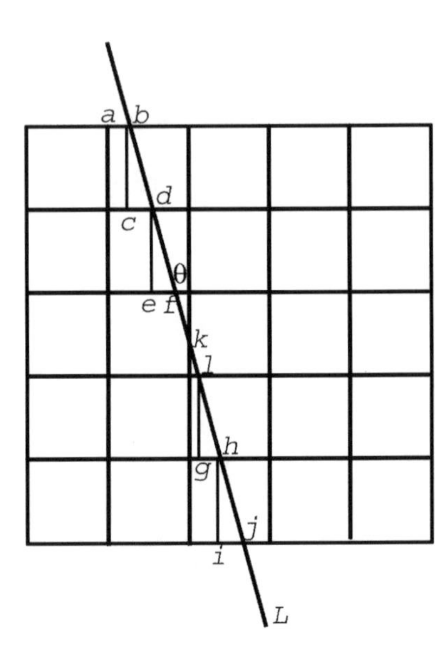

Fig. 4.7: A digital difference analyzer (DDA) for lines.

pixel in Fig. 4.7 (and hence also the distance between b and c, between d and e, between l and g, and between h and i) by δ. Let us abbreviate $\delta \tan\theta$ by τ and $\delta/\cos\theta$ by λ. Note that in Fig. 4.7, τ is the distance between c and d, between e and f, between g and h, and between i and j, while λ is the distance between b and d, between d and f, between l and h, and between h and j. In fact, λ is the length of intersection of L for four out of the six pixels that L intersects.

The control of the DDA is achieved by using a variable χ such that $0 \leq \chi < \delta$, which is initialized to be the distance between a and b. The DDA lists one-by-one each intersected pixel P, together with the length of intersection $l(P)$. The first P is the one that contains b.

The whole process can be understood by considering the general case of having a current value for χ and for P. We distinguish between two possibilities, and in either case the amount of computing that needs to be done is very little:

(i) $\chi + \tau < \delta$. In this case $l(P) = \lambda$, χ is replaced by $\chi + \tau$ and P is replaced by the pixel below it. The process stops if there is no such pixel.
(ii) $\chi + \tau \geq \delta$. In this case $l(P) = \lambda\frac{\delta-\chi}{\tau}$ and P is replaced by the pixel to the right of it. The process stops if there is no such pixel. For this new P,

$l(P) = \lambda \frac{\chi+\tau-\delta}{\tau}$. Now χ is replaced by $\chi + \tau - \delta$ and P is replaced by the pixel below it. The process stops if there is no such pixel.

Unless the process has stopped due to the nonexistence of a looked-for pixel, we are now back to the general case and the same two possibilities are considered again. Clearly, the total process can be programmed in a very efficient manner.

Notes and References

SNARK09 is described in detail in [61].

The linear attenuation coefficients of the various tissue types (except for bone) at the different energies were estimated from the values published by [219]. Values for bone were estimated based on the assumption that it is a mixture of calcium and fat.

Head phantoms, which are less realistic than the one discussed in Section 4.2, were proposed in [138] and [241]. The latter of these is usually referred to as the Shepp–Logan head phantom and it has been extremely widely used for evaluating reconstruction algorithms. Nevertheless its use for this purpose is not really advisable, since it lacks anatomical features (such as nearly straight edges of bones) that are likely to deteriorate the clinical usefulness of reconstructions. Many dozens of mathematically described phantoms of various parts of the human body have been proposed since these early works, much of it on the Internet. A particularly rich source of phantoms was produced by FORBILD (the Bavarian Center of Excellence for Medical Imaging and Image Processing), see http://www.imp.uni-erlangen.de/phantoms/.

The exact method for creating the "large tumor" of Fig. 4.5(b) is described in [121]. This large tumor also happens to be a ghost (as defined in Section 15.4); it is invisible for 22 projection directions.

A pioneering DDA-based practical algorithm for drawing lines using a digital plotter is due to Bresenham [30]. Both DDAs in general and Bresenham's algorithm in particular are referred to in a considerable body of literature; a relatively recent example is [66].

5

Data Collection and Reconstruction of the Head Phantom

In this chapter we give examples of simulating various errors and modes of data collection in CT. In each case we show the result of a reconstruction from the simulated data and make comparisons with the test phantom.

5.1 Methods of Picture Comparison

A reconstruction is a digitized picture. In case it is a reconstruction from simulated projection data of a test phantom, we can judge the quality of the reconstruction by comparing it with the digitization of the test phantom. Naturally, both the picture region and the grid must be the same size for the reconstruction and the digitized phantom. This section is devoted to a discussion of how one illustrates and measures the resemblance between a reconstruction and a phantom.

Visual evaluation is of course the most straightforward way. One may display both the phantom and the reconstruction and observe whether all features in which one is interested in the phantom are reproduced in the reconstruction and whether any spurious features have been introduced by the reconstruction process. A difficulty with such a qualitative evaluation is its subjectiveness, people often disagree on which of two pictures resembles a third one more closely.

A more quantitative way of evaluating pictures is the following. Select a column of pixels, which is such that it goes through a number of interesting features in the phantom. For example, in our digitized head phantom (described in Sections 4.3 and 4.4) the 131st of the 243 columns goes through the ventricles, both tumors, and the hematoma. In Fig. 5.1(a) we indicate this column. One way to evaluate the quality of a reconstruction is to compare the graphs of the 243 pixel densities for this column in the phantom (shown in Fig. 5.1(b)) and the reconstruction. This will be done for many reconstructions of the head phantom that we report on in this book.

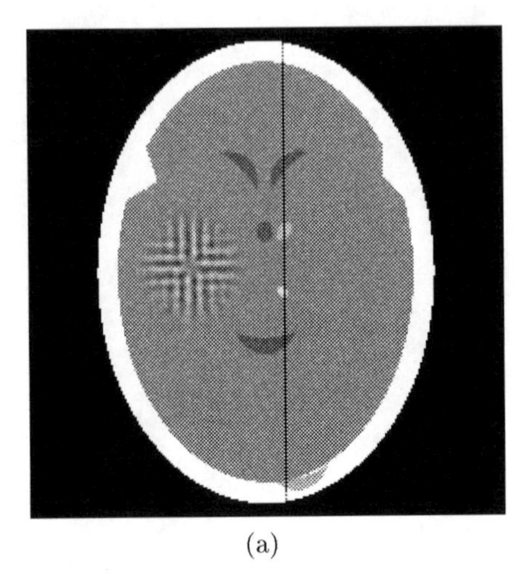

(a)

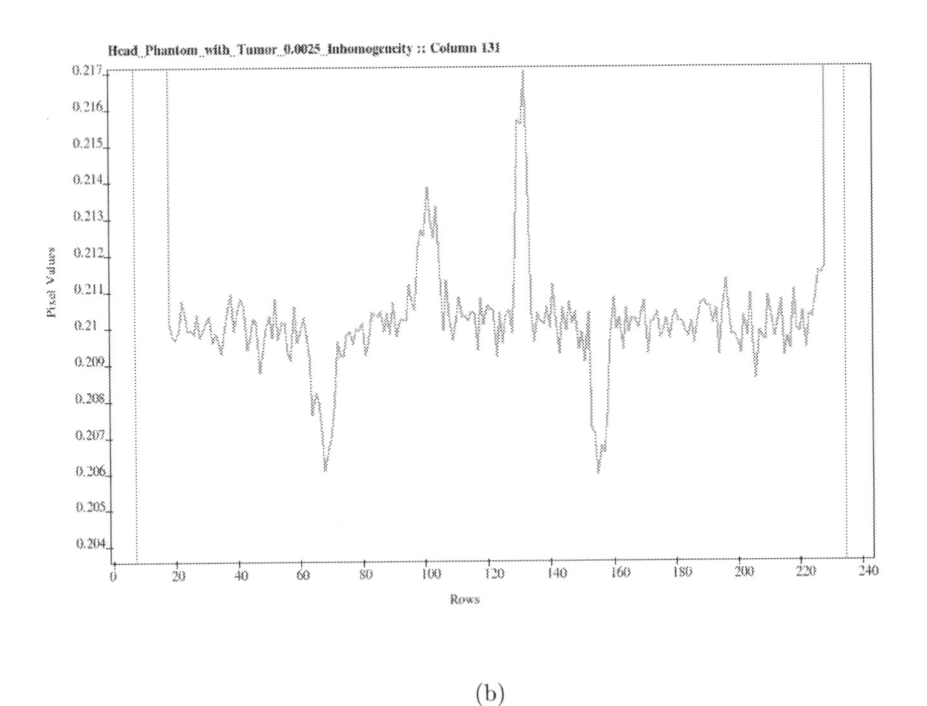

(b)

Fig. 5.1: (a) A head phantom with local inhomogeneities (the same as Fig. 4.6(a)) with the 131st of the 243 columns indicated by a vertical line. (b) The densities along this column in the phantom.

It also appears desirable to use a single value that provides a rough measure of the closeness of the reconstruction to the phantom. We now describe, and later on we use, two different methods of doing this. The reader must however be warned that a single number, or even collection of a few numbers, cannot possibly take care of all the ways in which two pictures may differ from each other. Rank ordering reconstructions based on a single measure of closeness to the phantom can be very misleading.

In this book we report on two *picture distance measures*. In our definition of these measure we use $t_{u,v}$ and $r_{u,v}$ to denote the densities of the vth pixel of the uth row of the digitized test phantom and the reconstruction, respectively, and $\bar{t}$ to denote the average of the densities in the digitized test phantom. We assume that both pictures are $\ell \times \ell$. The measures defined in the equations below are variants of often-used measures in the reconstruction literature.

$$d = \left(\sum_{u=1}^{\ell} \sum_{v=1}^{\ell} (t_{u,v} - r_{u,v})^2 / \sum_{u=1}^{\ell} \sum_{v=1}^{\ell} (t_{u,v} - \bar{t})^2 \right)^{1/2} . \tag{5.1}$$

$$r = \sum_{u=1}^{\ell} \sum_{v=1}^{\ell} |t_{u,v} - r_{u,v}| / \sum_{u=1}^{\ell} \sum_{v=1}^{\ell} |t_{u,v}| . \tag{5.2}$$

($|x|$ denotes the ***absolute value*** of x; it is x if $x \geq 0$ and it is $-x$ if $x < 0$.)

These measures emphasize different aspects of picture quality. The first one, d, is a *normalized root mean squared distance measure*. A large difference in a few places causes the value of d to be large. Note that the value of d is 1 if the reconstruction is a uniformly dense picture with the correct average density. The second one, r, is a *normalized mean absolute distance measure*. As opposed to d, it emphasizes the importance of a lot of small errors rather than of a few large errors. Note that the value of r is 1 if the reconstruction is a uniformly dense picture with zero density. Both measures are given for all reconstructions we report on in this book.

5.2 Task-Oriented Comparison of Algorithm Performance

A true measure of the appropriateness of a reconstruction procedure is its performance in a clinical diagnostic situation. Unfortunately, such a measure is difficult to quantify. One approach is by the use of *receiver operating characteristic* (ROC) curves, a topic beyond the scope of this book. We present instead a *statistical hypothesis testing* based methodology that allows us to evaluate the relative efficacy of reconstruction methods for a given task.

The evaluation methodology considers the following to be the relevant basic question: given a specific medical problem, what is the relative merit of two (or more) image reconstruction algorithms in presenting images that are helpful for solving the problem? (Compare this with the alternative essentially-unanswerable question: which is the best reconstruction algorithm?) Ideally, the evaluation should be based on the performance of human observers. However, that is costly and complex, since a number of observers have to be used, each has to read many images, conditions have to be carefully controlled, etc. Such reasons led us to use *numerical observers* instead of humans.

This evaluation methodology consists of four steps:

(i) Generation of random samples from a statistically described ensemble of images (phantoms) representative of the medical problem and computer simulation of the data collection by the device under investigation.
(ii) Reconstruction from the data so generated by each of the algorithms.
(iii) Assignment of a *figure of merit* (*FOM*) to each reconstruction. The FOM should be a measure of the helpfulness of the reconstructed image for solving the medical problem.
(iv) Calculation of *statistical significance* (based on the FOMs of all the reconstructions) by which the null hypothesis that the reconstructions are equally helpful for solving the problem at hand can be rejected.

We now discuss the details of each of these steps as used in this book. It must be emphasized that in order for such a methodology to be relevant to a particular medical task, the steps must be adjusted to that task. The task for which comparative evaluations of various pairs of reconstruction algorithms are reported in this book is that of detecting small low-contrast tumors in the brain based on reconstructions from x-ray CT projection data.

The ensemble of images generated for this task is based on the head phantom with a large tumor and local inhomogeneities, as specified in Section 4.4. Note that this by itself provides us a statistical ensemble because the local inhomogeneities are introduced using a Gaussian random variable. However there is an additional (for the task more relevant) variability within the ensemble that is achieved as follows. We specify a large number of pairs of potential tumor sites, the locations of the sites in a pair are symmetrically placed in the left and right halves of the brain. In any sample from the ensemble, exactly one of each pair of the sites will actually have a tumor placed there, with equal probability for either site. The tumors are circular in shape of radius 0.1 cm and with densities at each energy level assigned as for the meningioma in Table 4.1. In Fig. 5.2(a) we illustrate one sample from this ensemble. Once a sample has been picked, we generate projection data for it by simulating a CT scanner, in the manner that is specified for the "standard projection data" in Section 5.8 below. Further variability is introduced at this stage, since the data are generated by simulating noise due to photon statistics. In Fig. 5.2(b) we show a reconstruction from one such projection data set. The tumors are hard to see in this reconstruction, but that is exactly the point: we are trying to evaluate which of two reconstruction algorithms provides images in which the tumors are easier to identify. If we make the task too easy (by having large and/or high-contrast tumors), then all reasonable reconstruction algorithms

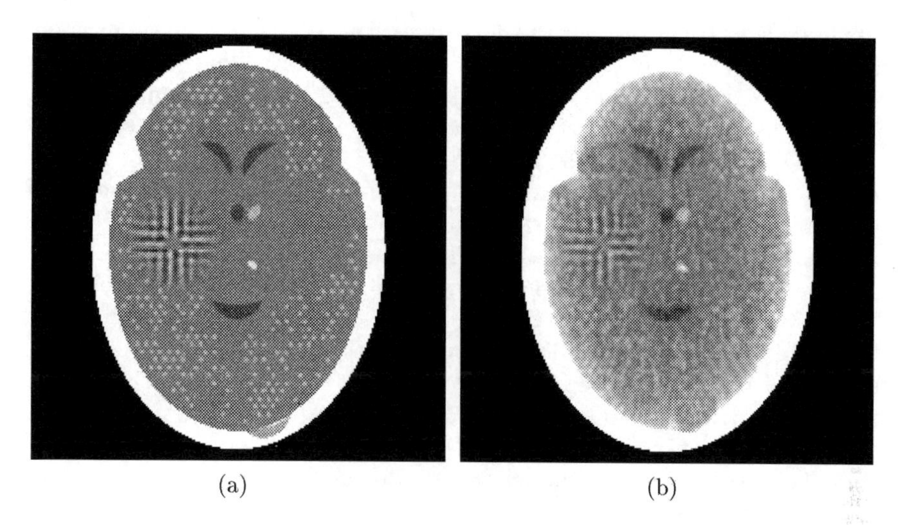

(a) (b)

Fig. 5.2: (a) A random sample from the ensemble of phantoms used in this book for the task-oriented comparison of reconstruction algorithms. (b) A reconstruction from noisy projection data taken of the phantom illustrated in (a).

would perform perfectly from the point of view of the task. On the other hand, if the task is too difficult (very small and very low-contrast tumors), then correct detection would become essentially a matter of luck, rather than of algorithm performance. Our ensemble was chosen to be in-between these extremes. The two FOMs that we chose to use are specific to the type of ensemble of phantoms that we have just specified.

Given a phantom and one of its reconstructions, as in Fig. 5.2, we define the *image-wise region of interest FOM* (*IROI*) of the reconstruction as follows. For any digitized picture and for any elemental object (see Fig. 4.1), let the *average density* in that picture for that elemental object be the sum over all pixels whose center falls within that elemental object of the pixel densities divided by the number of such pixels. Let us number the pairs of potential tumor sites (each tumor site is determined by a circular elemental object) from 1 to B, and let (for $1 \leq b \leq B$) $\alpha_t^p(b)$ (respectively, $\alpha_n^p(b)$) denote the average density in the phantom for the tumor site of the bth pair that has (respectively, has not) the tumor in it. We specify similarly $\alpha_t^r(b)$ (respectively, $\alpha_n^r(b)$), for the reconstruction. For this phantom-reconstruction pair we define

$$\mathrm{IROI} = \frac{\sum_{b=1}^{B} \left(\alpha_t^r(b) - \alpha_n^r(b)\right)}{\sqrt{\sum_{b=1}^{B} \left(\alpha_n^r(b) - \frac{1}{B}\sum_{b'=1}^{B} \alpha_n^r(b')\right)^2}} \Big/ \frac{\sum_{b=1}^{B} \left(\alpha_t^p(b) - \alpha_n^p(b)\right)}{\sqrt{\sum_{b=1}^{B} \left(\alpha_n^p(b) - \frac{1}{B}\sum_{b'=1}^{B} \alpha_n^p(b')\right)^2}}. \tag{5.3}$$

The first thing to note about this formula is that the numerator and the denominator in the big fraction are exactly the same except that the numerator refers to the reconstruction and the denominator refers to the phantom. Thus, if the reconstruction is perfect (in the sense of being identical to the phantom) then IROI $= 1$. Analyzing the contents of the numerator and the denominator, we see that they are (except for constants that cancel out) the mean difference between the average values at the tumor site and the corresponding non-tumor site divided by the standard deviation of the average values at the non-tumor sites. It has been found by experiments with human observers that this FOM correlates well with the performance of people.

The other FOM on which we report in this book is *hit ratio*. Using the notation of the previous paragraph, we consider that the reconstruction has a *hit* for the bth pair if $\alpha_t^r(b) > \alpha_n^r(b)$. Then the value HITR of the hit ratio for the reconstruction is the number of hits divided by the total number B of pairs. The justification for the relevance to diagnostic practice of this FOM is that for nearly symmetric structures, such as the brain, in order to make a decision as to the presence of a tumor at a suspicious site the radiologist is likely to compare it with the site in a symmetric location.

In order to obtain statistically significant results we need to sample the ensemble of phantoms and generate projection data a number (say C) of times. (For the experiments reported in this book we use $C = 30$.) Suppose that we wish to compare the task-oriented performance of two reconstruction algorithms. For $1 \le c \le C$, let $\mathrm{IROI}^1(c)$ and $\mathrm{IROI}^2(c)$ denote the values of IROI, as defined by (5.3), for the reconstructions by the two algorithms from projection data of the cth phantom. (The other of our FOMs, HITR, is treated in a strictly analogous fashion.) The *null hypothesis* that the two reconstruction methods are equally good for the task at hand translates into the statistical statement that each value of $\mathrm{IROI}^1(c) - \mathrm{IROI}^2(c)$ is a sample of a continuous random variable D whose mean μ_D is 0; see (1.8). We have no idea of the shape of the probability density function p_D of this random variable, but the central limit theorem comes to our rescue, by telling us that, for a sufficiently large C,

$$s = \sum_{c=1}^{C} \left(\mathrm{IROI}^1(c) - \mathrm{IROI}^2(c)\right) \tag{5.4}$$

can be assumed to be a sample from a Gaussian random variable S with mean 0 and variance $V_S = CV_D$; see (1.14). This fact combined with (1.9) and (1.14) allows us to say that, at least approximately, S is a Gaussian random variable whose mean is 0 and whose variance is

$$V_S = \sum_{c=1}^{C} \left(\mathrm{IROI}^1(c) - \mathrm{IROI}^2(c)\right)^2 . \tag{5.5}$$

It is a consequence of the null hypothesis that s is a sample from a zero-mean random variable. However, even if that were true, we would not expect our particular sample s to be exactly 0. Suppose for now that $s > 0$. This makes us suspect that in fact the first algorithm is better than the second one (for our task) and so the null hypothesis may be false. The question is: how significant is the observed value s for rejecting the null hypothesis? To answer this question we consider the so-called *P-value,* which is defined to be $P_S(s, \infty]$, see (1.7). The P-value is the probability of a sample of S being as large or larger than s. If the null hypothesis were correct, we would not expect to come across an s defined by (5.4) for which the P-value is very small. Thus, the smallness of the P-value is a measure of ***significance*** for rejecting the null hypothesis that the two reconstruction algorithms are equally good for our task in favor of the ***alternative hypothesis*** that the first one is better than the second one. This is for the case when $s > 0$. If $s < 0$, then the P-value is given by $P_S(-\infty, s]$ and the alternative hypothesis is that the second algorithm is better than the first one. For the task-oriented comparisons that were carried out for this book, we report on the average values of $\text{IROI}^1(c)$ and of $\text{IROI}^2(c)$, as well as of $\text{HITR}^1(c)$ and of $\text{HITR}^2(c)$, and also on the associated P-values.

5.3 An Illustration Using Selective Smoothing

In this section we illustrate the ideas introduced in the previous two sections. As an example we consider the difference between a reconstruction method and the same method when its output is selectively smoothed.

Selective smoothing may be useful in applications in which the images to be reconstructed are made up from regions within which the densities come from a relatively small range, but these ranges are clearly separated from each other. For our head phantoms there are three such regions: the outside of the skull, the skull itself, and the contents of the skull. Selective smoothing produces from a digitized picture another one as follows.

Let $v_1, \ldots, v_9$ denote the densities in a pixel p and its neighbors as indicated by the diagram

$$\begin{matrix} v_6 & v_2 & v_7 \\ v_3 & v_1 & v_4 \\ v_8 & v_5 & v_9 \end{matrix}$$

Let t, w_1, w_2, and w_3 be real nonnegative numbers with w_1 positive, called the *threshold* and *smoothing weights*, respectively. After the selective smoothing, the density in p is

$$\frac{w_1 v_1 + w_2 \sum_{i=2}^{5} f_i v_i + w_3 \sum_{i=6}^{9} f_i v_i}{w_1 + w_2 \sum_{i=2}^{5} f_i + w_3 \sum_{i=6}^{9} f_i}, \tag{5.6}$$

where

$$f_i = \begin{cases} 1, & \text{if } |v_i - v_1| \leq t, \\ 0, & \text{otherwise.} \end{cases} \tag{5.7}$$

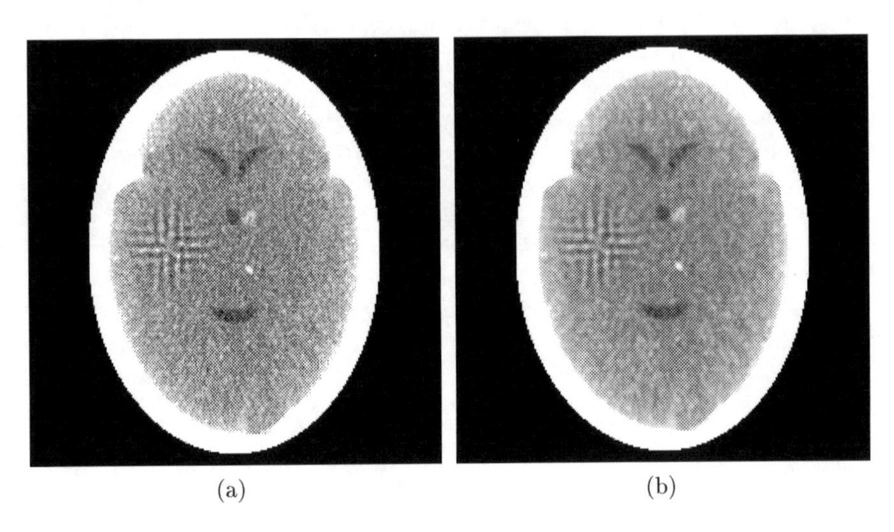

(a) (b)

Fig. 5.3: (a) A reconstruction from noisy projection data. (b) The result of selective smoothing of the reconstruction in (a).

If p is a border pixel, and so v_i is undefined for some of the is, then we set $f_i = 0$ for the corresponding is.

Figures 5.3 illustrates the effect of selective smoothing applied to the output of a reconstruction algorithm. The input to the algorithm was noisy projection data of a random sample of the ensemble of phantoms specified in the previous section. Another sample from this ensemble and its reconstruction by the same process that produced Fig. 5.3(b) are shown in Figs. 5.2(a) and (b), respectively. In both cases we used $t = 0.004$ and $w_1 = 9$, $w_2 = 4$, and $w_3 = 1$. Table 5.1 shows the improvements in the picture distance measures that are achieved by selective smoothing.

According to the picture distance measures, selective smoothing provides an improvement. Also, the digitized picture after selective smoothing in Fig. 5.3(b) is possibly more pleasing to the eye than the one before selective smoothing in Fig. 5.3(a). But does selective smoothing provide an improvement from the point of view of the task of detecting small low-contrast tumors in the brain based on reconstructions from x-ray CT projection data?

To answer this question, we performed a task-oriented comparison as described in the previous section, comparing the reconstructions produced by

Table 5.1: Picture distance measures for the reconstructions in Fig. 5.3.

reconstruction	d	r
before selective smoothing	0.0902	0.0414
after selective smoothing	0.0864	0.0364

a standard reconstruction algorithm with the results obtained by selectively smoothing those reconstructions. We found that the average (over the 30 reconstructions) of the IROIs before and after smoothing were 0.1698 and 0.1501, respectively. The significance by which we can reject the null hypothesis that selective smoothing makes no difference in favor of the alternative hypothesis that selective smoothing is bad for the stated task is extremely high: the P-value is less than 10^{-13}.

Let us discuss what is going on here. First of all, the P-value is this small because it turns out that, in this experiment, the IROI before smoothing is greater than the IROI after smoothing for all 30 samples from the ensemble. Let us therefore look more in detail at just one of the 30 samples, namely the one that produced the images in Fig. 5.3. To see why the IROI is greater before selective smoothing than after selective smoothing, we plotted in Fig. 5.4 values along column 131. The lighter graph in Fig. 5.4(a) is that for the phantom. We can identify five small tumors in this phantom that are traversed by column 131, two on the left side and three on the right side of the graph. The darker graph is of the selectively smoothed reconstruction values. We can see peaks in the reconstructed values at all the five locations of the small tumors. However, when we compare in Fig. 5.4(b) these increases with those that we get before selective smoothing, we see a reduction as a result of the selective smoothing. To consider the effect of this on IROI as defined in (5.3), we can ignore the denominator in that definition since that is determined by the phantom, which is the same in the two cases. The observed decreases in peak density values in Fig. 5.4(b) translate into the numerator of the numerator being smaller after selective smoothing than before selective smoothing. While the same is true for the denominator of the numerator, there the difference is much less since it is due entirely to smoothing of densities that, if it were not for the small inhomogeneities in the phantom and inaccuracies in the reconstruction, should all be the same.

To see how this works consider a simple situation in which all three smoothing weights have value 1 and the threshold is large enough so that the f_i are also always 1. In this case selective smoothing replaces each pixel density by the average of itself and the densities in the eight neighboring pixels. Thus if a pixel has density 9 and its neighbors have densities 0 (a very simplified tumor model), then after smoothing the density of the pixel will be only 1, a reduction by a factor of 9. As opposed to this, consider the situation when densities in a pixel and its eight neighbors are independent samples of a random variable of standard deviation 3 (a very simplified non-tumor model). It follows from (1.14) that after smoothing the density in the pixel will be a sample of a random variable of standard deviation 1, a reduction by a factor of only 3. This difference between the two factors indicates why in the numerator of (5.3) the numerator gets reduced more as a result of selective smoothing than the denominator.

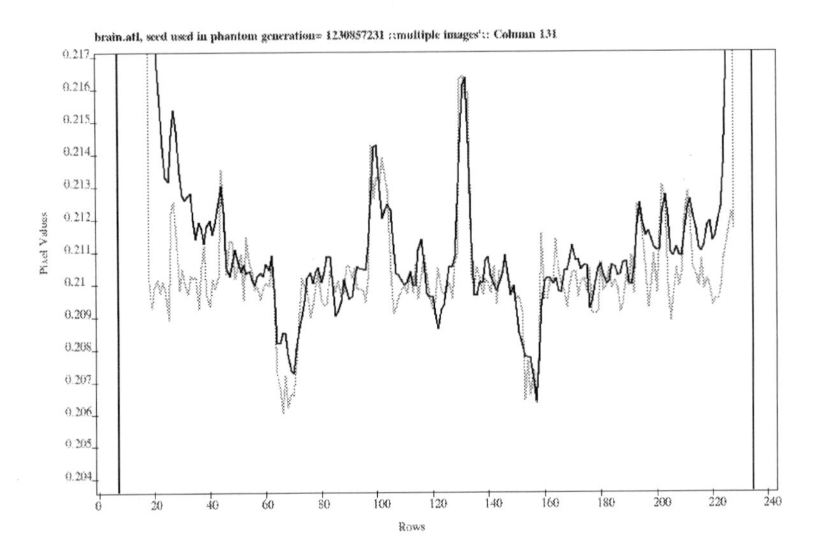
brain.atl, seed used in phantom generati
brain.atl, s_sig1: testin_DCON_0002_r_a
brain.atl, seed used in phantom generation= 1230857231 ::multiple images':: Column 131
Pixel Values
0.217
0.216
0.215
0.214
0.213
0.212
0.211
0.21
0.209
0.208
0.207
0.206
0.205
0.204
0
20
40
60
80
100
120
140
160
180
200
220
240
Rows

(a)

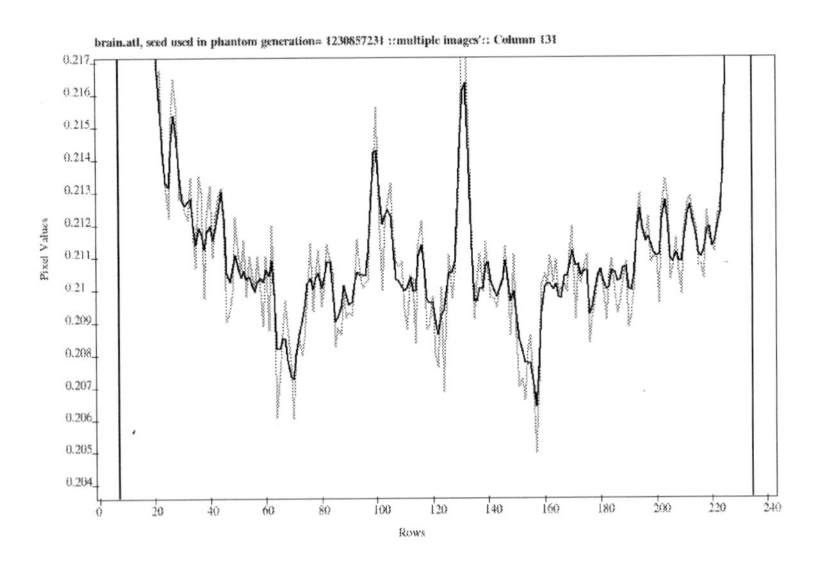
brain.atl, s_sig1: testin_DCON_0001_r_a
brain.atl, s_sig1: testin_DCON_0002_r_a
brain.atl, seed used in phantom generation= 1230857231 ::multiple images':: Column 131
Pixel Values
0.217
0.216
0.215
0.214
0.213
0.212
0.211
0.21
0.209
0.208
0.207
0.206
0.205
0.204
0
20
40
60
80
100
120
140
160
180
200
220
240
Rows

(b)

While the use of IROI is justified by its already mentioned correlation to human performance in detecting small low contrast tumor, the general methodology that is illustrated here does not depend in any essential way on using IROI as the figure of merit. The same basic statistical approach to task-oriented comparison of algorithm performance can be applied with any reasonable FOM that a user may wish to choose. Indeed, we also measured in the same experiment the FOM HITR, which reflects a different model of observer behavior. The results produced by this FOM lead to a conclusion different from the one based on the results produced by IROI: the average (over the 30 reconstructions) of the HITRs before and after smoothing were 0.9335 and 0.9563, respectively. The significance by which we can reject the null hypothesis that selective smoothing makes no difference in favor of the alternative hypothesis that selective smoothing is good for the stated task is also extremely high: the P-value is less than 10^{-10}. This shows clearly that the outcome of a task-oriented evaluation is strongly dependent on the assumed task, as reflected by the FOM.

Another phenomenon worth pointing out is that, in spite of the extremely high significance of the results for rejecting the null hypotheses, the actual values of the FOMs are not particularly reliable. We repeated the experiment reported above with everything being the same except for the random number sequence that determines the exact effect of the inhomogeneity, the placement of the pairs of potential tumors sites and the noise in the data. The new values obtained for IROI were 0.1724 and 0.1528 with P-value less than 10^{-13}, and for HITR were 0.9300 and 0.9520 with P-value less than 10^{-12}. The average FOMs are noticeably different from the values reported above. The reason for this is that the two data sets are quite different and the average FOMs depend quite a bit on the data sets for which they were evaluated. As opposed to this the statistical significances depend on these data sets less, because the comparisons in (5.4) are *pairwise*: IROI^1 and IROI^2 are evaluated for the same data c prior to a subtraction that mostly eliminates the component of the FOM that depends on the data, leaving us with the component that depends on the algorithms.

As a final issue in this section we point out that even though the null hypothesis of equal efficacy can be rejected by the reported experiment with extremely high significance, the difference between the average values of the IROI in the two cases is not all that large, it is less than 13% of either value. Whether or not such a difference is *relevant* cannot be discussed in the context

---

Fig. 5.4: Plots of density values along column 131 of the images in Fig. 5.3. (a) Comparison of values in the phantom (light) with the selectively smoothed reconstruction of Fig. 5.3(b) (dark). (b) Comparison of values in the reconstruction without selective smoothing of Fig. 5.3(a) (light) with the selectively smoothed reconstruction of Fig. 5.3(b) (dark).

of this book; it depends on whether or not the difference in the expected values of the two FOMs translates into a difference of any relevance to the outcome of medical care. As an analogy, consider a thought experiment in which cars of Model A consistently get 0.0001 more miles per gallon than cars of Model B. Because of the consistency, this result is statistically significant. But surely it is not relevant, even the most rational of human being may purchase a car of Model B because of its more pleasing color.

5.4 Reconstruction from Perfect Data

We now describe the basic geometry of data collection that we use throughout this book, except in those cases where the point to be illustrated needs a different geometry. Our basic geometry is based on the third scanning mode in Section 3.4, the fan beam spinning scanner shown in Fig. 3.3(c).

Schematically, the method of data collection is shown in Fig. 5.5. The source and the detector strip are on either side of the object to be reconstructed and they move in unison around a common center of rotation denoted by O in Fig. 5.5. The data collection (actual measurement) takes place in M distinct steps. The source and detector strip are rotated between two steps of the data collection by a small angle, but are assumed to be stationary while the measurement is taken. The M distinct positions of the source during the

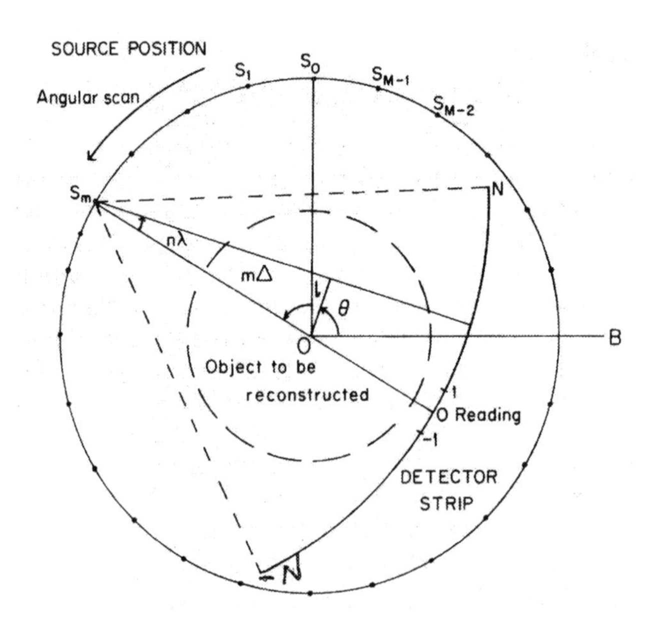

Fig. 5.5: Schematic of our standard method of data collection (divergent beam). This is consistent with the data collection mode for CT that is shown in Fig. 3.3(c).

M steps of the data collection are indicated by the points $S_0, \ldots, S_{M-1}$ in Fig. 5.5. In simulating this geometry of data collection, we assume that the source is a point source.

The detector strip consists of $2N + 1$ detectors, spaced equally on an arc whose center is the source position. The line from the source to the center of rotation goes through the center of the central detector. In this section we assume that each of the detectors is a point detector, the effect of using detectors that have non-negligible widths is shown in Section 5.7.

The object to be reconstructed is a picture such that its picture region is enclosed by the broken circle shown in Fig. 5.5. We assume that the origin of the coordinate system that is used to define the picture is the center of rotation, O, of the apparatus. In this section we also assume that we have perfect data, i.e., that we know exactly the integrals of the picture to be reconstructed along the $M(2N+1)$ lines that connect the source to the $2N+1$ detectors for each of the M source positions.

The algorithm we use for reconstruction from these data is the "divergent beam filtered backprojection (FBP) algorithm with the generalized Hamming window using $\alpha = 0.8$ and linear interpolation." The nature of this algorithm is explained in Chapter 10. The results on which we report are the ones obtained after the selective smoothing specified in the previous section. For the effects of the different problems associated with data collection to be clearly seen, we use in this chapter exactly the same reconstruction algorithm in all cases where it is applicable. The only exception is in Section 5.8 when illustrating reconstruction from data collected along sets of parallel lines.

Specifically, unless otherwise stated, we use in this book the following geometry of data collection. (We refer to it as the *standard geometry* of data collection.) The number of source positions, M, is 720. Consequently, the angle $m\Delta$ shown in Fig. 5.5 is $0.5m$ degrees. The source positions are equally spaced around a circle of radius 78 cm. The distance of the source from the detector strip is 110.735 cm. There are 345 detectors, and the distance between two detectors along the arc of the detector strip is 0.10668 cm.

The reconstruction algorithm estimates a digitization of the phantom from the projection data. Figure 5.6 shows the 243×243 digitization of the head phantom (same as Fig. 4.6(a)), the reconstruction from perfect projection data for the geometry just described, and the values of the digitized phantom and the reconstruction along the 131st column. The values of the picture distance measures for this reconstruction are

$$d = 0.0531, \qquad r = 0.0185. \tag{5.8}$$

Note that even though the data are perfect, the reconstruction is not. This is because a picture is not uniquely determined by its integrals along a finite number of lines (see Section 15.4). The best that a reconstruction algorithm can do is to *estimate* the picture from its projection data.

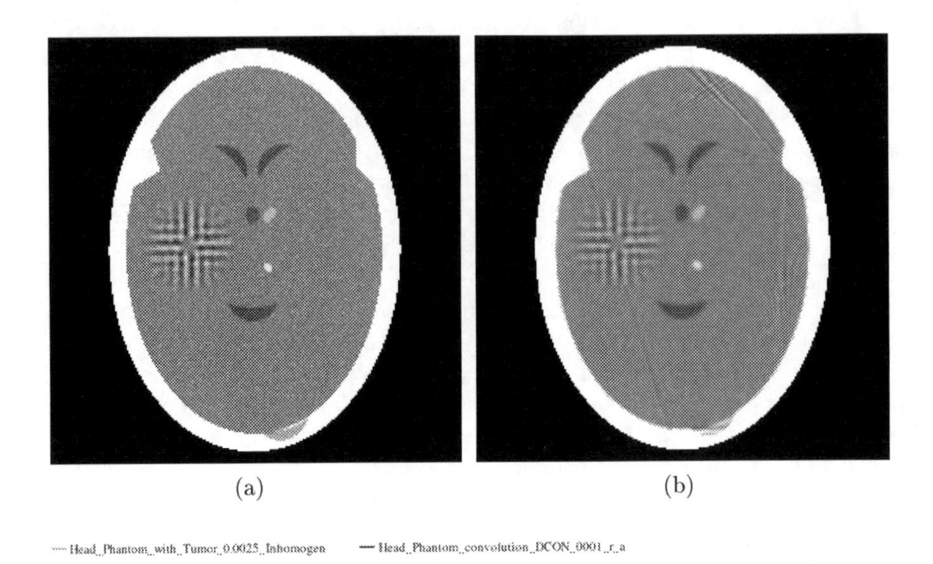

(a) (b)

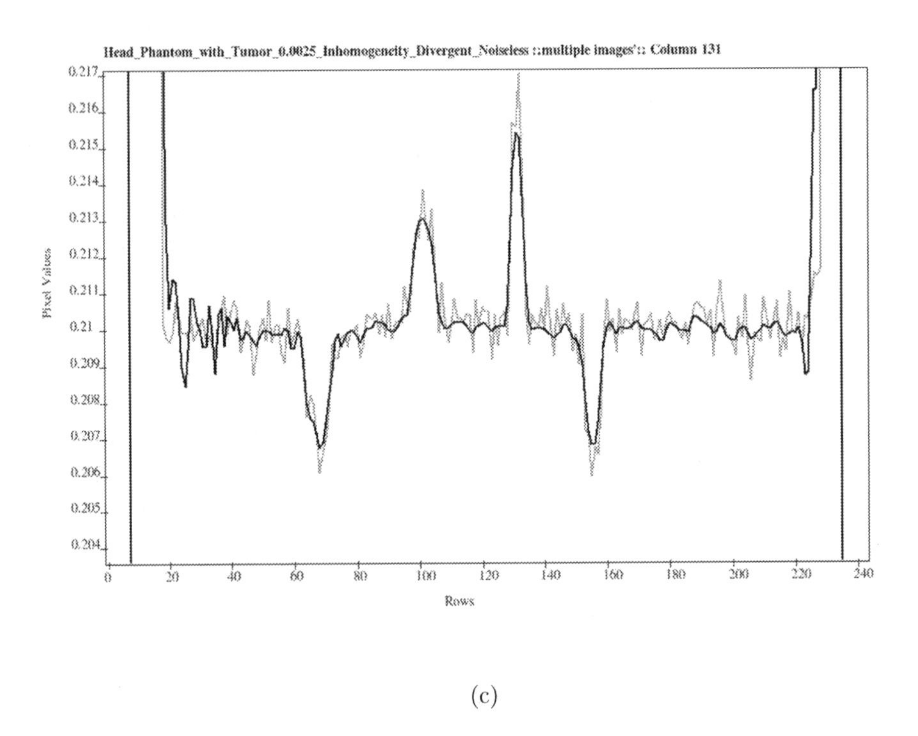

(c)

Fig. 5.6: (a) Head phantom (the same as Fig. 4.6(a)). (b) Its reconstruction from "perfect" data collected for the standard geometry. (c) Line plots of the 131st column of the phantom (light) and the reconstruction (dark).

There are interesting observations that one can make regarding this reconstruction. One is that, generally speaking, the brain appears smoother in it than in the phantom. This is because the algorithm that we use was designed to perform efficaciously on real data and it does some smoothing to counteract the effect of noise. Consequently, small variations due to inhomogeneity are also smoothed. The most noticeable features in the reconstruction that are not present in the phantom are the streaks that seem to emanate from straight interfaces between the skull and the brain. (Similar features are observable in the real reconstruction shown in Fig. 4.2.) Their presence can be explained by considering Radon's formula (2.5), which expresses the distribution of the linear attenuation coefficient in terms of its line integrals. Consider an ℓ and a θ such that $m(\ell, \theta)$ is the integral along a line that is very near to a straight edge between the skull and the brain. Due to the fact that attenuation is much larger for bone than for brain, numerical estimation of the partial derivative $m_1(\ell, \theta)$ from the discretely sampled projection data is likely to be inaccurate, introducing errors into the calculated reconstruction. As mentioned already in the Notes and References for the previous chapter, phantoms that lack such anatomical features should not be used for algorithm evaluation, since the resulting reconstructions do not indicate the errors that will occur in a real application in which the object to be reconstructed is likely to have such straight interfaces. This is illustrated in Fig. 5.7.

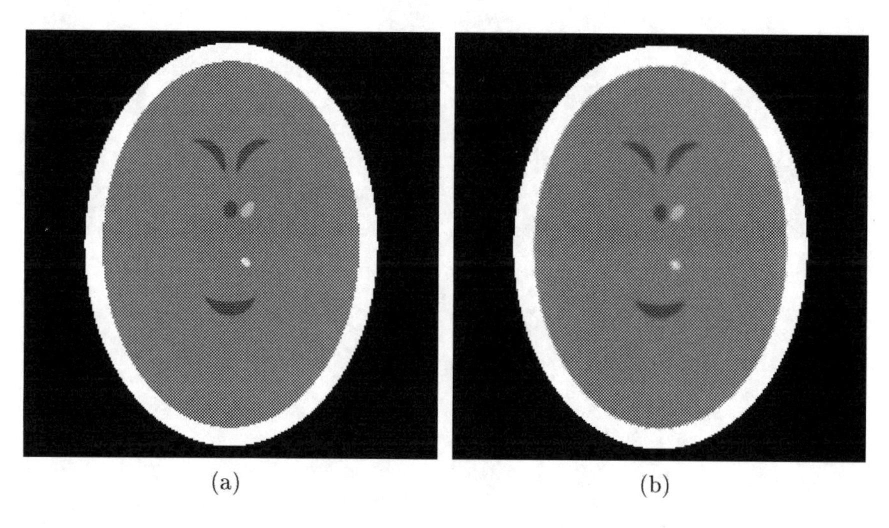

(a) (b)

Fig. 5.7: (a) A simple head phantom without any straight edges between bone and brain. (b) Its reconstruction from "perfect" data collected for the standard geometry. In this reconstruction there are no false features of the kind that emanate from the straight edges between the bone and the brain in Fig. 5.6(b).

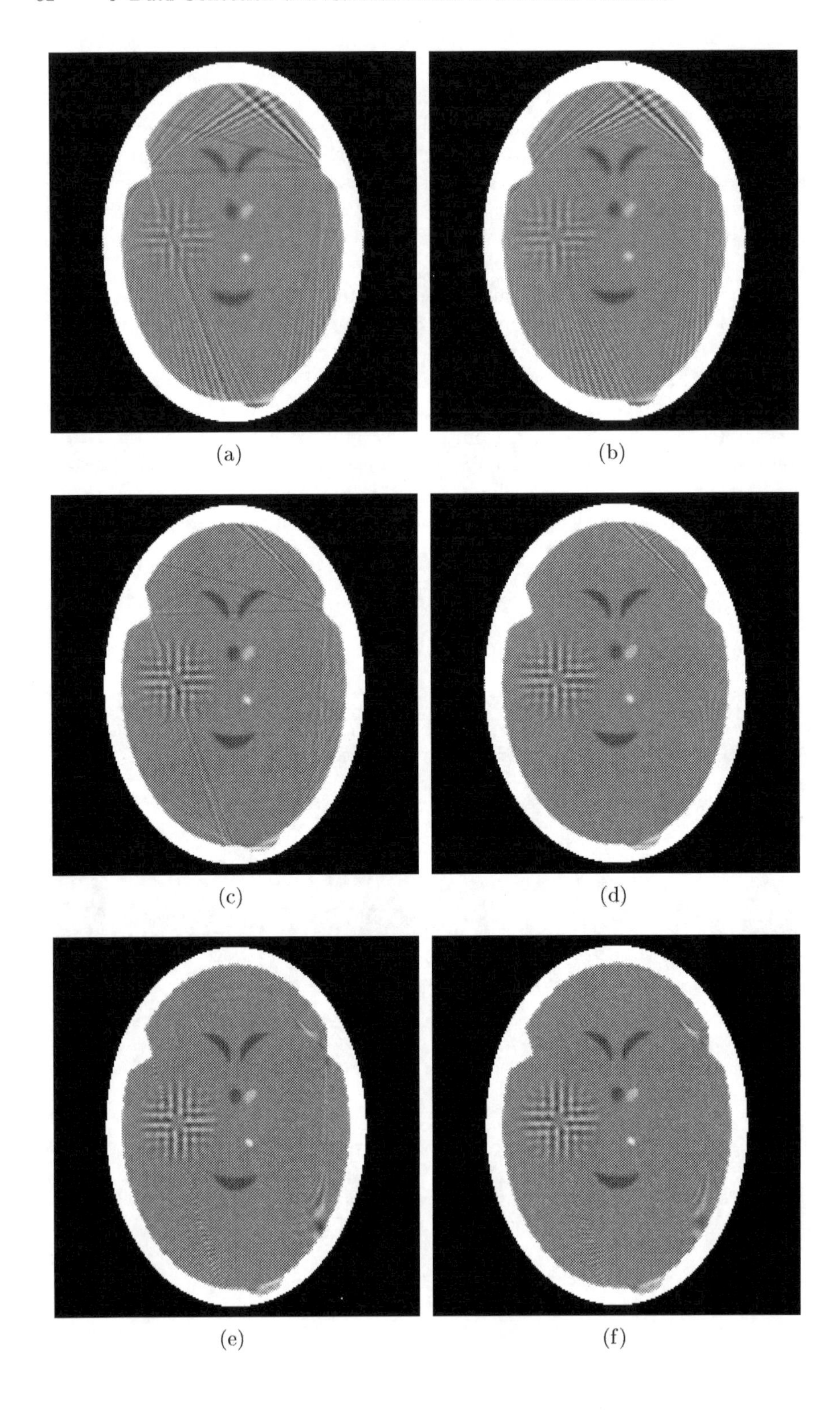
(a)
(b)
(c)
(d)
(e)
(f)

Table 5.2: Picture distance measures for reconstructions from perfect data for various values of M and N in Fig. 5.5.

reconstruction in	M	$2N+1$	d	r
Fig. 5.8(a)	360	173	0.1308	0.0496
Fig. 5.8(b)	720	173	0.1309	0.0496
Fig. 5.8(c)	360	345	0.0530	0.0190
Fig. 5.8(d)	1,440	345	0.0523	0.0181
Fig. 5.8(e)	720	691	0.0189	0.0091
Fig. 5.8(f)	1,440	691	0.0176	0.0071

To show how the quality of the reconstruction is affected by the sampling of the line integrals, we carried out six further experiments with perfect data: three with fewer and three with more samples than our standard geometry. (The arc between the first and the last detector was kept constant.) Table 5.2 shows the resulting picture distance measures. The reconstructions are shown in Fig. 5.8. We see that the nature of the streaks emanating from bone edges in the reconstructions changes with the sampling of the line integrals, but the streaks do not disappear (at least with the algorithm that we use here) for any of the tried sampling methods. Also, at least for our phantom, the number of detectors influences the results more than the number of source positions.

5.5 Effects of Photons Statistics

The projection data for reconstructions shown in this section were generated according to the principles explained in Section 4.5, under the assumptions of a point source, point detector, monochromatic x-rays, and no scatter. For any source–detector pair the calculated monochromatic ray sum is

$$m = -\ln \frac{A_0/A_r}{C_0/C_r}, \tag{5.9}$$

where A_0, A_r, C_0, C_r are samples of Poisson random variables with means λ_a, λ_r, λ_c, λ_c, respectively. Here, λ_a, is related to λ by the equation

$$\lambda_a = \lambda \exp\left(-\sum_{j=1}^{J} \ell_j d_j\right), \tag{5.10}$$

Fig. 5.8: The effect of M and N in Fig. 5.5 on the reconstruction from perfect data. (a) $M = 360$, $2N+1 = 173$. (b) $M = 720$, $2N+1 = 173$. (c) $M = 360$, $2N+1 = 345$. (d) $M = 1,440$, $2N+1 = 345$. (e) $M = 720$, $2N+1 = 691$. (f) $M = 1,440$, $2N+1 = 691$.

where d_j is the density of the jth elemental object at the fixed monochromatic energy level, as can be seen from (4.6) in the monochromatic case of $I = 1$.

What we are interested in is the effect of the choice of λ and λ_c on the quality of the reconstruction. We also compare the effects of errors in the calibration measurements in the third and fourth scanning modes (see the discussions in Sections 3.4 and 4.5). Altogether four experiments are presented to demonstrate the effects of photon statistics.

In the experiment that is most realistic from the point of view of CT scanners, we used $\lambda = 10^6$ and $\lambda_c = 720 \times 10^6$. This means that we assume that during the actual measurement approximately a million photons are counted by the reference detector and that about the same number of photons would be counted by the detector if the object to be reconstructed were removed from the reconstruction region. For our phantom, this results in the values of λ_a being between 40,000 and 1,000,000, depending on how much and what type of tissue the line in question goes through. Thus, the standard deviation of the random variable of which the photon counts are samples is always less than 0.5% of the mean. The figure for λ_c was arrived at by considering the standard practice of calibrating the CT scanner by going through a complete scan of some reference material. Since in our standard geometry we assume 720 views, we get $\lambda_c = 720\lambda$.

In our other experiments we took smaller values of λ and λ_c than customary, in order to indicate the effect of low photon counts. Table 5.3 reports on the picture distance measures. The reconstructions are shown in Fig. 5.9. These results demonstrate the following.

For accurate reconstruction it is important to keep λ high, as can be seen in the deterioration of reconstruction quality from $\lambda = 10^6$ to $\lambda = 10^5$, when λ_c is kept at the value 720×10^6. Unfortunately, to reduce the potentially harmful x-ray dose to the patient it is important to keep λ low. The resolution of this dilemma (reconstruction efficacy versus radiation damage) is one of the most important practical problems in CT. It appears that, for our data collection geometry, $\lambda = 10^6$ is high enough as can be seen by comparing Fig. 5.6(b) with Fig. 5.9(a), as well as the first two lines of Table 5.3.

Errors in calibration are unlikely to come from photon limitations, since there is no damage to patients during the calibration process. However, in-

Table 5.3: Picture distance measures for reconstructions from data with photon statistics for various values of λ and λ_c and scanning modes.

reconstruction in	λ	λ_c	scanning mode	d	r
Fig. 5.6(b)	∞	∞	3 or 4	0.0531	0.0185
Fig. 5.9(a)	10^6	720×10^6	3	0.0533	0.0192
Fig. 5.9(b)	10^5	720×10^6	3	0.0546	0.0231
Fig. 5.9(c)	10^6	10^5	3	0.0573	0.0209
Fig. 5.9(d)	10^6	10^2	4	0.0533	0.0193

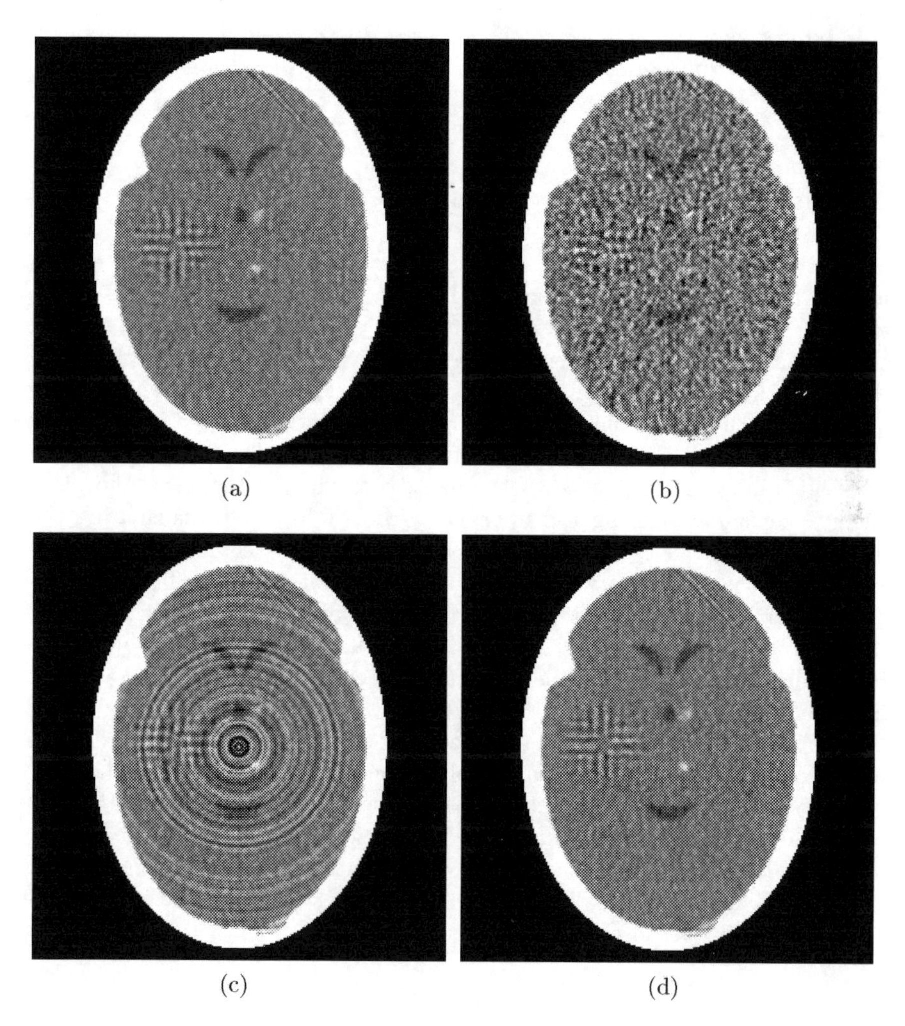

Fig. 5.9: Reconstructions of the head phantom of Fig. 5.6(a) using data with photon noise only. (a) $\lambda = 10^6$, $\lambda_c = 720 \times 10^6$. (b) $\lambda = 10^5$, $\lambda_c = 720 \times 10^6$. (c) $\lambda = 10^6$, $\lambda_c = 10^5$. (d) $\lambda = 10^6$, $\lambda_c = 10^2$. The third scanning mode shown in Fig. 3.3(c) was used in producing (a), (b) and (c) and the fourth scanning mode shown in Fig. 3.3(d) was used to produce (d).

accuracy in calibration may occur for other reasons, e.g., lack of stability in the detector. The effects of such inaccuracies can be simulated by low values of λ_c. As can be seen, using the third scanning mode, this leads to very noticeable ringlike artifacts on the reconstruction (Fig. 5.9(c)), while the fourth scanning mode is hardly affected even if λ_c is very low (Fig. 5.9(d)). This was one of the major motivations for introducing the fourth scanning mode. However, improvements in detection technology and the development of computer algorithms for ring removal resulted in CT devices, using the third scanning mode, which produce pictures without the ring artifact (see Fig. 1.5(d)).

5.6 Effect of Beam Hardening

To illustrate the effect of beam hardening, we collected polychromatic projection data of the head phantom using (4.6). The number of discrete energy levels, I, is five and the t_is (the probabilities that a photon counted during the calibration measurement is at energy level i) are provided by Table 5.4. In the real x-ray situation the spectrum is continuous; Table 5.4 gives a discrete approximation of a continuous spectrum typical of what is used in CT.

In applying (4.6), Table 4.2 was used for the size and location of the elemental objects, with the $d_{j,i}$ (the density of the jth elemental object at energy i) calculated using the information in Table 4.1. In calculating the polychromatic projection data, a point source, a point detector, and no scatter and no photon statistics were assumed. We are interested in how well the phantom (based on linear attenuation coefficients at 60 keV) reconstructs from the polychromatic projection data, and in the improvement in the quality of reconstruction that can be achieved using correction techniques, such as those mentioned in Section 3.2.

Table 5.5 reports on picture distance measures. Note that these are much worse for the reconstruction from polychromatic projection data than for the reconstructions from monochromatic projection data (5.8). Figure 5.10(a) shows the reconstruction from the polychromatic data. The reader should observe the "cupping" of the reconstructed linear attenuation coefficients inside the skull. This is a characteristic beam hardening artifact for head reconstructions, it can also be observed in Fig. 5.11(a).

Table 5.4: Spectrum (t_i) of the polychromatic x-ray beam used in the experiments. The linear attenuation coefficients of the various tissues in the head phantom at the various energy levels are given in Table 4.1.

i	energy (keV)	t_i
1	41	0.1
2	52	0.3
3	60	0.3
4	84	0.2
5	100	0.1

Table 5.5: Picture distance measures for reconstructions from polychromatic projection data without and with various corrections.

reconstruction in	data	d	r
Fig. 5.10(a)	polychromatic projection data	0.1159	0.0556
Fig. 5.10(b)	polynomial correction	0.1022	0.0522
Fig. 5.10(c)	iteration 1	0.0815	0.0390
Fig. 5.10(d)	iteration 2	0.0777	0.0361

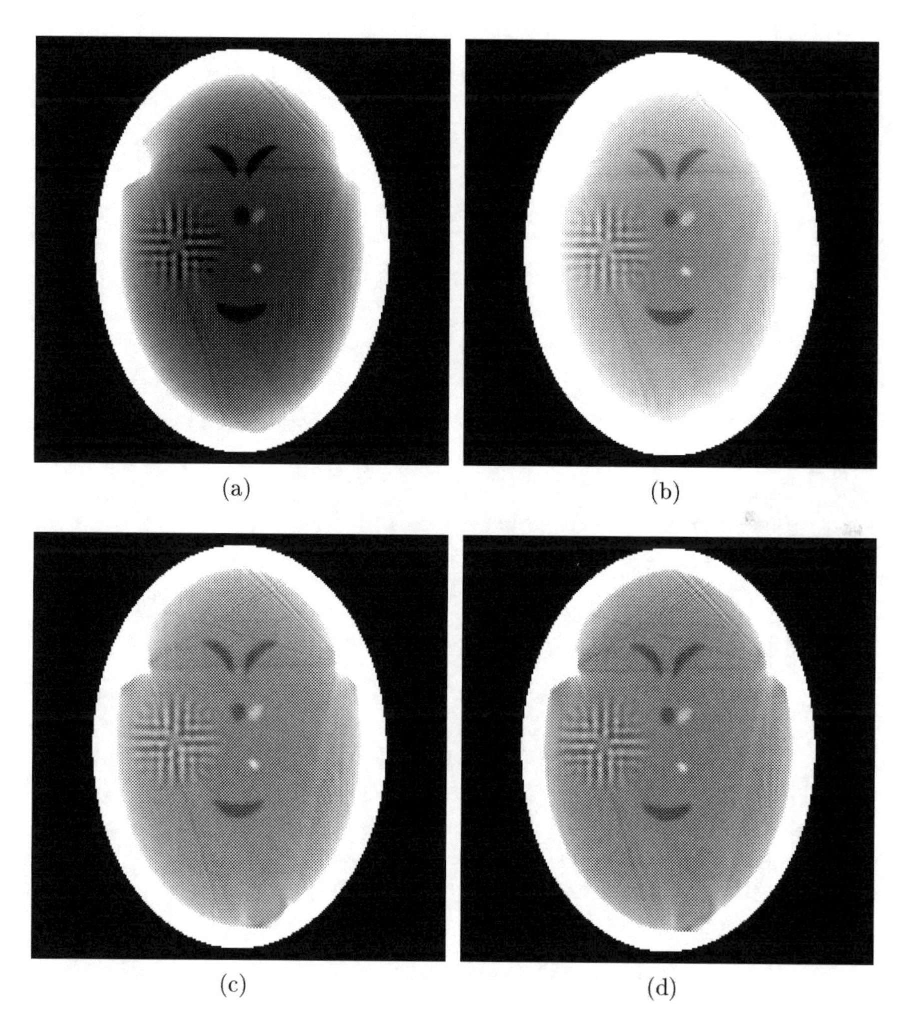

Fig. 5.10: Reconstructions of the head phantom of Fig. 5.6(a) using polychromatic data (with no other sources of error) collected according to the standard geometry: (a) from uncorrected data, (b) from polynomially corrected data, (c) from data obtained after one iteration of the iterative data refinement process, and (d) from data obtained after two iterations of the iterative data refinement process.

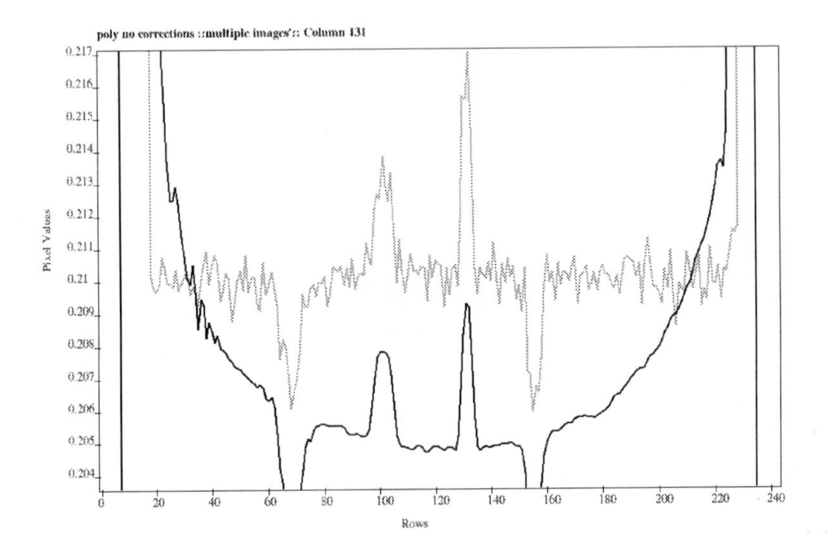
poly no corrections
poly no corr_FBP on uncor_DCON_0001_r_a
poly no corrections ::multiple images'':: Column 131
Pixel Values
Rows

(a)

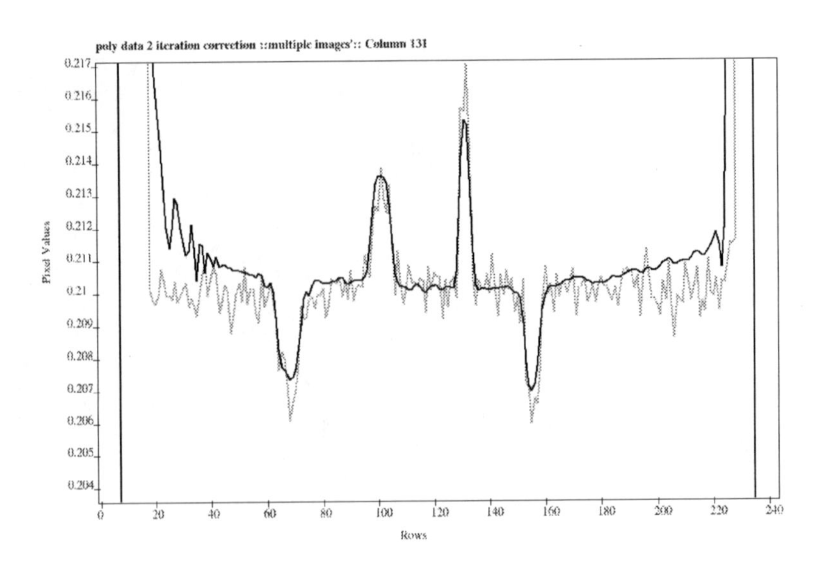
poly data 2 iteration correction
poly data 2_FBP on 2 its_DCON_0001_r_a
poly data 2 iteration correction ::multiple images'':: Column 131
Pixel Values
Rows

(b)

The simple correction method of (3.14), which assumes that there are only two types of material in the reconstruction region, is not appropriate for the head phantom and so we say no more about it here. We first discuss instead the method of ***polynomial correction***, expressed in (3.15). We used the following methodology to estimate, for any positive integer n, the coefficients $a_0, \ldots, a_n$ that are appropriate for phantoms such as our head phantom.

We randomly generated five versions of our head phantom with a large tumor and local inhomogeneities with $\sigma_X = 0.1$. (Note that this is ten times as large as the σ_X used to generate Fig. 4.6(b).) In fact, since we are dealing with the polychromatic situation here, this was done (independently) for each of the five energy levels listed in Table 5.4. For each of the five phantoms, we generated both the monochromatic and the polychromatic data for the standard geometry. In the standard geometry there are 720 source positions and 345 detectors, providing us with a total of 248,400 lines. Let us order these lines in some fashion and let m_j^t and p_j^t denote the monochromatic and polychromatic ray sums for the jth line ($1 \leq j \leq 248,400$) of the tth phantom ($1 \leq t \leq 5$). Then for any n, we calculated the coefficients $a_0, \ldots, a_n$ of the polynomial q of (3.15) so that the *mean square error*

$$\sqrt{\frac{\sum_{j=1}^{248,400} \left(m_j^t - q(p_j^t)\right)^2}{248,400}} \tag{5.11}$$

is minimized. The remarkable thing is that the values of the resulting minimum mean square errors is hardly dependent on either t or n; as we varied n from 1 to 15 the minimum mean square error stayed within the range 0.0383 to 0.0399, for all t. So there is not much point in using high order polynomials and in fact we found that by selecting

$$q(p) = 1.028p \tag{5.12}$$

the value of the mean square error as defined by (5.11) was still between 0.0392 and 0.0399, for $1 \leq t \leq 5$. Figure 5.10(b) shows the reconstruction from the corrected polychromatic projection data using (5.12). In this reconstruction the CT numbers very nearly reflect the actual tissue linear attenuation coefficients in the central region. However, it is impossible for such a polynomial to correct for the cupping, as it can only "lift" the CT numbers multiplicatively in all pixels. Given that the polynomial correction failed to correct for

---

Fig. 5.11: Plots of the reconstructions of the head phantom of Fig. 5.6(a) using polychromatic data collected according to the standard geometry. (a) Reconstruction from uncorrected data. (b) Reconstruction from data obtained after two iterations of the iterative data refinement process.

cupping, the task is to find an improved correction method. We now illustrate an iterative procedure, which is a special case of a general approach that goes under the name of *iterative data refinement.*

If one could obtain estimates m' and p' of the monochromatic and polychromatic ray sums such that $m' - q(p')$ closely resembles $m - q(p)$, where q is the correcting polynomial, then one could obtain an approximation to the monochromatic ray sum by

$$m \simeq m' - q(p') + q(p). \tag{5.13}$$

An approach is outlined in the following.

Represent the reconstruction, which is a digitized picture, by a vector x (its dimension, J, is the number of pixels) such that the jth component, x_j, of x is the estimate of the relative linear attenuation in the jth pixel at energy $\bar{e}$. We estimate m' and p' based on x. Let r be the J-dimensional vector whose jth component, r_j, is the length of intersection of the line with the jth pixel. Then we define the *pseudo monochromatic ray sum*, m', by

$$m' = \sum_{j=1}^{J} r_j x_j. \tag{5.14}$$

Let, for $1 \leq i \leq I$ and $1 \leq j \leq J$, $\mu_{i,j}$ denote the average relative linear attenuation at the ith energy level in the jth pixel. Suppose that we can produce, based on physical information, I functions g_i such that, for $1 \leq i \leq I$,

$$g_i(x_j) \simeq \mu_{i,j}. \tag{5.15}$$

Using t_i to denote the probability that a photon counted during the calibration measurement is at energy level i, we define the *pseudo polychromatic ray sum*, p', by

$$p' = -\ln \sum_{i=1}^{I} t_i \exp\left(-\sum_{j=1}^{J} r_j g_i(x_j)\right). \tag{5.16}$$

By comparing (5.14) with (2.4) and (5.16) with (3.10), we see that if x provides a good approximation to the digitization of the picture to be reconstructed, then (5.13) is likely to be valid. The right-hand side of (5.13) provides us with a new estimate of the monochromatic projection data, which then can be used as an input to the reconstruction algorithm. Figure 5.10(c) shows the reconstruction produced from such an input. The central area, which was already well corrected before this iterative step, is largely unaffected, but much of the cupping is eliminated and the skull–brain boundary is much better defined.

Given that the new reconstruction in Fig. 5.10(c) is better than the old one in Fig. 5.10(b), one would expect that recalculating m' and p' from the new reconstruction and using (5.13) one would get an even better reconstruction.

Such a reconstruction is shown in Fig. 5.10(d) with the plots of the 131st column in Fig. 5.11(b). There is only a slight improvement over the previous reconstruction. In view of the cost, further iterations of the process were not considered worthwhile.

5.7 The Effects of Detector Width and Scatter

As has been discussed in Section 3.3, there are a number of other reasons, besides photon statistics and beam hardening, why physical measurements can only provide us with approximations of the line integrals of the relative linear attenuation. In this section we show the effects of two of these: the width of detectors and the scattering of photons.

The mathematics of reconstruction, at least as embodied in (2.5), assumes the availability of line integrals of the relative linear attenuations. The non-negligible size of the focal spot of the x-ray source and of the detector gives rise to the partial volume effect, discussed in Section 3.3. We simulated this effect for our head phantom and standard geometry by assuming a point source but a wide detector. In fact, we assumed that each one of our detectors is 0.10668 cm wide; i.e., that there is no gap between adjacent detectors on the detector strip (see Fig. 5.5). This makes the width of the detectors as large as they can possibly be for the assumed mode of data collection.

As mentioned in Chapter 4, SNARK09 simulates such a situation by calculating A_0 as the weighted average of (4.6) for a number of lines between the point source and the detector. In our simulation we placed eleven points on the detector (one-eleventh of the detector width apart from each other), and gave equal weights to the lines between the source and each of the eleven points. We assumed no photon statistics, monochromatic x-rays, and no scatter.

Reconstruction from the data so obtained is shown in Fig. 5.12(a), with line plots for the 131st column in Fig. 5.12(c). The values of the picture distance measures for this reconstruction are

$$d = 0.0613, \qquad r = 0.0166. \tag{5.17}$$

It may appear surprising that this reconstruction compares very well with the reconstruction from perfect data, reproduced in Fig. 5.12(b). That this is reasonable will become clearer from our discussion of the implementation of reconstruction algorithms. For now the following summary explanation has to suffice. The estimation of the partial derivative $m_1(\ell, \theta)$ in the Radon inversion formula (2.5) is difficult from the discrete samples of $m(\ell, \theta)$ if the value changes significantly from one sample to the next. The finite detector width "smoothes" the discrete data, and thereby improves our ability to estimate $m_1(\ell, \theta)$. This, to some extent, counteracts the partial volume effect.

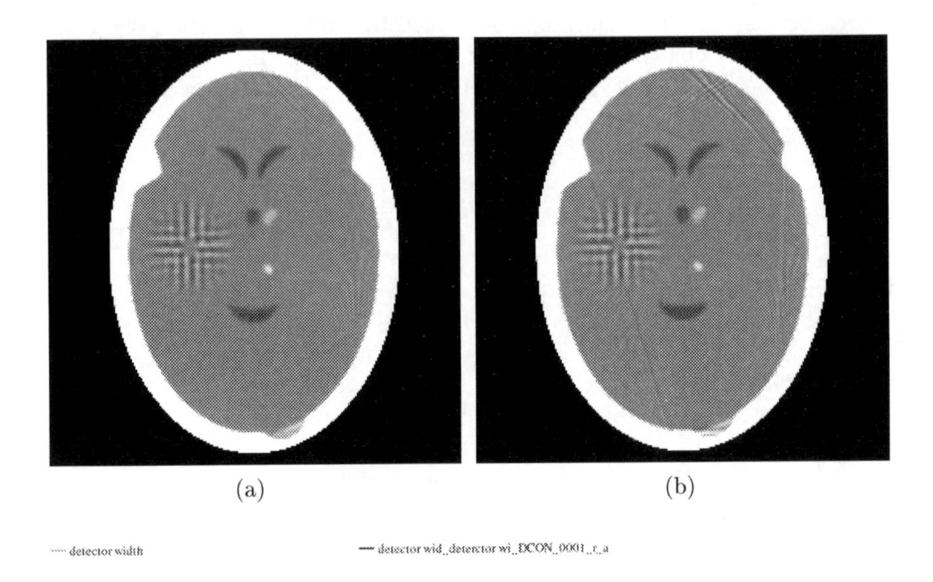

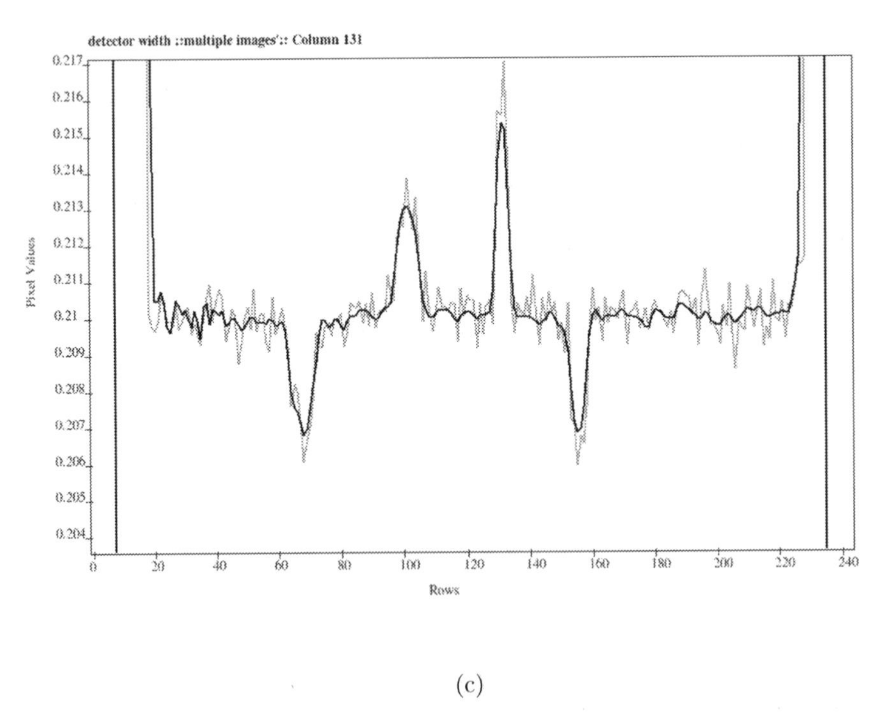

(c)

Fig. 5.12: (a) Head phantom reconstruction from data containing the effect of detector width. (b) Reconstruction from "perfect" data collected for the standard geometry. (c) Plots of the 131st column of the phantom (light) and the reconstruction from data containing the effect of detector width (dark).

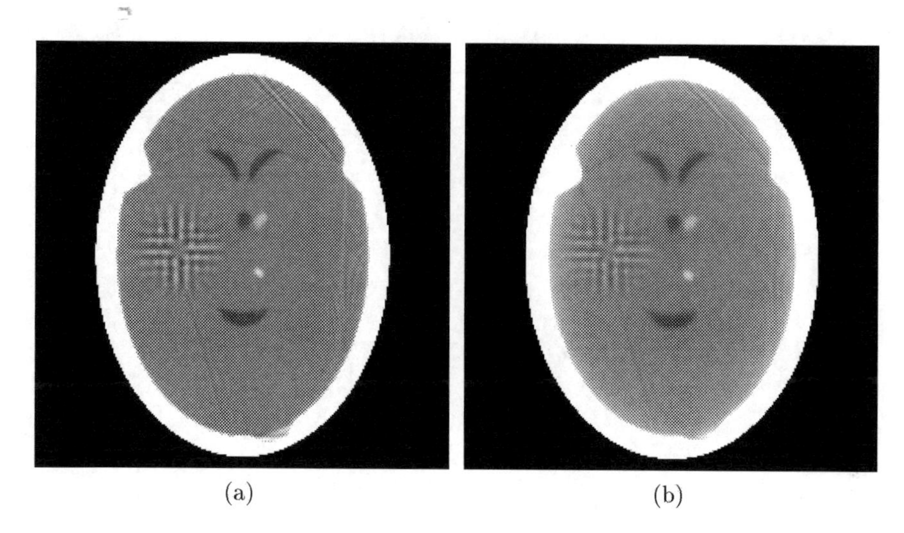

Fig. 5.13: The effect of scatter on reconstructions. (a) 5% scatter. (b) 100% scatter.

The same argument applies to a limited amount of scatter. We consider two different situations, one with high scatter and one with low scatter. In the high scatter case we assume 100% scatter, by which we mean that the number of photons counted by the detectors that have been scattered is the same as the number of photons counted by the detectors that have not been scattered; in the low scatter case we assume 5% scatter. In either case, we assume that scatter can affect the readings of four detectors on either side of the detector towards which the photons were originally moving, with a preference for the smaller angular changes in the direction of movement as a result of scatter. The case of 100% scatter is extreme. Careful engineering, combined with mathematical correction (to eliminate the effect of scatter) applied to the raw photon counts, makes 5% scatter more realistic.

Using the scatter model of SNARK09 we simulated projection data for both low and high scatter, with no other sources of error. Figure 5.13 shows the reconstructions and Fig. 5.14 shows line plots of the 131st column. As can be seen, the reconstruction obtained from data with low scatter compares well with reconstructions from perfect data, but high scatter has a significant blurring effect on the reconstruction. The associated picture distance measures are shown in Table 5.6.

Table 5.6: Picture distance measures for reconstructions from data with scatter.

data	d	r
5% scatter	0.0579	0.0204
100% scatter	0.1234	0.0432

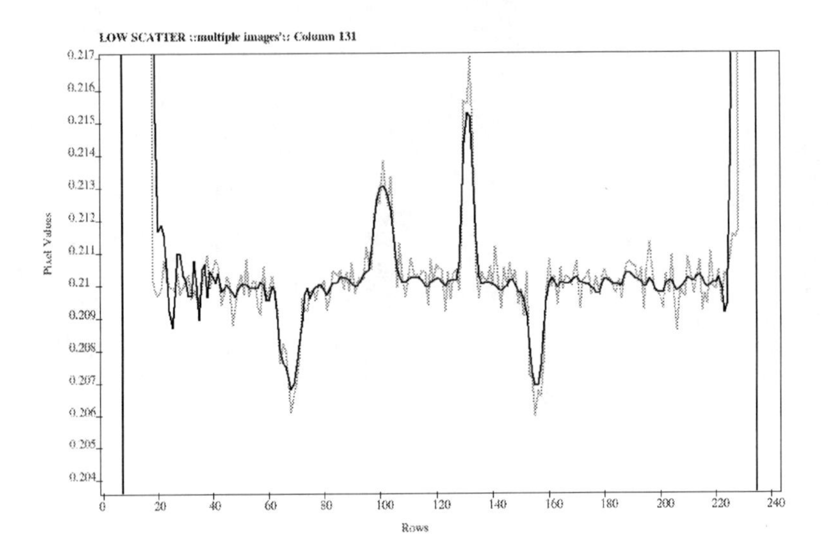

···· LOW SCATTER
— LOW SCATTER_convolution_DCON_0001_r_a
LOW SCATTER ::multiple images':: Column 131
Pixel Values
Rows

(a)

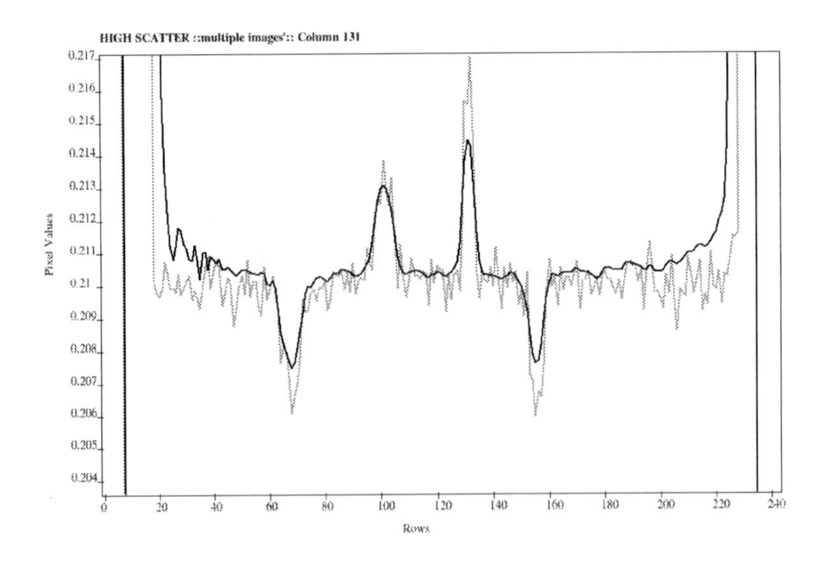

···· HIGH SCATTER
— HIGH SCATTER_convolution_DCON_0001_r_a
HIGH SCATTER ::multiple images':: Column 131
Pixel Values
Rows

(b)

We do not give examples of the effects of other important sources of error discussed in Section 3.3.

5.8 Simulation of Different Scanning Modes

When data are collected by an actual CT scanner all the different sources of error that we have discussed in the last four sections are present simultaneously. In testing reconstruction algorithms we want realistic projection data. We now define the *standard projection data*, which will be used for most of the remaining experiments in this book.

The data are collected for the head phantom with standard geometry as described in Section 5.4. For photon statistics we choose $\lambda = 10^6$ and $\lambda_c = 720\times10^6$ (see Section 5.5). The spectrum of the polychromatic x-ray beam is given by Table 5.4. The focal spot of the x-ray source is assumed to be a point, but the detectors are assumed to have width of 0.10668 cm (i.e., there are no gaps between the detectors). It is assumed that the number of scattered photons that are counted during the actual measurements is 5% of the number of unscattered photons that are counted during the actual measurement, and that the nature of the scatter is as described in Section 5.7. The data so obtained are corrected using (5.13) twice, to provide us with an estimate of the monochromatic projection data. The outcome of this correction is what we refer to as the standard projection data.

Figure 5.15(a) shows the reconstruction from the standard projection data using the divergent beam FBP algorithm used for all earlier experiments in this chapter. Figure 5.16(a) shows the line plot for the 131st column. The associated picture distance measures are reported in in Table 5.7.

The two basic modes of data collection for cross-sectional reconstruction are the parallel beam (Figs. 3.3(a) and (b)) and the divergent beam (Figs. 3.3(c) and (d)). While many reconstruction algorithms are applicable to both basic methods of data collection, some are restricted to only one of them. We therefore define the *standard parallel projection data*, which is used for illustrating the reconstruction algorithms that assume parallel x-ray beams. We attempt to make the standard parallel projection data have characteristics similar to the standard (divergent) projection data, so that reconstructions from the two data sets are comparable.

For the standard projection data we assume that the 720 source positions are equally spaced around the circumference of a circle (see Fig. 5.5); i.e., that the apparatus makes a full 360° rotation in 0.5° steps (see also Fig. 3.3(c)).

Fig. 5.14: Plots of the reconstructions of the head phantom of Fig. 5.6(a) using monochromatic data collected according to the standard geometry with (a) 5% scatter and (b) 100% scatter.

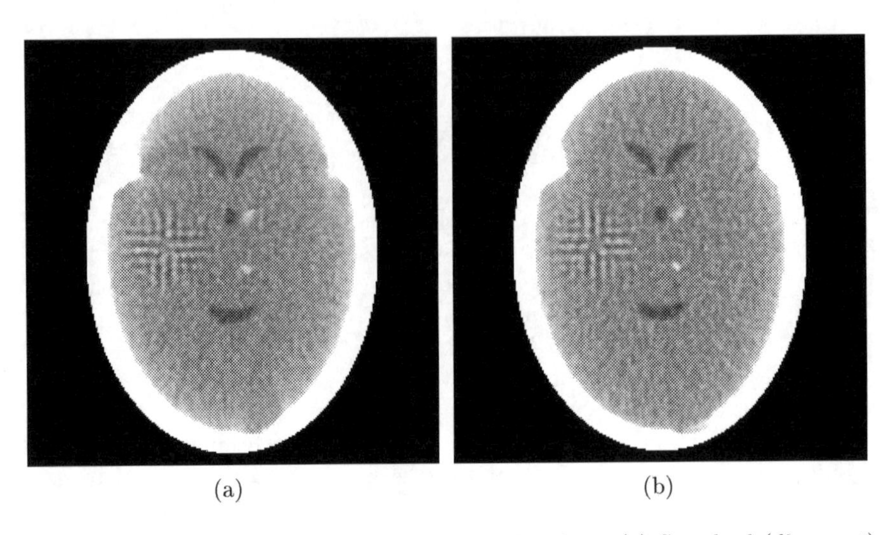

Fig. 5.15: Reconstructions from realistic projection data. (a) Standard (divergent) projection data. (b) Standard parallel projection data.

Observing Figure 3.3(a), we see that, at least in principle, there is no need to rotate the incremental scanner by more than 180° around the patient, since additional rotation would only collect ray sums along the same lines. Hence in the standard parallel projection data, we assume 360 incremental rotations with 0.5° between them. The distance between the parallel lines in a single set of parallel lines was chosen to be 0.0752 cm, which is about the distance between points on two neighboring diverging lines near the center of rotation in the standard (divergent) geometry. This distance also happens to equal the length of the side of a pixel in the head phantom. In any single set of parallel lines there are 345 lines covering the reconstruction region. Thus the total number of lines is half as many as in the standard geometry.

Table 5.7: Picture distance measures for the reconstructions in Fig. 5.15.

reconstruction from	d	r
standard (divergent) projection data	0.0864	0.0363
standard parallel projection data	0.0766	0.0288

Fig. 5.16: Plots of the reconstructions shown in Fig. 5.15. (a) Standard (divergent) projection data. (b) Standard parallel projection data.

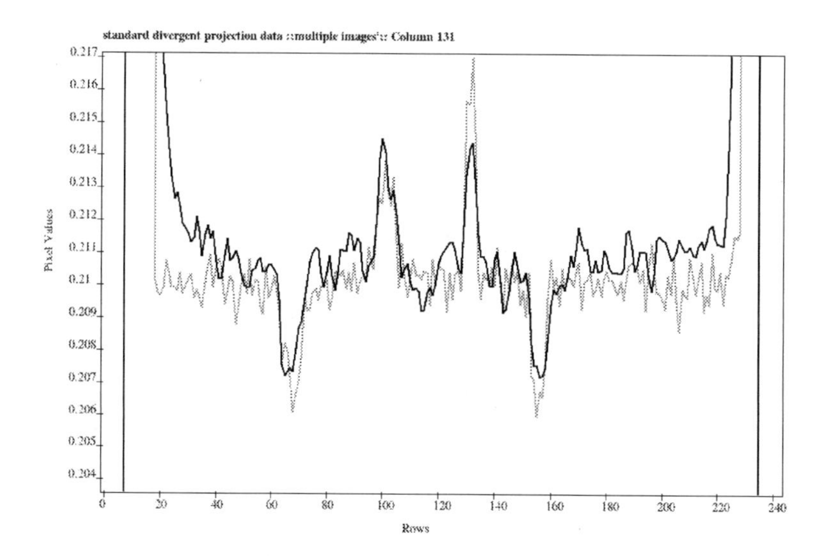
standard head phantom
standard pro_divergent st_DCON_0001_r_a
standard divergent projection data ::multiple images':: Column 131
Pixel Values
0.217
0.216
0.215
0.214
0.213
0.212
0.211
0.21
0.209
0.208
0.207
0.206
0.205
0.204
0
20
40
60
80
100
120
140
160
180
200
220
240
Rows

(a)

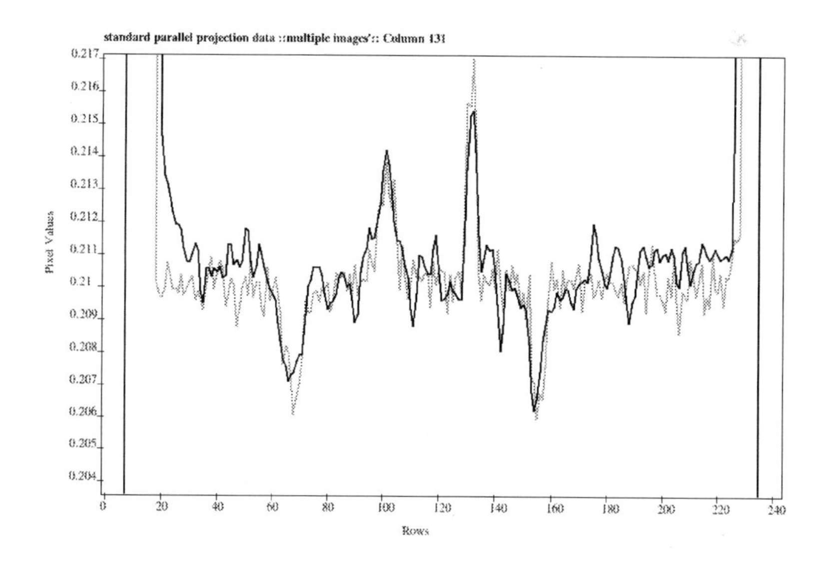
standard parallel projection data
standard par_parallel sta_CONV_0001_r_a
standard parallel projection data ::multiple images':: Column 131
Pixel Values
0.217
0.216
0.215
0.214
0.213
0.212
0.211
0.21
0.209
0.208
0.207
0.206
0.205
0.204
0
20
40
60
80
100
120
140
160
180
200
220
240
Rows

(b)

The data are collected for the head phantom. In order to keep the total exposure of the patient to x-rays the same as in the standard data set, for photon statistics we choose $\lambda = 2 \times 10^6$ and $\lambda_c = 720 \times 10^6$ (see Section 5.5). Thus the numbers of photons used in obtaining the standard divergent and standard parallel data are the same. The spectrum of the polychromatic x-ray beam is given by Table 5.4. Both the focal spot of the x-ray source and the detectors are assumed to have width of 0.0752 cm (that is, the strips between successive positions of the source and detector are abutting). It is assumed that the number of scattered photons that are counted during the actual measurements is 5% of the number of unscattered photons that are counted during the actual measurement, and that the nature of the scatter is as described in Section 5.7. (This means that our parallel data reflect the nature of the second scanning mode, see Fig. 3.3(b), rather than the first one, where there is no scatter from adjacent detector positions, see Fig. 3.3(a). This makes our two data sets more similar. As we have seen in Section 5.7, such low level of scatter makes very little difference to the reconstruction.) The data so obtained are corrected using (5.13) twice to provide us with an estimate of the monochromatic projection data. The outcome of this correction is what we refer to as the standard parallel projection data.

Figure 5.15(b) shows the reconstruction from the standard parallel projection data using the parallel beam FBP algorithm (see Chapter 8) with its parameters adjusted so that they match those that we used with the divergent beam FBP algorithm in this chapter. Figure 5.16(b) shows the line plot for the 131st column. Note that while the two reconstructions differ in some details, the overall quality is not very different, as is further borne out by Table 5.7.

Notes and References

The use of line plots to compare phantoms with reconstructions was introduced into the reconstruction literature by [241]. Variants of the two picture distance measures in Section 5.1 have been used by a large number of research workers; their first combined appearance is in [108], which discusses these and other measures and gives references to earlier work on picture comparison.

There are many publications on the role of receiver operating characteristics (ROC) curves in the evaluation of medical imaging techniques; see, for example, [202, 254]. Their use for image reconstruction algorithm evaluation is discussed, for example, in [97].

The task-oriented comparison methodology as reported in this chapter follows the description given in [116], which was based on the approach proposed in [107, 137, 144]. It has been used to compare reconstruction algorithms in diverse applications such as positron emission tomography [160, 198] and electron microscopy [195, 249]. The relevance of statistically significant differences between reconstruction algorithms was first discussed in [197].

The IROI figure of merit is based on the presentation in [210], where it was found to provide a better correlation with human observers than eight other numerical observers from the previously published literature. The hit ratio (not one of the eight mentioned in the previous sentence) was proposed as a figure of merit for image reconstruction in [137]. SNARK09 [61] has both IROI and HITR implemented in it, as well as other FOMs described in [116, 137], and provides automation of the task-oriented comparison methodology described in Section 5.2.

Our standard geometry of data collection is similar in nature to that of the five second fan beam CT scanner described in [50], but with a larger number of detectors and source positions, to reflect the direction of changes in the design of such scanners in consequent years.

Much of the material in Section 5.6 closely follows [140]. Technical details can be found in [112]. The general approach of iterative data refinement was proposed in [44] and has been applied in a variety of disciplines. Two relatively recent applications are in electron microscopic reconstruction [250] and in positron emission tomography [59].

6

Basic Concepts of Reconstruction Algorithms

With this chapter we begin our systematic study of reconstruction algorithms. We introduce the notation used in the rest of the book. We categorize reconstruction methods into two groups: transform methods and series expansion methods. We explain the nature of the algorithms in the two groups and indicate the desirable characteristics of reconstruction algorithms.

6.1 Problem Statement

Until now we have always used rectangular (Cartesian) coordinates for describing a function of two variables. Thus, we have used $\mu_{\bar{e}}(x, y)$ to denote the relative linear attenuation at the point (x, y), where (x, y) was in reference to a rectangular coordinate system, see Fig. 2.4. However, in the more mathematical work that follows it is more convenient to use polar coordinates (r, ϕ), which are related to the rectangular coordinates (x, y) by the formulas $r = \sqrt{x^2 + y^2}$, $\phi = \tan^{-1}(y/x)$, $x = r \cos \phi$, $y = r \sin \phi$. We use the phrase a *function of two polar variables* to describe a function f whose values $f(r, \phi)$ represent the value of some physical parameter (such as the relative linear attenuation) at the geometrical point whose polar coordinates are (r, ϕ). The mathematically distinguishing feature of a function f of two polar variables is that $f(0, \phi_1) = f(0, \phi_2)$, for all values of ϕ_1 and ϕ_2. This reflects the fact that the physical parameter represented by f can have only one value at the origin. Furthermore, we do not restrict the domain of the polar variables, that is, we allow r and ϕ to have any real values; hence a function f of two polar variables must also satisfy the condition $f(r, \phi) = f(-r, \phi + \pi)$.

In Section 4.1 we have defined a picture as a function of two variables whose value is zero outside the picture region, which is a square (of size $\sqrt{2}E \times \sqrt{2}E$, say) whose center is at the origin of the coordinate system. In what follows, we use f to denote the function of two polar variables r and ϕ, which is used to define the picture to be reconstructed. We know that

$$f(r, \phi) = 0, \quad \text{if } |r \cos \phi| > E/\sqrt{2} \text{ or } |r \sin \phi| > E/\sqrt{2}. \tag{6.1}$$

In particular, $f(r, \phi) = 0$ if $r > E$.

A possible physical interpretation of the picture function f is that the picture region is the reconstruction region of Fig. 2.4 and $f(r, \phi)$ is the relative linear attenuation at the point (r, ϕ). The remaining discussion is independent of such an interpretation. Reconstruction algorithms are applicable whatever physical property $f(r, \phi)$ is supposed to represent (see Section 1.1).

One important difference between studying f simply as a function and studying it as a representation of the distribution of some physical property is the way the mathematics is handled. Reconstruction algorithms are often based on mathematical theorems of the form: "If f has the property that ..., then ... ." We do not hesitate to use the conclusion of such a theorem, whenever the premise appears to be reasonable on physical grounds.

In particular, we shall not hesitate to assume, whenever needed, that pictures satisfy certain integrability conditions. (We use integrals without precise definition. While just about all that we say is valid for any standard definition of an integral; those who wish to make our approach mathematically watertight should use integrals in the sense of Lebesgue.) One of our assumptions is that any picture function f is *square integrable*; i.e., that

$$\int_0^{2\pi} \int_0^E (f(r, \phi))^2 \, r \, dr \, d\phi \tag{6.2}$$

exists. (Existence here means that the integral can be evaluated and its value is a real number.) It follows from this assumption that, for any two picture functions f_1 and f_2, the *distance*

$$d(f_1, f_2) = \sqrt{\int_0^{2\pi} \int_0^E (f_1(r, \phi) - f_2(r, \phi))^2 \, r \, dr \, d\phi}, \tag{6.3}$$

between them also exists. Clearly, (6.3) is related to the picture distance measure defined by (5.1).

We now define the *Radon transform* of a function f of two polar variables. First we introduce a notational convention that is used throughout the book. The Radon transform is an example of an *operator*; when acting on a function it produces another function. We use capital script letters to denote operators; for example, we use $\mathscr{R}$ to denote the Radon transform. If f is a function, then the function that is its Radon transform is denoted by $\mathscr{R}f$. The value of $\mathscr{R}f$ at a point (ℓ, θ) in its domain is denoted by $[\mathscr{R}f](\ell, \theta)$. The Radon transform of f is defined for real number pairs (ℓ, θ) as follows:

$$\begin{aligned} [\mathscr{R}f](\ell, \theta) &= \int_{-\infty}^{\infty} f\left(\sqrt{\ell^2 + z^2}, \theta + \tan^{-1}(z/\ell)\right) dz, \quad \text{if } \ell \neq 0, \\ [\mathscr{R}f](0, \theta) &= \int_{-\infty}^{\infty} f(z, \theta + \pi/2) \, dz. \end{aligned} \tag{6.4}$$

Observing Fig. 2.4, we see that $[\mathscr{R}f](\ell,\theta)$ is the line integral of f along the line L. (Note that the dummy variable z in (6.4) does not exactly match the variable z as indicated in Fig. 2.4. In (6.4) $z = 0$ corresponds to the point where the perpendicular dropped on L from the origin meets L.) The existence of the Radon transform for any ℓ and θ is another one of our integrability assumptions.

Observe that

$$[\mathscr{R}f](\ell,\theta) = [\mathscr{R}f](-\ell,\theta+\pi) = [\mathscr{R}f](\ell,\theta+2\pi) \tag{6.5}$$

and that, as a consequence of (6.1),

$$[\mathscr{R}f](\ell,\theta) = 0, \qquad \text{if} \quad |\ell| \geq E. \tag{6.6}$$

In view of these equations, the function $\mathscr{R}f$ is completely determined by its values at the points (ℓ,θ) with $-E < \ell < E$ and $0 \leq \theta < \pi$.

There is an important difference between the domains of the functions f and $\mathscr{R}f$. The picture function f is defined for pairs of real numbers (r,ϕ), which represent the polar coordinates of points in the plane. Hence the value of $f(0,\phi)$ is the same for all values of ϕ, since $(0,\phi)$ always represents the origin. This is not the case for $\mathscr{R}f$. Its value for the pair $(0,\theta)$ is the line integral of f along a line through the origin making an angle θ with the positive y axis. Hence, unless f is circularly symmetric about the origin, $[\mathscr{R}f](0,\theta)$ depends on θ. The pair of real numbers (ℓ,θ) in the domain of $\mathscr{R}f$ is not to be interpreted as polar coordinates of a point in the plane.

Roughly speaking, the operator $\mathscr{R}$ associates with a function f over the (r,ϕ) space another function $\mathscr{R}f$ over the (ℓ,θ) space. We can think of a single point in the (ℓ,θ) space as corresponding to a line L (at a distance ℓ from the origin making an angle θ with the positive y axis) in the (r,ϕ) space, since $[\mathscr{R}f](\ell,\theta)$ is the integral of f along L.

To further emphasize the relationship between the two spaces consider Fig. 6.1. It shows the loci in the (ℓ,θ) space of the points corresponding to two sets of lines in the (r,ϕ) space: (i) a set of parallel lines and (ii) a set of lines going through a fixed point.

Consider first the line K that makes an angle θ' with the baseline B (the positive x axis) in Fig. 6.1(a). Any line perpendicular to K makes an angle θ' with the positive y axis. Hence the locus of the set of points in the (ℓ,θ) space that corresponds to lines perpendicular to K is the straight line $\theta = \theta'$; see Fig. 6.1(b).

Consider next the point (r,ϕ) in Fig. 6.1(a). The distance ℓ from the origin of the line through it that makes an angle θ with the positive y axis is

$$\ell = r\cos(\theta - \phi). \tag{6.7}$$

Hence the locus of the set of points in (ℓ,θ) space that corresponds to lines through the point (r,ϕ) is the curve whose equation is (6.7), see Fig. 6.1(b).

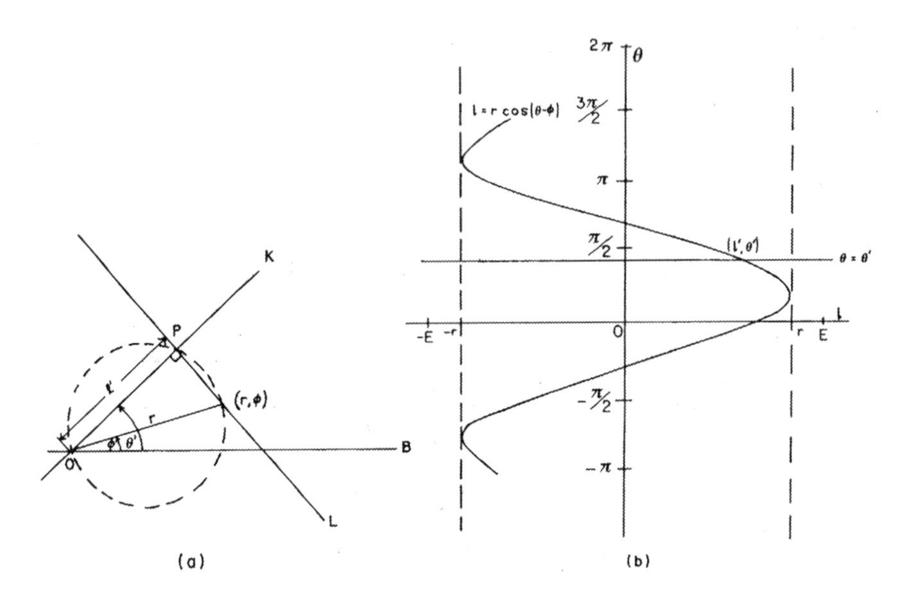

Fig. 6.1: The relationship between the (r, ϕ) space and the (ℓ, θ) space. (a) In the (r, ϕ) space, K is the line through the origin O making an angle θ' with the baseline B. The point (r, ϕ) is considered given and L is the line through (r, ϕ) orthogonal to K. L meets K at the point P, which is at a distance ℓ' from O. (b) In the (ℓ, θ) space, the points that correspond to the lines perpendicular to K in the (r, ϕ) space lie on the straight line $\theta = \theta'$. The points that correspond to the lines through (r, ϕ) in the (r, ϕ) space lie on the sinusoidal $\ell = r\cos(\theta - \phi)$. The point corresponding to L, namely (ℓ', θ'), is the intersection of these two curves. (Reproduced from [115], Copyright 1981.)

The point in (ℓ, θ) space that corresponds to the line L that is both perpendicular to K (and so makes an angle θ' with the positive y axis) and goes through the point (r, ϕ) is the point $(\ell', \theta') = (r\cos(\theta' - \phi), \theta')$.

The input data to a reconstruction algorithm are estimates (based on physical measurements) of the values of $[\mathscr{R}f](\ell, \theta)$ for a finite number of pairs (ℓ, θ); its output is an estimate, in some sense, of f. The main purpose of this chapter is to make this brief description precise.

Suppose that estimates of $[\mathscr{R}f](\ell, \theta)$ are known for I pairs: $(\ell_1, \theta_1), \ldots, (\ell_I, \theta_I)$. For $1 \le i \le I$, we define $\mathscr{R}_i f$ by

$$\mathscr{R}_i f = [\mathscr{R}f]\,(\ell_i, \theta_i). \tag{6.8}$$

$\mathscr{R}_i$ is a *functional*; when acting on a function, it produces a real number. In what follows we use, unless otherwise stated, y_i to denote the available estimate of $\mathscr{R}_i f$ and we use y to denote the I-dimensional column vector whose ith component is y_i. We refer to the vector y as the *measurement vector*.

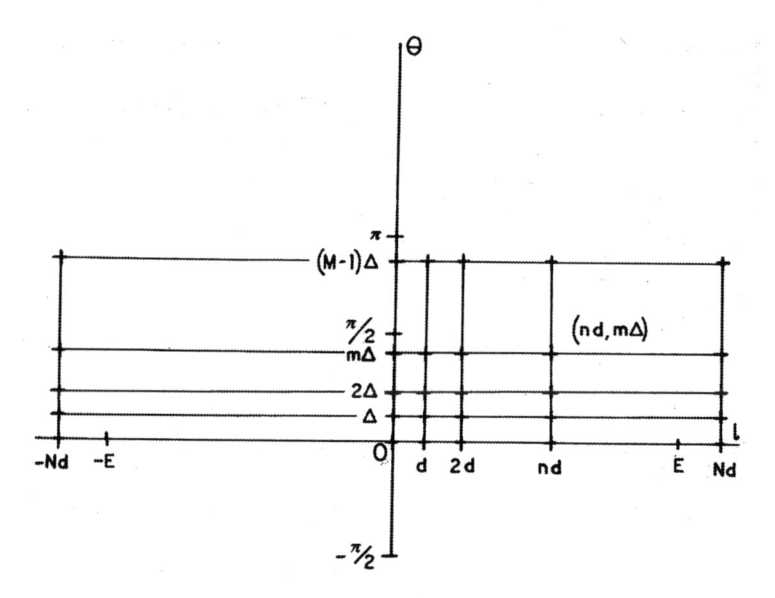

Fig. 6.2: The locations in the (ℓ, θ) space of the points that correspond to lines for which measurements have been collected in the parallel mode of data collection. It is assumed that a single source and a single detector move parallel to each other in $2N+1$ steps of size d, with $Nd > E$, the radius of the circular region containing the object to be reconstructed. After the data have been collected for these $2N+1$ lines (one view), the whole apparatus is rotated by an angle Δ, and the data are again collected for the $2N+1$ lines of the next view. This is repeated for a total of M views, where $M\Delta = \pi$. Thus, for a complete set of views, the apparatus rotates around to nearly cover a semicircle. A typical point in the (ℓ, θ) space is $(nd, m\Delta)$, which lies in the intersection of two straight lines $\ell = nd$ and $\theta = m\Delta$, with $-N \leq n \leq N$ and $0 \leq m \leq M-1$. (Reproduced from [115], Copyright 1981.)

When designing a reconstruction algorithm we assume that the method of data collection, and hence the set $\{(\ell_1, \theta_1), \ldots, (\ell_I, \theta_I)\}$, is fixed and known. Roughly stated, the reconstruction problem is

given the data y, **estimate** the picture f.

In the next two sections we discuss the basic approaches for estimating f. We shall usually use f^* to denote the estimate of the picture f.

$\mathscr{R}_i f$ is the value of $\mathscr{R} f$ at the point (ℓ_i, θ_i) in the (ℓ, θ) space. Any geometry of data collection provides us with a finite set of points (ℓ_i, θ_i) at which an estimate of $\mathscr{R}_i f$ is known. For example, Fig. 6.2 shows the arrangement of such points (ℓ_i, θ_i) for the parallel modes of data collection shown in Figs. 3.3(a) and (b); this arrangement forms a rectangular grid. The corresponding arrangements for the divergent modes of data collection (Figs. 3.3(c) and (d)) are more complicated; they are discussed in Chapter 10.

6.2 Transform Methods

One way of defining the estimate f^* of f is to give a formula that expresses the value of $f^*(r,\phi)$ in terms of r, ϕ, y_1, ..., y_I. Such a formula may be a "discretized" version of a Radon inversion formula, which expresses f in terms of its Radon transform $\mathscr{R}f$. We refer to reconstruction methods based on such an approach as *transform methods*. In the rest of this section we give a more detailed explanation of what has been said in this paragraph.

The Radon transform associates with a function f of two polar variables another function $\mathscr{R}f$ of two variables. What we are looking for is an operator $\mathscr{R}^{-1}$, which is an *inverse* of $\mathscr{R}$ in the sense that $\mathscr{R}^{-1}\mathscr{R}f$ is f (i.e., $\mathscr{R}^{-1}$ associates with the function $\mathscr{R}f$ the function f). Just as (6.4) describes how the value of $\mathscr{R}f$ is defined at any real number pair (ℓ,θ) based on the values f assumes at points in its domain, we need a formula that for functions p of two real variables defines $\mathscr{R}^{-1}p$ at points (r,ϕ). Such a formula is

$$\left[\mathscr{R}^{-1}p\right](r,\phi) = \frac{1}{2\pi^2}\int_0^{\pi}\int_{-E}^{E}\frac{1}{r\cos(\theta-\phi)-\ell}p_1(\ell,\theta)\,d\ell\,d\theta, \tag{6.9}$$

where $p_1(\ell,\theta)$ denotes the partial derivative of $p(\ell,\theta)$ with respect to ℓ; it is of interest to compare this formula with (2.5). We prove in Section 15.3 that, for any picture function f of two polar variables (satisfying some physically reasonable conditions), $\mathscr{R}^{-1}\mathscr{R}f = f$, in the sense that, for all points (r, ϕ),

$$\left[\mathscr{R}^{-1}\mathscr{R}f\right](r,\phi) = f(r,\phi). \tag{6.10}$$

In order to understand the nature of the operator $\mathscr{R}^{-1}$, we express it as a sequence of simpler operators.

We use $\mathscr{D}_Y$, to denote *partial differentiation* with respect to the first variable of a function of two real variables. Thus, for any function p of two real variables and for any real number pair (ℓ, θ),

$$\left[\mathscr{D}_Y p\right](\ell,\theta) = \lim_{\Delta\ell\to 0}\frac{p(\ell+\Delta\ell,\theta)-p(\ell,\theta)}{\Delta\ell}, \tag{6.11}$$

assuming of course that the limit on the right-hand side exists.

In our application, the function p that is operated on by $\mathscr{D}_Y$ is the Radon transform of a picture. It is quite easy to describe pictures f such that $\mathscr{D}_Y\mathscr{R}f$ is not defined for all (ℓ,θ). An example is the picture that has value one everywhere inside the picture region. There are mathematically rigorous ways of extending the definition $\mathscr{D}_Y$, so that it makes sense even in such cases. Here we simply assume that for any picture f that we may wish to reconstruct, the right-hand side of (6.11) is defined for $p = \mathscr{R}f$.

The next operator we wish to define is the *Hilbert transform* $\mathscr{H}_Y q$ with *respect to the first variable* of a function q of two variables. For any real number pair (ℓ,θ), we define

$$[\mathscr{H}_Y q](\ell', \theta) = -\frac{1}{\pi} \int_{-\infty}^{\infty} \frac{q(\ell, \theta)}{\ell' - \ell} \, d\ell. \tag{6.12}$$

Note that this is an *improper integral* since its integrand becomes infinite at $\ell = \ell'$. It is to be evaluated in the *Cauchy principal value* sense; i.e.,

$$[\mathscr{H}_Y q](\ell', \theta) = -\frac{1}{\pi} \lim_{\varepsilon \to 0} \left(\int_{-\infty}^{\ell' - \varepsilon} \frac{q(\ell, \theta)}{\ell' - \ell} \, d\ell + \int_{\ell' + \varepsilon}^{\infty} \frac{q(\ell, \theta)}{\ell' - \ell} \, d\ell \right). \tag{6.13}$$

In our application, q is $\mathscr{D}_Y \mathscr{R} f$ for some picture f. We again assume that for pictures that we wish to reconstruct the limit on the right-hand side of (6.13) exists.

Finally, we introduce an important operator called *backprojection*. Given a function t of two variables, $\mathscr{B}t$ is another function of two polar variables, whose value at any point (r, ϕ) is defined by

$$[\mathscr{B}t](r, \phi) = \int_0^{\pi} t\,(r \cos(\theta - \phi), \theta) \, d\theta. \tag{6.14}$$

Observing Fig. 6.1(b), we see that the value at point (r, ϕ) of the backprojection of a function t is obtained by integrating t on a segment of the curve (from $\theta = 0$ to $\theta = \pi$) whose equation is (6.7).

The reason for the name backprojection is the following. Look at the line K in Fig. 6.1(a). It makes an angle θ' with the positive x axis (the baseline B). The "projection" of a function of two variables onto the line K is the function of one variable obtained from the line integrals of f along lines perpendicular to K. In other words, it is $[\mathscr{R} f](\ell, \theta')$, considered as a function of ℓ alone. The line L that goes through a point (r, ϕ) and is perpendicular to K meets the line K at a point P that is at a distance $\ell' = r \cos(\theta' - \phi)$ from the origin.

Now consider the reverse process. Rather than producing $\mathscr{R} f$ from f by integrating (projecting) along lines such as L, produce from a given function t of two variables another function $\mathscr{B}t$ by spreading (backprojecting) the values of t along such lines. For a fixed θ' (determining the line K), the contribution of t to $\mathscr{B}t$ is the same for all points (r, ϕ) lying on the same line L perpendicular to K; and the value of this contribution is proportional to $t(\ell', \theta')$, where ℓ' is the distance of L from the origin. More precisely, given a point (r, ϕ), we evaluate the value of $\mathscr{B}t$ at (r, ϕ) by summing up (integrating), as θ' varies, the values of $t(\ell', \theta')$ for the ℓ' that is the distance of the line L from the origin. Since L goes through (r, ϕ) and K goes through the origin, the locus of the points P where these perpendicular lines meet as θ' varies is the circle with its diameter from the origin to the point (r, ϕ).

Combining (6.11), (6.12), and (6.14) we get that, for a function p of two variables and for any point (r, ϕ),

$$[\mathscr{B} \mathscr{H}_Y \mathscr{D}_Y p](r, \phi) = -\frac{1}{\pi} \int_0^{\pi} \int_{-\infty}^{\infty} \frac{p_1(\ell, \theta)}{r \cos(\theta - \phi) - \ell} \, d\ell \, d\theta. \tag{6.15}$$

The identity, except for a multiplicative constant, of the right-hand sides of (6.9) and (6.15) can be concisely described by stating the operator equation:

$$\mathscr{R}^{-1} = -\frac{1}{2\pi}\mathscr{B}\mathscr{H}_Y\mathscr{D}_Y. \tag{6.16}$$

In words, the inverse Radon transform $\mathscr{R}^{-1}p$ of a function p of two variables can be obtained by the following sequence of operations:

(i) partial differentiate p with respect to its first variable to obtain a function q,
(ii) Hilbert transform q with respect to its first variable to obtain a function t,
(iii) backproject t, and
(iv) multiply the value of the resulting function by $-(1/2\pi)$. This is sometimes called *normalization*.

Such a process assumes that the exact values of $p(\ell,\theta)$ are known for all ℓ and θ and that the required operations can be carried out precisely. Neither of these assumptions is satisfied when we use a computer to estimate a function from its experimentally obtained projection data. Transform methods for image reconstruction are based on (6.16), or on alternative expressions for the inverse Radon transform $\mathscr{R}^{-1}$, but they have to perform on finite and imperfect data using the not unlimited capabilities of computers. How this is done is explained in the following chapters. The essence of what needs to be done is to find *numerical procedures* (i.e., ones that can be implemented on a digital computer), which estimate the value of a double integral, such as appears on the right-hand side of (6.9), from given values of $p(\ell_i,\theta_i)$, $1 \le i \le I$.

6.3 Series Expansion Methods

In the approach to the image reconstruction problem that is summarized in the preceding section, the techniques of mathematical analysis are used to find an inverse of the Radon transform. The inverse transform is described in terms of operators on functions defined over the whole continuum of real numbers. For implementation of the inverse Radon transform on a computer we have to replace these continuous operators by discrete ones that operate on functions with a finite number of arguments. This is done at the very end of the derivation of the reconstruction method.

The series expansion approach is basically different. The problem itself is discretized at the very beginning: estimating the function is translated into finding a finite set of numbers. This is done as follows.

For any specified picture region, we fix a set of J *basis functions* $\{b_1,\dots,b_J\}$, each of which is a picture function with the specified picture region. These ought to be chosen so that, for any picture f with the specified picture region that we may wish to reconstruct, there exists a linear combination of the basis functions that we consider an adequate approximation to f.

An example of such an approach is the $n \times n$ digitization discussed in Section 4.1. In that case $J = n^2$. We number the pixels from 1 to J, and define

$$b_j(r,\phi) = \begin{cases} 1, & \text{if } (r,\phi) \text{ is inside the } j\text{th pixel,} \\ 0, & \text{otherwise.} \end{cases} \tag{6.17}$$

Then the $n \times n$ digitization of the picture f is the picture $\hat{f}$ defined by

$$\hat{f}(r,\phi) = \sum_{j=1}^{J} x_j b_j(r,\phi), \tag{6.18}$$

where x_j is the average value of f inside the jth pixel. A shorthand notation we use for equations of this type is $\hat{f} = \sum_{j=1}^{J} x_j b_j$. Note that since the values of f are linear attenuation coefficients that have dimensionality inverse length as shown in Section 15.1, the dimensionality of each x_j is inverse length, while the b_j are dimensionless.

There are other ways of choosing the basis functions; some of these are discussed later on. Once the basis functions are fixed, any picture $\hat{f}$ that can be represented as a linear combination of the basis functions b_j is uniquely determined by the choice of the coefficients x_j, $1 \le j \le J$, in the formula (6.18). We use x to denote the column vector whose jth component is x_j and refer to x as the *image vector*.

This approach restricts the general problem of "estimating a picture f" to the more specific problem of "finding an image vector x such that the $\hat{f}$ defined by (6.18) is as near to f as possible using the given basis functions." To make the notion of "nearness" precise, we use the definition (6.3) of distance between two picture functions.

It follows from standard results of mathematical analysis that, irrespective of how the basis functions are chosen, for any picture f there is one, and only one, picture $\hat{f}$ with the following properties:

(i) $\hat{f}$ is a linear combination of the basis functions,

(ii) if $\hat{\hat{f}}$ is a linear combination of the basis functions, then

$$d\left(f,\hat{f}\right) \le d\left(f,\hat{\hat{f}}\right). \tag{6.19}$$

Furthermore, if the basis functions are chosen so that they are *linearly independent* (i.e., none of them can be expressed as a linear combination of the others), then there is a unique image vector x that has the relationship expressed in (6.18) to this $\hat{f}$. For example, if the basis functions are defined by (6.17), then the $n \times n$ digitization of f is the $\hat{f}$ satisfying (i) and (ii), and the associated image vector x is unique.

Ideally, the series expansion approach should aim at finding the image vector that gives rise to the $\hat{f}$ nearest to f. However, since our data do not uniquely determine f, usually we try to find an image vector x that satisfies a less efficacious, but achievable, optimization criterion. Such criteria are discussed in the next section.

In order to show how the image reconstruction problem translates into a discrete problem using the series expansion approach we need to observe two properties of the functionals $\mathscr{R}_i$ defined by (6.8). The first property is that they are *linear*. This means that for all pictures f_1 and f_2, for all real numbers c_1 and c_2, and for $1 \leq i \leq I$,

$$\mathscr{R}_i(c_1 f_1 + c_2 f_2) = c_1 \mathscr{R}_i f_1 + c_2 \mathscr{R}_i f_2. \tag{6.20}$$

This is easily proved using the definitions of $\mathscr{R}_i$ and $\mathscr{R}$. The other property is mathematically less rigorous. We would like to be able to say that "if f_1 and f_2 are near each other, then so are $\mathscr{R}_i f_1$ and $\mathscr{R}_i f_2$." Unfortunately, using the distance for functions given in (6.3), a mathematically precise version of this statement would not be always true. Nevertheless, it is reasonable to argue, based on the definition of $\mathscr{R}_i$, that if $\hat{f}$ is defined so that the previously stated properties (i) and (ii) hold, then $\mathscr{R}_i \hat{f}$ will be approximately the same as $\mathscr{R}_i f$. This property is called *continuity*. A basic weakness of the series expansion approach is that this assumption is sometimes violated. Combining these properties we can state that, for $1 \leq i \leq I$,

$$\mathscr{R}_i f \simeq \mathscr{R}_i \hat{f} = \sum_{j=1}^{J} x_j \mathscr{R}_i b_j. \tag{6.21}$$

Since the b_j are user-defined functions, usually the $\mathscr{R}_i b_j$ can be easily calculated by analytical means. For example, in the case when the b_j are defined by (6.17), $\mathscr{R}_i b_j$ is just the length of intersection with the jth pixel of the line of the ith position of the source–detector pair. (More precisely, of the line at a distance ℓ_i from the origin making angle θ_i with the positive y axis; see (6.8) and Fig. 2.4. In this case, for any given i, a list of all the j such that $\mathscr{R}_i b_j \neq 0$ and the values of these $\mathscr{R}_i b_j$ can be efficiently calculated using a DDA; see Section 4.6.) When using alternate basis functions, it can happen that the ith line misses the picture region, but nevertheless $\mathscr{R}_i b_j \neq 0$; causing a violation of (6.21). It is strongly advisable to remove the measurements associated with such lines from the projection data sets, and we have done this in all the relevant experiments on which we report in this book. Unless otherwise stated, we use $r_{i,j}$ to denote our calculated value of $\mathscr{R}_i b_j$. Hence,

$$r_{i,j} \simeq \mathscr{R}_i b_j. \tag{6.22}$$

Recall also that we use y_i to denote the physically obtained estimate of $\mathscr{R}_i f$. Combining this with (6.21) and (6.22), we get that, for $1 \leq i \leq I$,

$$y_i \simeq \sum_{j=1}^{J} r_{i,j} x_j. \tag{6.23}$$

Note that in CT the $r_{i,j}$ have dimensionality length, since they are line integrals of a dimensionless function. Since the x_j have dimensionality inverse length, the right-hand side of (6.23) is dimensionless, as it should be to match its dimensionless left-hand side.

Let R denote the matrix whose (i, j)th element is $r_{i,j}$. We refer to this matrix as the *projection matrix*. Let e be the I-dimensional column vector whose ith component, e_i, is the difference between the left- and right-hand sides of (6.23). We refer to this as the *error vector*. Then (6.23) can be rewritten as

$$y = Rx + e. \tag{6.24}$$

The series expansion approach leads us to the following *discrete reconstruction problem*: based on (6.24),

given the data y, **estimate** the image vector x.

If the estimate that we find as our solution to the discrete reconstruction problem is the vector x^*, then the estimate f^* to the picture to be reconstructed is given by

$$f^* = \sum_{j=1}^{J} x_j^* b_j. \tag{6.25}$$

We make the following important observation. Our justification for the series expansion approach did *not* need that the functionals $\mathscr{R}_i$ be defined by (6.8). It only needed that the $\mathscr{R}_i$s satisfy the property expressed by (6.21). Many different ways of defining the $\mathscr{R}_i$s will have this property: integration along curved rather than straight lines or even areas (such as strips) rather than lines are potentially relevant to the general reconstruction problem. A major advantage of the series expansion methods over the transform methods is that they are immediately applicable to such more general ways of data collection.

6.4 Optimization Criteria

In this section we discuss optimization criteria by which the image vector of the series expansion approach is estimated. Although this will not be explicitly indicated, much of what we say is also relevant to estimating pictures using transform methods.

In (6.24), the vector e is unknown. The very most we can hope for is that we can specify a random variable of which e is a sample, and in most cases even this is impossible. The simple approach of trying to solve (6.24) by first assuming that e is the zero vector is dangerous: $y = Rx$ may have no solutions, or it may have many solutions, possibly none of which is any good for the practical problem at hand. Some criteria have to be developed, indicating which x ought to be chosen as a solution of (6.24).

The criteria that have been used for the reconstruction problem are usually of the form: choose as the "solution" of (6.24) an image vector x for which the value of some function $\phi_1(x)$ is minimal, and if there is more than one x that minimizes $\phi_1(x)$ choose among these one for which the value of some other function $\phi_2(x)$ is minimal. In this section we survey some of the choices for ϕ_1 and ϕ_2 that have been proposed.

A theoretically attractive approach is the following. Consider both the image vector x and the error vector e to be samples of random variables, denoted by X and E, respectively. Since our discussion in Section 1.2 was restricted to continuous random variables whose samples are real numbers, while here we deal with column vectors of real numbers, further explanation is needed. (A reader who is not desirous to learn about the foundations of Bayesian estimation may safely skip to (6.33).)

In fact, there is an additional subtle point that needs to be appreciated, especially because ignoring it can have some undesirable consequences. As discussed after (6.18), the dimensionality of the components of the image vector x is inverse length. As opposed to this, it follows from the discussion after (6.23) that the components of the error vector e are dimensionless. Because of this, any formulas involving samples from both X and E have to be formulated with the unit of length in mind.

The random variable X has an associated probability density function p_X, which is a real number valued function on J-dimensional vectors of real numbers (the possible samples of X). This function p_X is defined so that, for any J pairs (ℓ_j, u_j) of numbers such that $\ell_1 < u_1, \ldots, \ell_J < u_J$, the probability that a sample x of X will have the property that $\ell_j \leq x_j \leq u_j$, for $1 \leq j \leq J$, is

$$\int_{\ell_1}^{u_1} \cdots \int_{\ell_J}^{u_J} p_X(x)\, dx_J \cdots dx_1. \tag{6.26}$$

For notational convenience we sometimes abbreviate such integrals as

$$\int_{\ell}^{u} p_X(x)\, dx. \tag{6.27}$$

Since the probability expressed in (6.26) is dimensionless, it follows from the dimensionality of the J components x that $p_X(x)$ has to have dimensionality length to the Jth power.

Corresponding to the concepts of mean and variance of a continuous random variable as defined in (1.8) and (1.9), we have the concepts of *mean vector* μ_X and *covariance matrix* V_X, defined as

$$\mu_X = \int_{-\infty}^{\infty} x p_X(x)\, dx, \tag{6.28}$$

$$V_X = \int_{-\infty}^{\infty} (x - \mu_X)(x - \mu_X)^T p_X(x)\, dx, \tag{6.29}$$

where x^T denotes the row vector that is the *transpose* of the column vector x (i.e., a row vector whose ith component is x_i). These integrals are to be interpreted component by component. For example, using $(x - \mu_X)_i$ to denote the ith component of the vector $x - \mu_X$, the (i,j)th entry of V_X is given by

$$(V_X)_{i,j} = \int_{-\infty}^{\infty} (x - \mu_X)_i (x - \mu_X)_j p_X(x)\, dx. \tag{6.30}$$

It follows from these formulas that the dimensionality of the components of μ_X is inverse length, while the dimensionality of the entries of V_X is inverse length squared. Note that V_X is a *symmetric matrix* since it is clear from (6.30) that $(V_X)_{i,j} = (V_X)_{j,i}$.

The discussion in the previous two paragraphs has a simpler analog for the distribution E of the error vectors. In that case all numbers (the values of $p_E(e)$ and the components of μ_E and of V_E) are dimensionless. Similarly, the discussion of the next paragraph concerning X has a simpler dimensionless analog concerning E.

Let μ denote a J-dimensional vector of real numbers with dimensionality inverse length and let V denote a $J \times J$ symmetric matrix of real numbers with dimensionality inverse length squared. Let us further assume that V is *positive definite*, which means that $x^T V x$ is positive for any J-dimensional vector x with at least one nonzero component. Using elementary matrix algebra it can be shown that V has an inverse (denoted by V^{-1}) and its determinant (denoted by $\det V$) is positive. Furthermore, the dimensionality of the entries of V^{-1} is length squared and the dimensionality of $\det V$ is inverse length to the $2J$th power. Using such a μ and V, we can define a function p_X over the set of all J-dimensional vectors of real numbers of dimensionality inverse length by

$$p_X(x) = \frac{1}{(2\pi)^{J/2}(\det V)^{1/2}} \exp\left(-\frac{1}{2}(x - \mu)^T V^{-1} (x - \mu)\right). \tag{6.31}$$

It is not difficult to check that this p_X is a probability density function on the set of all J-dimensional vectors of real numbers of dimensionality inverse length and, using (6.28) and (6.29), that $\mu_x = \mu$ and $V_X = V$. A random variable X defined in such a fashion is called a *multivariate Gaussian random variable*. The probability density function of a multivariate Gaussian random variable peaks at its mean vector.

The importance of multivariate Gaussian random variables rests on two facts. One is that many random variables occurring in practice are approximately multivariate Gaussian. The other is that the assumption that an unknown random variable is multivariate Gaussian usually makes the mathematical treatment of the problem much easier than it would be otherwise.

Let us return now to the random variables X and E associated with x and e of (6.24). In this case p_X is referred to as the *prior probability density function*, since $p_X(x)$ indicates the likelihood of coming across an image vector similar to x. In CT it makes sense to adjust p to the area of the body we are imaging; the probabilities of the same picture representing a cross section of the head or of the thorax should be different. Our treating X and E separately is by itself a simplifying assumption, since in practice E is not independent of X, as can be seen from the discussion in Section 3.1. The theory that we are describing can be developed without making this assumption, but it becomes more complicated.

At last we are in position to state an optimization criterion (it assumes that p_X and p_E are known): given the data y, choose the image vector x for which the value of

$$p_E(y - Rx)p_X(x) \tag{6.32}$$

is as large as possible. Note that the second term in the product is large for vectors x that have large prior probabilities, while the first term is large for vectors x that are consistent with the data (at least if p_E peaks at the zero vector). The relative importance of the two terms depends on the nature of p_X and p_E. If p_X is flat (many image vectors are equally likely) and p_E is highly peaked near the zero vector, then our criterion will produce an image vector x^* that fits the measured data y in the sense that Rx^* will be nearly the same as y. On the other hand, if p_E is flat (large errors are nearly as likely as small ones) but p_X is highly peaked, our having made our measurements will have only a small effect on our preconceived idea as to how the image vector should be chosen. The x^* that maximizes (6.32) is called the *Bayesian estimate*.

A difficulty with using Bayesian estimation is that it presupposes knowledge of p_X and p_E. Precise knowledge of the true distributions of the image vector and of the error vector is usually not available. A second difficulty is that, for many p_X and p_E, the estimation of x that maximizes (6.32) may be far from trivial.

If we assume that both X and E are multivariate Gaussian, the optimization problem becomes much simpler. In that case it is easy to see from (6.31) that, assuming that μ_E is the zero vector, the x that maximizes (6.32) is the same x that minimizes

$$(y - Rx)^T V_E^{-1} (y - Rx) + (x - \mu_X)^T V_X^{-1} (x - \mu_X) . \tag{6.33}$$

Note that both terms in this sum are dimensionless.

A less sophisticated approach is to aim at finding a *least squares solution* of (6.24), i.e., an x that minimizes

$$\|e\|^2 = \|y - Rx\|^2 = \sum_{i=1}^{I} \left(y_i - \sum_{j=1}^{J} r_{i,j} x_j \right)^2 . \tag{6.34}$$

Such a criterion does not necessarily determine x; there may be more than one vector x that minimizes (6.34). In such a case one has to select an x by a second criterion, choices for which are described in the following.

Another reason why a least squares solution is not necessarily very good is that the criterion expressed in (6.34) does not contain any information regarding the nature of a "desirable" solution x. In the Bayesian approach of (6.33) such information is incorporated into the prior covariance matrix V_X.

It can be reasonably argued that a desirable property of the solution of (6.24) is that the variance

$$\sum_{j=1}^{J} (x_j - \bar{x})^2, \tag{6.35}$$

where

$$\bar{x} = \frac{1}{J} \left(\sum_{j=1}^{J} x_j \right) \tag{6.36}$$

should be small. If the basis functions are chosen according to (6.17), then $\bar{x}$ is the average density in the digitized picture. It can be shown that if $\bar{x}$ is considered fixed for all acceptable solutions to (6.24), then the x that minimizes (6.35) is the same x that minimizes the (*Euclidean*) *norm* $\|x\|$ of x, where

$$\|x\|^2 = \sum_{j=1}^{J} x_j^2. \tag{6.37}$$

In other words, in such a case the *minimum variance* and *minimum norm* solutions are the same.

The criteria expressed in (6.35) and (6.37) are not to be used as "primary" criteria in image reconstruction. That is, in terms of the notation introduced at the beginning of this section, it is not reasonable to define $\phi_1(x)$ by (6.35). That would lead to the "solution" in which all components of x are the same, namely $\bar{x}$. The use of (6.35) is either as a secondary criterion, or as a component of the primary criterion, where the other components force the "solution" to be consistent with the measurements, or express other properties of desirable solutions of (6.24).

For example, in the case when the basis functions are chosen according to (6.17) it may be considered "desirable" that the values x_j assigned to neighboring pixels should be close to one another on the average. Such a criterion can be expressed (see Section 12.3) by saying that we desire to minimize $x^{\mathrm{T}}Bx$, where B is an appropriately chosen matrix. This, in conjunction with the desire to minimize (6.34) and (6.37) at the same time, leads us to state that the sought solution x of (6.24) is the one that minimizes

$$a \|y - Rx\|^2 + x^T(bB + U)x, \tag{6.38}$$

where a and b are appropriately chosen positive numbers, indicating the relative importance we attach to minimizing the various expressions previously discussed, and U is the identity matrix. Here is where the potential for making a mistake by ignoring dimensionality lies. By stating that U is the identity matrix, we are implicitly assuming that its entries are dimensionless, otherwise changing units could turn U into a matrix other than the identity. Hence bB also has to be dimensionless and the dimensionality of the second term is inverse length squared. In order to keep the two terms of (6.38) physically consistent, we need to use an a that has dimensionality of inverse length squared. In other words, a cannot be a fixed number that is independent of the unit of length used. Also the expression in (6.38) (which has dimensionality of inverse length squared) is a different kind of thing from the expression in (6.33) (which is dimensionless), but this is a minor technical matter: by dividing both terms in (6.38) by the positive a, we get a dimensionless expression and an x^* minimizes this expression if, only if, it minimizes (6.38).

The approaches indicated by (6.33), (6.34), (6.35), (6.37), and (6.38) are special cases of a *quadratic optimization* problem that can be stated as follows. Find an x that minimizes

$$a\left(y - Rx\right)^T A\left(y - Rx\right) + \left(x - x_0\right)^T \left(bB + cC^{-1}\right)\left(x - x_0\right), \qquad (6.39)$$

where A is a symmetric $I \times I$ matrix, B and C are $J \times J$ matrices, a, b, and c are nonnegative real numbers, and x_0 is a J-dimensional vector. (Further details on the nature of these matrices, constants, and vectors are given in Section 12.1, which also contains the reasons for writing the matrix in the second term in the cumbersome form $bB + cC^{-1}$.) There may be more than one x that minimizes (6.39), in which case we need a second criterion for selecting one of them. As indicated in the last paragraph, in order to avoid making mistakes careful attention needs to be paid to the dimensionalities that occur in (6.39).

There are alternative ways of incorporating prior information about pictures of interest into the process of selecting a solution to (6.24). One example is to use the knowledge that x_j must lie within a certain range. In many applications, all pictures $f(r,\phi)$ that may occur have only nonnegative values. Then it is reasonable to demand that we accept an image vector x based on the digitization process of (6.17) as a solution to (6.24) only if $x_j \geq 0$, for $1 \leq j \leq J$. In fact, one may go further and demand also that for any solution of (6.24), the error should be within a certain bound, i.e., specify positive numbers $\varepsilon_1, \ldots, \varepsilon_I$, and accept as solutions only those x_js that have the property

$$-\varepsilon_i \leq y_i - \sum_{j=1}^{J} r_{i,j} x_j \leq \varepsilon_i, \qquad (6.40)$$

for $1 \leq i \leq I$. Other inequality constraints may also be introduced.

Using such arguments, we can replace the system of equations (6.24) with the unspecified e and possibly with inequality side conditions, by a system of inequalities of the form

$$\sum_{j=1}^{J} n_{i,j} x_j \leq q_i, \qquad (6.41)$$

which may be written in matrix notation as

$$Nx \le q, \tag{6.42}$$

and restate the reconstruction problem as a search for an image vector x that satisfies (6.42). One must bear in mind here that there may be no x that satisfies all inequalities in (6.42), and if there is one such x, then usually there are many others as well. Just as in the case when there is more than one minimizing vector of (6.39), we need a secondary criterion to select one of these vectors as the desired solution. There have been several secondary optimization criteria proposed in the reconstruction literature.

One of these is based on the minimization of the norm $\|x\|$, which we already discussed above. More generally, a unique solution will be ensured, if among all the image vectors that satisfy the primary criterion we choose the one that minimizes

$$\left\|D^{-1}x\right\|, \tag{6.43}$$

where D is a positive definite symmetric $J \times J$ matrix. (Recall that this implies that $x^{\mathrm{T}}Dx > 0$ for all nonzero vectors x.) As discussed below, some reconstruction techniques minimize (6.43) for various Ds.

An alternative secondary criterion is applicable if the average value $\bar{x}$ of the x_js is known. In such a case there is at most one vector x for which $x_j \ge 0$, for $1 \le j \le J$, whose average value is $\bar{x}$ and that maximizes

$$-\sum_{j=1}^{J} (x_j/J\bar{x}) \ln (x_j/J\bar{x}) . \tag{6.44}$$

This has been referred to as the *maximum entropy* criterion. The use of this criterion is usually justified by arguments (which are too long to be reproduced here) aimed at showing that of all the pictures that satisfy the primary criterion the maximum entropy solution has the smallest information content, and so it is least likely to mislead the user by the presence of spurious features.

The reason why one may assume that $\bar{x}$ is known is the following. Consider Fig. 2.4. For any source–detector pair, the ray sum divided by the length of intersection of the line with the picture region (reconstruction region) gives an estimate of the average relative linear attenuation for that line. If we have many such lines that provide a fairly uniform and dense covering of the reconstruction region, then the sum of all the ray sums divided by the sum of the lengths of intersections is a reasonable estimate of $\bar{x}$. For example, for our standard head phantom $\bar{x} = 0.1315$. The estimate of $\bar{x}$ obtained from the standard projection data (Section 5.8) by the method described above is 0.1307. This is in spite of the fact that the standard projection data are contaminated with errors due to photon statistics, beam hardening, scatter, etc. Similarly, the estimate of $\bar{x}$ obtained from the standard parallel projection data is 0.1312. Such experiments justify the use of the method described above for the estimation of $\bar{x}$ in conjunction with optimization criteria, such as maximum entropy or minimum variance.

A third secondary criterion that has been gaining popularity in recent years is *total variation (TV) minimization.* We restrict our discussion of this to a special case in which the basis functions are chosen according to (6.17). Let T denote the set of all indices of pixels that are not in the rightmost column or in the bottom row of the $n \times n$ digitization and, for any pixel with index i in T, let $r(i)$ and $b(i)$ denote the index of the pixel to its right and below it, respectively. Then the *total variation* of the image vector x is defined as

$$TV(x) = \sum_{i \in T} \sqrt{\left(x_{r(i)} - x_i\right)^2 + \left(x_{b(i)} - x_i\right)^2}. \tag{6.45}$$

A widely studied optimization criterion in the field of image reconstruction from projections is provided by the concept of *maximum likelihood estimation.* This is a quite general concept that can be described in our context as follows. Assume that we have a statistical model that provides us, for any image vector x, with a probability density function p_Y^x of the multivariate random variable Y associated with the process that generates the measurement vector y. In practice we choose such a model based on our understanding of the nature of our application and how the data are collected in that application. For example, if we already know the probability density function p_E associated with the error vector e that we discussed earlier, then we can define

$$p_Y^x(y) = p_E(y - Rx). \tag{6.46}$$

Then, having observed the measurement vector y, a *maximum likelihood estimate* of the image vector is an x that maximizes $p_Y^x(y)$. (Note that the name of this estimator has an unjustified positive connotation: a maximum likelihood estimator x is not really a "most likely" one, but rather it is the case that among all possible image vectors there are none for which the likelihood of observing y is greater than the likelihood of observing y when x is the image vector.) Comparing (6.46) with (6.32) that is used to define the Bayesian estimate, we see that the essential difference is that the formula for the maximum likelihood estimate does not make use of an assumed prior probability density function p_X for the distribution of the image vectors.

Such an approach is likely to be useful in applications in which the nature of p_Y^x is reasonably well understood, but there is uncertainty regarding the nature of p_X. For example, in positron emission tomography (see Section 1.1), one may assume that, for $1 \le i \le I$, y_i is a sample from the Poisson random variable with parameter $\sum_{j=1}^{J} r_{i,j} x_j$ and that these I samples are independent. Under these assumptions it follows from (3.1) that

$$p_Y^x(y) = \prod_{i=1}^{I} \frac{\left(\sum_{j=1}^{J} r_{i,j} x_j\right)^{y_i} \exp\left(-\sum_{j=1}^{J} r_{i,j} x_j\right)}{y_i!}. \tag{6.47}$$

Since the natural logarithm is a monotonically increasing function, finding the x that maximizes this $p_Y^x(y)$ is the same as finding the x that minimizes

$$\sum_{i=1}^{I}\left(\left(\sum_{j=1}^{J} r_{i,j}x_j\right) - y_i \ln\left(\sum_{j=1}^{J} r_{i,j}x_j\right)\right). \tag{6.48}$$

In practice it has been found that the image vector that minimizes (6.48) is often very noisy looking, as if some salt-and-pepper type of noise had been superimposed on what is basically a good reconstruction. To counteract this, the criterion is often *regularized*, for example, by replacing it with

$$\sum_{i=1}^{I}\left(\left(\sum_{j=1}^{J} r_{i,j}x_j\right) - y_i \ln\left(\sum_{j=1}^{J} r_{i,j}x_j\right)\right) + bx^T Bx, \tag{6.49}$$

where B is the already mentioned smoothing matrix (compare this with (6.38) and see also Section 12.3). We could have derived the same formula using Bayesian estimation based on (6.32), combined with (6.46) and (6.47) and using a multivariate Gaussian p_X with μ_X the zero vector and $V_X^{-1} = bB$; compare with (6.33).

6.5 Blob Basis Functions

Generalized Kaiser–Bessel window functions, which are also known by the simpler name *blobs*, form a large family of functions that can be defined in a Euclidean space of any dimension. Here we restrict ourselves to a subfamily in the two-dimensional plane, whose elements have the form

$$b_{a,\alpha,\delta}(r,\phi) = \begin{cases} C_{a,\alpha,\delta}\left(1-\left(\frac{r}{a}\right)^2\right) I_2\left(\alpha\sqrt{1-\left(\frac{r}{a}\right)^2}\right), & \text{if } 0 \le r \le a, \\ 0, & \text{otherwise,} \end{cases} \tag{6.50}$$

where I_k denotes the modified Bessel function of the first kind of order k, a stands for the nonnegative radius of the blob and α is a nonnegative real number that controls the blob's taper (the shape of the blob). The multiplying constant $C_{a,\alpha,\delta}$ is defined below. Note that such a blob is circularly symmetric, since its value does not depend on ϕ. It has the value zero for all $r \ge a$ and its first derivatives are continuous everywhere. In this sense (and in a deeper mathematical sense that we do not detail here) blobs are very "smooth" functions, see Fig. 6.3. Their smoothness can be controlled by the choice of the parameters a, α and δ, as we demonstrate shortly.

For now let us consider the parameters a, α and δ, and hence the function $b_{a,\alpha,\delta}$, to be fixed. This fixed function gives rise to a set of J basis functions $\{b_1, \ldots, b_J\}$ as follows. We define a set $G = \{g_1, \ldots, g_J\}$ of *grid points* in the

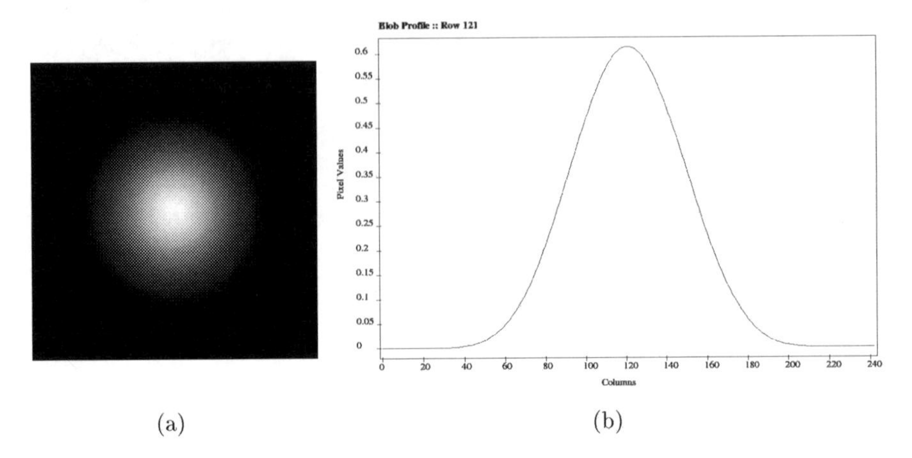

(a) (b)

Fig. 6.3: (a) A 243×243 digitization of a blob. (b) Its values on the central row.

picture region. Then, for $1 \le j \le J$, b_j is obtained from $b_{a,\alpha,\delta}$ by shifting it in the plane so that its center is moved from the origin to g_j. This definition leaves a great deal of freedom in the selection of G, but it was found in practice advisable that it should consists of those points of a set (in rectangular coordinates)

$$G_\delta = \left\{ \left(\frac{m\delta}{2}, \frac{\sqrt{3}n\delta}{2} \right) \middle| \, m \text{ and } n \text{ are integers and } m+n \text{ is even} \right\} \tag{6.51}$$

that are also in the picture region. Here δ has to be a positive real number and G_δ is referred to as the *hexagonal grid with sampling distance* δ. Having fixed δ, we complete the definition in (6.50) by

$$C_{a,\alpha,\delta} = \frac{\sqrt{3}\delta^2 \alpha}{4\pi a^2 I_3(\alpha)}. \tag{6.52}$$

The Radon transform (6.4) maps a picture into its line integrals. Its inversion in practice tends to amplify errors in the measured data. One way of reducing this is to seek a smoothed version of the theoretical solution. This is often done by a regularization term (see, for example, (6.49)), but it can be also tackled by using smooth basis functions.

Pixel-based basis functions (6.17) have a unit value inside the pixels and zero outside. Blobs on the other hand, have a bell-shaped profile that tapers smoothly in the radial direction from a high value at the center to the value 0 at the edge of their supports (i.e., at $r = a$ in (6.50)); see Fig. 6.3. The smoothness of blobs suggests that reconstructions of the form (6.18) are likely to be resistant to noise in the data. This has been shown to be particularly useful in fields in which the projection data are noisy, such as positron emission tomography and electron microscopy, which were discussed in Section 1.1.

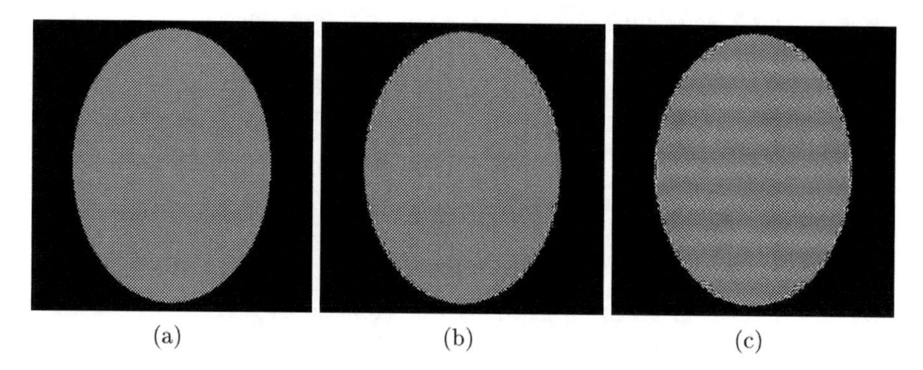

Fig. 6.4: (a) A 243×243 digitization of a solid bone "head" cross section. (b) Its approximation with default blob parameters and (c) with slightly different parameters. The display window is extremely narrow for better indication of errors.

For blobs to achieve their full potential, the selection of the parameters a, α and δ is important. The mathematical analysis of how they should be chosen is beyond the scope of this book. In SNARK09, the software automatically calculates good ***default blob parameters*** based on the geometry of the digitized picture that is being produced as output. For example, for the 243×243 digitizations used in this book, the default values (to four decimal place accuracy) are $a = 0.1551$, $\alpha = 11.2829$ and $\delta = 0.0868$. Using these default parameters, one can approximate homogeneous regions very well, in spite of the bell-shaped profile of the individual blobs. This is illustrated in Fig. 6.4(b), in which a cross section through solid bone shown in Fig. 6.4(a) is approximated by a linear combination of the blob basis functions with the default parameters. There are some inaccuracies very near the sharp edges, but the interior of the bone is approximated with great accuracy. On the other hand, if we change the parameters ever so slightly to $a = 0.16$, $\alpha = 11.28$ and $\delta = 0.09$, then the best approximation that can be obtained by a linear combination of the blob basis functions is shown in Fig. 6.4(c), which is clearly inferior.

Based on the mathematical formulas (6.50), (6.51) and (6.52) one can calculate, for any line i and for any blob basis function b_j, the value of $r_{i,j} \simeq \mathscr{R}_i b_j = [\mathscr{R} f](\ell_i, \theta_i)$. In fact, because blobs are circularly symmetric, these integrals are not dependent on the orientation θ_i of the line of integration but only on the distance of the line from the center g_j of the basis function b_j. In practice, for any fixed blob parameters, the values of the integrals as a function of distance from the blob center can be precalculated and stored on the computer and so, during any particular reconstruction using such blobs, the computation of the integral is efficiently achieved by the retrieval of a precalculated value. This combined with a DDA-like mechanism that indicates which blobs may possibly be intersected by the given line, allows one to calculate rapidly the right-hand side of (6.23) for any given image vector x.

6.6 Computational Efficiency

In the succeeding chapters we show reconstructions of our head phantom from the standard projection data (or from the standard parallel projection data) using many different methods. We also show plots of the 131st column and give picture distance measures defined in Section 5.1 and statistical performance comparisons of the kind discussed in Section 5.2.

In addition, we indicate the cost of the reconstruction in terms of computer time. All the algorithms are implemented in the SNARK09 programming system (see Chapter 4), and the times reported are the number of seconds when using a computer with an AMD Athlon™ 64 Processor 3500+, 2.2 GHz, 1GB DDR Memory, running Linux Fedora 9.

While these timings are given for the sake of completeness, they are not to be taken too seriously. A general framework of computer programs containing many different algorithms, such as SNARK09, is by necessity not as efficient for any single algorithm as a program specially written for that purpose. Thus the absolute, and even the relative, values of computer times quoted below may be misleading. Implementations of algorithms used in actual CT scanners usually involve low (i.e., assembly or machine) level programming and even special-purpose hardware, making the execution of reconstructions orders of magnitude faster than what is possible using SNARK09. (The reason for using SNARK09 is ease of implementation; it would be quite beyond the capability of an individual to implement all algorithms to be reported on in this book by special-purpose programming.)

This attitude towards timing reflects the fact that electronic hardware used for calculations is getting cheaper and cheaper at an amazing rate. It is unlikely that an efficacious reconstruction algorithm would for long remain unused solely because of computational considerations.

Notes and References

Much of the material in this chapter is based on a survey paper on iterative reconstruction algorithms [127]. That paper contains discussions of and references to many earlier publications concerning reconstruction algorithms based on the series expansion approach and optimization criteria. There are many more recent texts discussing reconstruction algorithms; a good treatment from a more mathematical point of view is given in [211].

A good coverage of Lebesgue integrals and square integrable functions, operators, and linear functionals is given by [161].

Our treatment of the inverse Radon transform adapted the approach and notation of [234]. A thorough mathematical discussion of Hilbert transforms can be found in [37]. References to literature on derivations of the Radon inversion formula without assuming properties such as differentiability are given at the end of Chapter 15.

Our treatment of multivariate random variables is based on [235]. That book also contains a discussion of Bayes' theorem, which provides the mathematical justification for the use of the Bayesian estimate. The equivalence of the minimum norm and minimum variance criteria is shown in [130].

The maximum entropy formalism is a general scientific approach; there are whole books devoted to the subject; see, e.g., [180]. The suggestion that it be used for image reconstruction first appeared in the open literature in [99]. It has been extensively used in the related field of digital image restoration; see, e.g., [8]. As examples of works on the computation of maximum entropy solutions, see [74] and [203]. Total variation minimization has become something of a fad at the time of writing this edition; for a critical discussion with background references see [121]. TV minimization has been applied in a variety of fields, for an example in IMRT see [280].

The maximum likelihood formalism was introduced to the image reconstruction community by L.A. Shepp and A. Vardi [242]. The idea of combining the likelihood function with one that expresses assumed prior knowledge about the space of pictures that we are likely to come across in a reconstruction application was presented in [181]. Original implementations of such approaches tended to be slow, many faster variants have been developed over the years, for example, in [34, 122, 147]. The last of these references seems to have found great popularity in the emission tomography community. It achieves its efficiency by using essentially the same idea that was proposed much earlier in [73] for finding the minimizer of (6.39): divide the system of equations, such as (6.23) or (6.24) into subsets (also called blocks) and get an overall solution by repeatedly cycling through the blocks, one at a time. A recent interesting application of the maximum likelihood formalism to image reconstruction from projections is reported in [237]: several conformations of a molecule are simultaneously reconstructed from a heterogeneous mixture of their electron microscopic projections taken at unknown orientations.

There are many additional optimization criteria proposed in the literature include, for instance, maximum signal-to-noise power ratio [255].

Generalized Kaiser–Bessel window functions (blobs) were first proposed for image reconstruction by R.M. Lewitt [183, 184]. They are also applicable, if anything more significantly so, in the reconstruction of 3D objects from 2D projections. The blob basis functions have proved to be more suitable than the pixel basis functions (in 2D) and the voxel basis functions (in 3D). It has been shown that the use of blobs as basis functions can produce superior results for different types of applications, such as positron emission tomography [160, 198] and electron microscopy [194, 195]. The choice of the hexagonal grid and the selection of the default blob parameters is justified by the material in [199, 200].

Optimization using parallel (and hence fast) computations is discussed in [48] with special reference to series expansion reconstruction methods. A recent development along this line is [80]. For methods of using standard hardware to speed up reconstruction algorithms, see [206, 274] and their references.

7

Backprojection

Backprojection methods of reconstruction do not produce as good images as the more sophisticated techniques discussed in the succeeding chapters. They are studied mainly because they indicate the nature of parts of the more sophisticated reconstruction procedures (both for transform methods and for some of the series expansion methods), and the need for the other steps in such procedures.

7.1 Continuous Backprojection

The simplest algorithm for reconstruction is to estimate the density at a point by adding all the ray sums of the lines through that point. This has been called both the *summation method* and the *backprojection method.*

Note that traditional tomography (see Section 2.2) is essentially a backprojection method. In Fig. 2.2, the linear attenuation at A is estimated by the summing up (integration) of the total density along the path from X_t to A_t as t (the time) varies. Note that A_t is always the same point on the moving photographic plate P, and that A is the only point that two paths from X_t to A_t have in common at different times t. All forms of traditional tomography involving such coordinated movements of x-ray source and film are three-dimensional versions of the backprojection method.

As explained in Section 6.2, given a function p of two variables, the backprojection operator $\mathscr{B}$ produces another function $\mathscr{B}p$ of two polar variables, such that $[\mathscr{B}p](r, \phi)$ is obtained by integrating, as θ varies, the values of $p(\ell, \theta)$ with $\ell = r\cos(\theta - \phi)$. For fixed r, θ and ϕ, $\ell = r\cos(\theta - \phi)$ denotes the distance from the origin of the line L through (r, ϕ) perpendicular to the line K making angle θ with the x axis (see Fig. 6.1). If $p(\ell, \theta)$ is the ray sum associated with the line L, we see that the mathematical idealization of the summation method described at the beginning of this section is to associate with the projection data p the estimated reconstruction $\mathscr{B}p$.

We first discuss basic objections to such a procedure as a method of reconstruction and then (in Section 7.2) we look at implementations of the procedure from the type of finite data we have to deal with in practice.

We have discussed in Section 6.2 the fact that the inverse Radon transform can be obtained by a series of operations: differentiation, Hilbert transform, backprojection, and normalization. Using only backprojection for reconstruction has little justification and is likely to produce blurred pictures. To see how this blurring occurs, consider the following intuitive argument.

Let us take a number of views of an object consisting of a single point. The result of the reconstruction from these projections by the summation method is a star-shaped object whose center is the original point (Fig. 7.1). Let us take equally-spaced projections of a point from a full range of directions. As we increase the number of views, the reconstruction comes to resemble a density distribution proportional to $1/r$, where r is the distance from the point. This is because the limiting case of superposition of a number of equally-spaced straight lines through a common point is equivalent to the rotation of a line about the point. The weight of each point of the straight line is distributed during rotation along the length of a circumference $2\pi r$. This intuitive argument indicates that any implementation of the backprojection method is likely to blur out sharp features in the picture to be reconstructed.

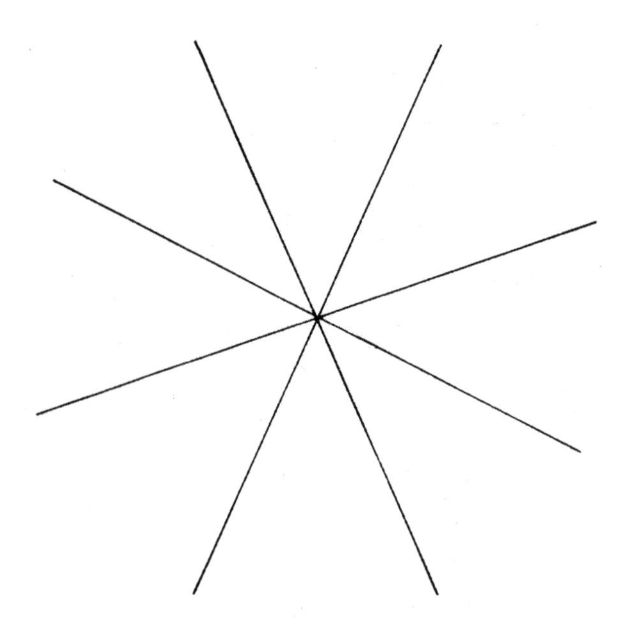

Fig. 7.1: Reconstruction of a single point using the backprojection method. Each line is due to the a projection of the point in the corresponding direction.

However, there is an even more basic, physical reason why backprojection alone cannot possibly be an acceptable method of reconstruction in CT.

To understand this reason some knowledge of elementary physics is required. Essentially the reason is that the value produced by backprojection is of the wrong *dimensionality*. The relative linear attenuation (reconstruction of which is what we are after in CT) has dimensionality inverse length. That means that the value of relative linear attenuation is inversely proportional to the unit of length used; if it is 0.192 cm^{-1}, then it is 19.2 m^{-1}. As opposed to this, ray sums have no dimensionality, they are just numbers. The result of summing up ray sums, or even integrating with respect to angle as in (6.14), will also be a dimensionless quantity. Hence, the result of the backprojection method does not depend on the unit of length used. If it happens to be a reasonable estimator of the distribution of the relative linear attenuation when the unit of length used is a centimeter, then it will be off by a factor of 100 when the unit of length is a meter. (In the next section we show that correct dimensionality can be reintroduced by a certain normalization.)

To see that the same objection cannot be raised to the inverse Radon transform $\mathscr{R}^{-1}$, consider the dimensionality of the output of each step in the sequence of operations shown in (6.16) of the last chapter. If p is dimensionless, $\mathscr{D}_Y p$ has dimensionality inverse length, see (6.11). Neither $\mathscr{H}_Y$, nor $\mathscr{B}$, nor normalization changes the dimensionality, see (6.13) and (6.14). Hence $\mathscr{R}^{-1}p$ has the same dimensionality as $\mathscr{D}_Y p$, which is the correct dimensionality for the relative linear attenuation.

7.2 Implementation of the Backprojection Operator

The summation method can be implemented by various "analog" devices. For example, an oscilloscope screen can be used on which we successively display lines whose positions correspond to lines for which the ray sums have been measured. The oscilloscope pattern is integrated on a photographic film, with the brightness (alternatively length of display) of a line modulated by the ray sum. The resulting picture on the film will be a backprojection reconstruction.

We shall not be concerned with such analog techniques. Our interest is in calculating the value of $[\mathscr{B}p](r,\phi)$ from the data y, where $y_i = p(\ell_i, \theta_i)$ for $1 \le i \le I$ (see Sections 6.1 and 6.2). We restrict our discussion to the parallel mode of data collection, with M equally-spaced views and $2N+1$ equally-spaced parallel lines in each view. We use Δ to denote the angles between the views (thus $\Delta = \pi/M$) and d to denote the distance between the parallel lines. We assume that $Nd > E > r$. Figure 7.2 is essentially a superimposition of Figs 6.2 and 6.1(b); it shows both the points at which the values of p are known and the curve along which p has to be integrated to obtain

$$[\mathscr{B}p](r,\phi) = \int_0^\pi p(r\cos(\theta-\phi),\theta)\,d\theta. \tag{7.1}$$

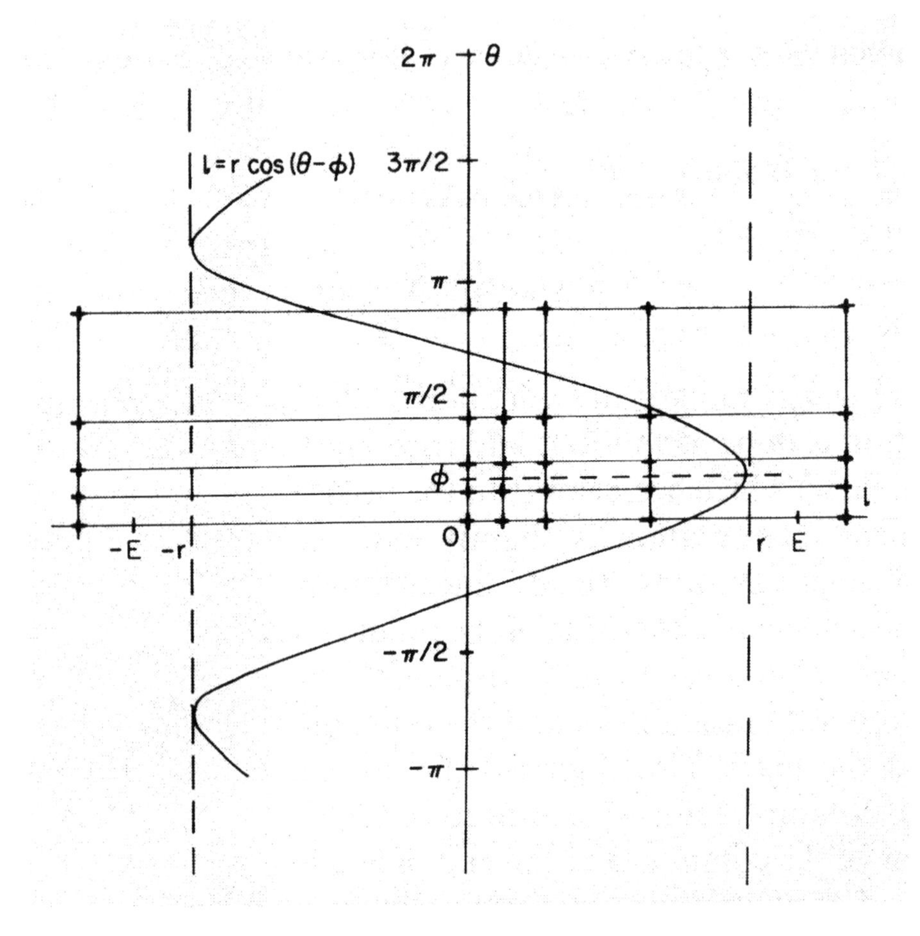

Fig. 7.2: Numerical evaluation of the backprojection operator is done by estimating the line integral along $\ell = r\cos(\theta-\phi)$ from the known values at the locations marked by a $+$.

A commonly used technique for numerically evaluating this integral is the following. The integral on the right-hand side of (7.1) is approximated by

$$\Delta \sum_{m=0}^{M-1} p\,(r\cos(m\Delta - \phi), m\Delta)\,. \tag{7.2}$$

(This is called a *Riemann sum* for the integral.) In order to do this, we need to approximate, for each m, the value of $p(r\cos(m\Delta - \phi), m\Delta)$ from the known values $p\,(nd, m\Delta)$ $(-N \le n \le N)$ by *interpolation*.

Two commonly used methods of interpolation in CT are the *nearest neighbor* and the *linear* interpolations. The nearest neighbor interpolation approximates $p\,(r\cos(m\Delta - \phi), m\Delta)$ by the value of $p(nd, m\Delta)$ where n is chosen so that $|nd - r\cos(m\Delta - \phi)|$ is as small as possible. In linear interpolation, we select n so that $nd \leq r\cos(m\Delta - \phi) < (n+1)d$ and approximate $p(r\cos(m\Delta - \phi), m\Delta)$ by

$$\frac{(n+1)d - r\cos(m\Delta - \phi)}{d} p(nd, m\Delta) + \frac{r\cos(m\Delta - \phi) - nd}{d} p\left((n+1)d, m\Delta\right). \tag{7.3}$$

Thus, numerical evaluation of $[\mathscr{B}p](r, \phi)$ using nearest neighbor interpolation is done as follows: add together the ray sums of the lines in each view that are nearest to the point (r, ϕ) and multiply the result by Δ. Linear interpolation is slightly more complicated; instead of single ray sums, we add linear interpolates of the ray sums of the lines that lie on either side of the point.

In order to produce a digitized picture, this calculation is repeated for the central point of each pixel and the outcome is assigned as the estimated density to the pixel. This digitized picture can be represented as a J-dimensional column vector x^*; see Section 6.3.

In view of the comments at the end of Section 7.1, it is clear that this method may produce a digitized picture x^* whose average density $\bar{x}^*$ is very different from the average density $\bar{x}$ of the digitization x of the picture to be reconstructed. Since we usually have a good estimate $\bar{\bar{x}}$ of $\bar{x}$ (see the discussion below (6.44)), we can correct for this by *normalization*, which may be *additive* or *multiplicative*. Additive normalization produces a digitized picture x^{**}, whose jth component is

$$x_j^{**} = x_j^* + (\bar{\bar{x}} - \bar{x}^*). \tag{7.4}$$

Multiplicative normalization produces a picture x^{**}, whose jth component is

$$x_j^{**} = x_j^* \, (\bar{\bar{x}} / \bar{x}^*), \tag{7.5}$$

assuming that $\bar{x}^* \neq 0$. Note that in both cases the average density of x^{**} is $\bar{\bar{x}}$.

An interesting property of multiplicative normalization is that the correct dimensionality is reintroduced. This is because $\bar{\bar{x}}$ itself has dimensionality inverse length (it is a sum of dimensionless quantities divided by a sum of lengths) and so x_j^{**} has the correct dimensionality. On the other hand, (7.4) makes little physical sense: $\bar{\bar{x}} - \bar{x}^*$ is the difference between the quantity $\bar{\bar{x}}$ measured in inverse length and the dimensionless quantity $\bar{x}^*$. For this reason, multiplicative rather than additive normalization is recommended.

We applied the summation method with linear interpolation and multiplicative normalization to the standard parallel projection data. The result is shown in Fig. 7.3. Clearly, this technique is not acceptable for examining the contents of the head. The image in Fig. 7.3(a) appears black, due to our convention of displaying values 0.204 cm^{-1} or less as black (see Section 4.3). We display the same image in Fig. 7.3(b) but replacing 0.204 by 0.11, and we use the same setting for producing the plots in Fig. 7.3(c).

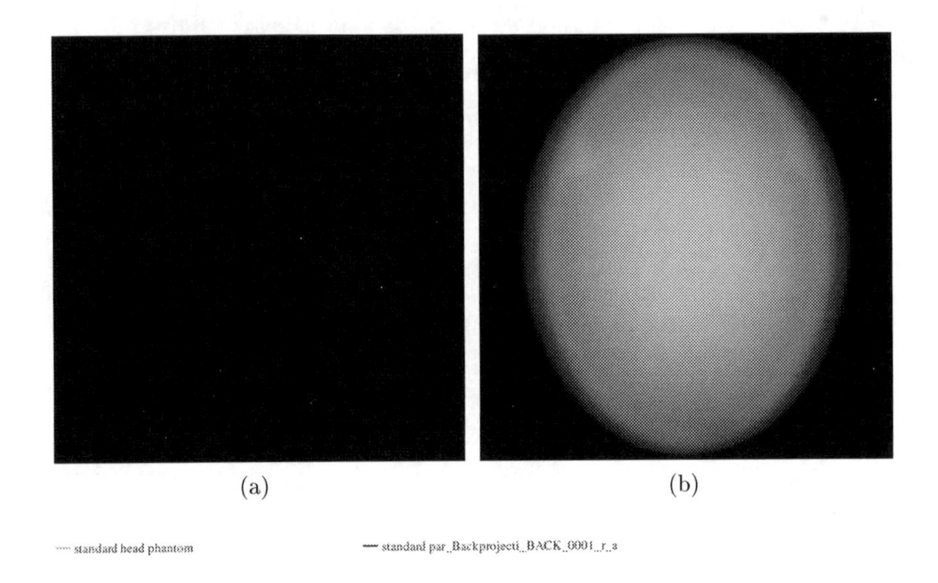

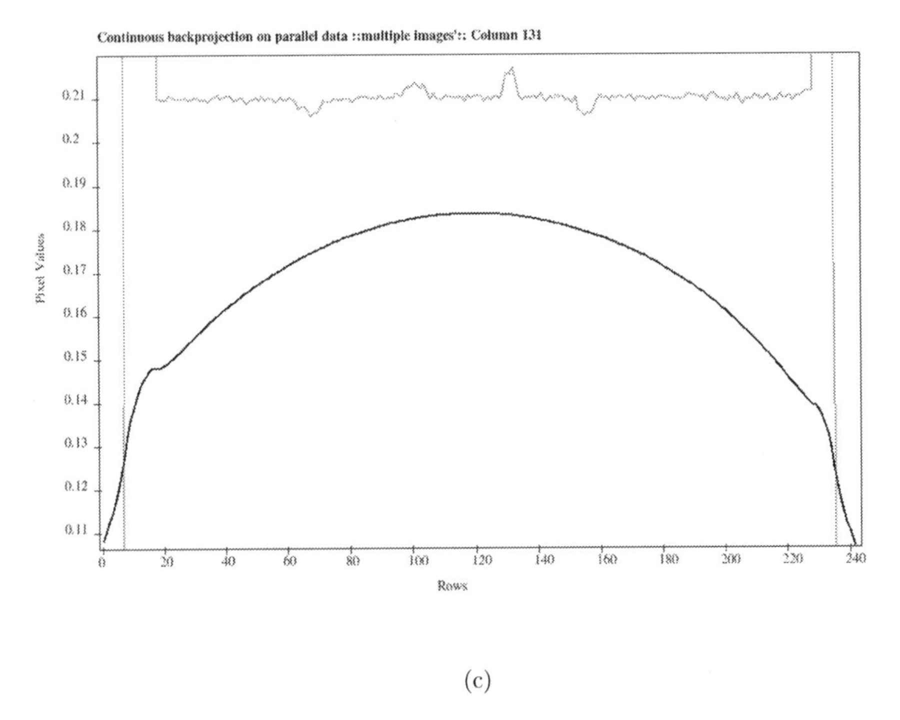

(c)

Fig. 7.3: (a) Reconstruction of the head phantom from the standard parallel projection data using continuous backprojection with linear interpolation and multiplicative normalization. (b) The same as (a), but with the display window changed to bring out features in the reconstruction. (c) Plots of the 131st column of the phantom (light) and the reconstruction (dark), using the display window of (b).

The picture distance measures and the time in seconds needed to perform the reconstruction are

$$d = 0.8082, \qquad r = 0.6818, \qquad t = 0.7. \tag{7.6}$$

7.3 Discrete Backprojection

In the last section we have produced a digitized picture by numerically evaluating the integral in (7.1) for the center points of the pixels. An alternative approach is provided by the series expansion method.

Consider the basis functions (6.17) that have value 1 within a pixel and 0 outside. In this case $r_{i,j}$ is the (calculated) length of intersection of the ith line with the jth pixel. The following basic criteria describe what we intuitively expect from an implementation of the backprojection method that uses pixels.

(i) A line should contribute to those pixels that it intersects and to no others. (For any line, these pixels can be rapidly identified using a DDA, see Section 4.6.)
(ii) The contribution of the ith line to a pixel should be proportional to y_i (the measured ray sum for the ith line).
(iii) The contribution of the ith line to the jth pixel should be proportional to $r_{i,j}$. (These can also be rapidly calculated by a DDA.)

All these criteria are satisfied if we estimate the density x_j^* in the jth pixel by

$$x_j^* = \sum_{i=1}^{I} r_{i,j} y_i. \tag{7.7}$$

This can be expressed in matrix notation as

$$x^* = R^T y, \tag{7.8}$$

where R^T (the *transpose* of the matrix R) is the matrix whose (i, j)th element is $r_{j,i}$. (Implementational details are deferred until Section 11.1.)

The argument given above does not depend in any essential way on the basis functions being pixels. We consider, in general, (7.8) to be the backprojection solution of the discrete reconstruction problem with projection matrix R. In particular, we refer to multiplication of an (I-dimensional) vector by R^T as *discrete backprojection.*

Just as in the case of continuous backprojection, the average density of x^* may be quite different from that of the picture to be reconstructed. In such a case the additive or multiplicative normalization procedures, see (7.4) and (7.5), can be applied to advantage. This of course only makes sense if the series expansion is a digitization.

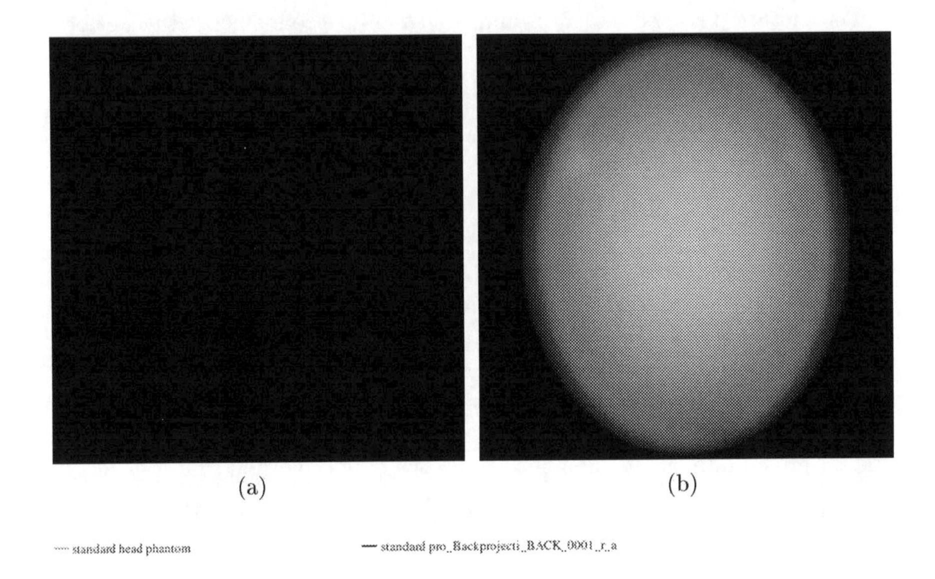

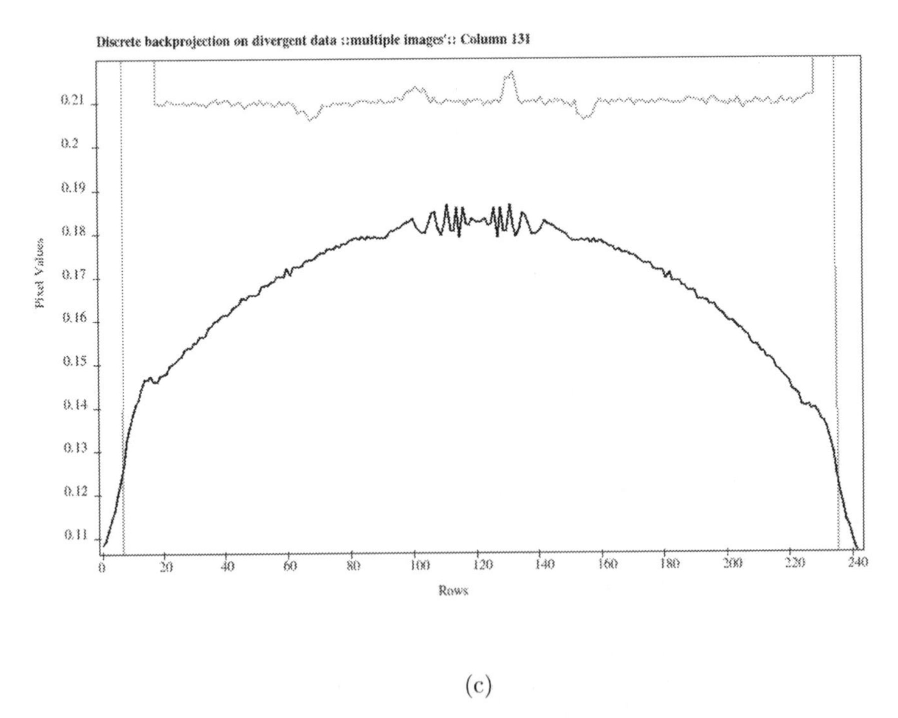

Fig. 7.4: (a) Reconstruction of the head phantom from the standard projection data using discrete backprojection with multiplicative normalization. (b) The same as (a), but with the display window changed to bring out features in the reconstruction. (c) Plots of the 131st column of the phantom (light) and the reconstruction (dark), using the display window of (b).

Discrete backprojection, as expressed by (7.8), is applicable to any method of data collection. When applied to the standard (divergent) projection data it produces the reconstructions shown in Fig. 7.4(a) and (b), with line plots for the 131st column in Fig. 7.4(c). The picture distance measures and the timing are

$$d = 0.8091, \qquad r = 0.6828, \qquad t = 2.8. \tag{7.9}$$

Notes and References

The backprojection method in various analog and digital implementations has been proposed by a number of authors. For a history, see [100]. The particular analog technique described in Section 7.2 is taken from [164].

Numerical evaluation of integrals, and in particular Riemann sums, are discussed in detail in [62]. A discussion of alternative modes of numerical evaluation of the integral in (7.1) is given by [33]. A particularly efficient method for backprojection is employed by the so-called linogram method, which will be discussed in detail in Section 9.3.

Interpolation methods other than the ones we have mentioned have been studied by a number of authors in conjunction with the backprojection operator. An exhaustive evaluation of the Lagrange interpolation methods is provided in [234]. An alternative is to use the so-called modified cubic splines; these are evaluated in [139]. A further discussion regarding the choices for interpolation and their consequences is provided in Section 8.5.

8

Filtered Backprojection for Parallel Beams

The most commonly used methods in CT for parallel beam projection data are the filtered backprojection (FBP) methods. (In some of the earlier literature these methods are also referred to as "convolution methods.") The reason for this is ease of implementation combined with good accuracy. These methods are transform methods, where the taking of the derivative and the Hilbert transform is approximated by the use of a single convolution.

8.1 Convolutions, Hilbert Transforms, Regularization

Given two real-valued functions ϕ and ψ over the real numbers, their *convolution* $\phi * \psi$ is another real-valued function over the real numbers, defined by

$$[\phi * \psi](v) = \int_{-\infty}^{\infty} \phi(u)\psi(v-u)\,du. \tag{8.1}$$

Note that it is possible that, for certain values of v, $[\phi * \psi](v)$ is not defined (because the integral on the right-hand side of (8.1) does not exist). According to our earlier convention we shall not worry about such mathematical niceties; for now we assume that $[\phi * \psi](v)$ is defined whenever we need it.

Note that convolution is an operator that, acting on two functions ϕ and ψ, produces a third function $\phi * \psi$. It is easy to show that $\phi * \psi = \psi * \phi$, in the sense that, for all v,

$$[\phi * \psi](v) = [\psi * \phi](v). \tag{8.2}$$

We have already come across an example of convolution: the *Hilbert transform* $\mathscr{H}\phi$ of a function ϕ can be defined as the convolution of ϕ with the function ρ such that

$$\rho(u) = -(1/\pi u). \tag{8.3}$$

In other words, we may write

$$\mathscr{H}\phi = \phi * \rho, \tag{8.4}$$

where ρ is defined by (8.3). Combining (8.1), (8.3), and (8.4) we get

$$[\mathscr{H}\phi](v) = -\frac{1}{\pi}\left(\int_{-\infty}^{\infty} \frac{\phi(u)}{v-u}\,du\right). \tag{8.5}$$

The right-hand side of (8.5) is what is called an *improper integral* both of the *first kind* and of the *second kind.* It is an improper integral of the first kind because the limits of the integration are $-\infty$ and ∞. This does not worry us in image reconstruction, since the values of $\phi(u)$ are zero outside a finite range. This can be seen by comparing (8.5) with (6.12). We see that Hilbert transforms arise in image reconstruction with $\phi(u) = q(u, \theta)$, for some fixed θ, where

$$\phi(u) = q(u,\theta) = [\mathscr{D}_Y p](u,\theta) = [\mathscr{D}_Y Rf](u,\theta) = 0 \tag{8.6}$$

if $|u| \geq E$; see (6.12), (6.11), and (6.6). The right-hand side of (8.5) is also an improper integral of the second kind, since the integrand becomes infinite at $u = v$. We interpret the integral in its Cauchy principal value sense, i.e.,

$$[\mathscr{H}\phi](v) = -\frac{1}{\pi}\lim_{\varepsilon\to 0}\left(\int_{-\infty}^{v-\varepsilon} \frac{\phi(u)}{v-u}\,du + \int_{v+\varepsilon}^{\infty} \frac{\phi(u)}{v-u}\,du\right). \tag{8.7}$$

Even if this integral exists, its numerical evaluation may be far from straightforward. One approach is the method of *regularization*. This method consists of defining a set $\{\rho_A \mid A > 0\}$ of functions on the real numbers, where the subscript A is a positive real number. Roughly speaking, the idea is that ρ_A should be chosen so that, for the ϕs that we are interested in,

$$\lim_{A\to\infty} \phi * \rho_A = \mathscr{H}\phi, \tag{8.8}$$

and for any fixed A the convolution on the left-hand side is easy to evaluate.

To make this more precise we have to define the class of functions ϕ for which (8.8) is true. In Section 15.7 we define precisely the terminology "the function ϕ is *reasonable* at the point v." For now we may simply assume that the functions ϕ we are dealing with are reasonable at all points. We call a set $\{\rho_A \mid A > 0\}$ of functions a *regularizing family*, if, for any function ϕ over the real numbers and any real number v such that ϕ is reasonable at v,

$$\lim_{A\to\infty} [\phi * \rho_A](v) = [\mathscr{H}\phi](v). \tag{8.9}$$

Numerical evaluation of $[\mathscr{H}\phi](v)$ can now be carried out by numerical evaluation of $[\phi * \rho_A](v)$, with A chosen sufficiently large so that the left-hand side of (8.9) is near enough to its right-hand side for our purpose. If the ρ_A have some nice properties (e.g., boundedness, differentiability, etc.), then $[\phi * \rho_A](v)$ may be quite easy to evaluate numerically. In particular, if ϕ is the derivative of another function, one may use integration by parts to evaluate $[\phi * \rho_A](v)$. This is in fact the case in our application, as can be seen in (8.6).

The preceding discussion hinges on the existence of a regularizing family. In fact, there is a large variety of regularizing families, as can be seen from the following result, which is proved in Section 15.7. We refer to this result as the *regularization theorem*, which can be stated as follows.

For each real number A, let F_A be a real-valued integrable function such that, for $U \geq 0$,

(i) $0 \leq F_A(U) \leq 1$, $F_A(U) = 0$ if $U \geq A/2$,
(ii) $F_A(U)$ is a monotonically nonincreasing function of U,
(iii) $\lim_{A \to \infty} F_A(U) = 1$.

Let

$$\rho_A(u) = -2 \int_0^{A/2} F_A(U) \sin(2\pi U u)\, dU. \tag{8.10}$$

Then $\{\rho_A \mid A > 0\}$ is a regularizing family of functions.

For reasons that become clear later, the F_A in this result is often referred to as a *window* with *bandwidth* A. Note that the function ρ_A, as defined by (8.10), is *antisymmetric*; i.e., $\rho_A(-u) = -\rho_A(u)$.

It is easy to produce families of windows satisfying conditions (i)–(iii). In Table 8.1 we give a few examples, together with names commonly used for them. In all cases the expression for $F_A(U)$ in the table is valid only for $0 \leq U \leq A/2$, since for $U \geq A/2$, $F_A(U) = 0$, according to (i). Note that the bandlimiting window is the same as the generalized Hamming window with parameter $\alpha = 1$. When $\alpha = 0.54$, the generalized Hamming window is called just the *Hamming window*, and when $\alpha = 0.5$, the generalized Hamming window is called the *hanning window*. The shapes of some windows are shown in Fig. 8.1 together with the corresponding ρ_A. In the plots of $F_A(U)$ (Figs. 8.1(a), (c) and (e)), the U axis is labelled as "frequency" and the $F_A(U)$ axis is labelled as "amplitude," and $F_A(U)$ is defined for negative values of U by assuming that F_A is *symmetric*; i.e., $F_A(-u) = F_A(u)$. In the plots of $\rho_A(u)$ (Figs. 8.1(b), (d) and (f)), the u axis is labelled as "distance" and the $\rho_A(u)$ axis is labelled as "value."

Table 8.1: Definitions of some commonly used windows.

name of window	$F_A(U)$
bandlimiting	1
cosine	$\cos(\pi U/A)$
sinc	$\dfrac{\sin(\pi U/A)}{(\pi U/A)}$
generalized Hamming with parameter α $(0.5 \leq \alpha \leq 1.0)$	$\alpha + (1-\alpha)\cos(2\pi U/A)$

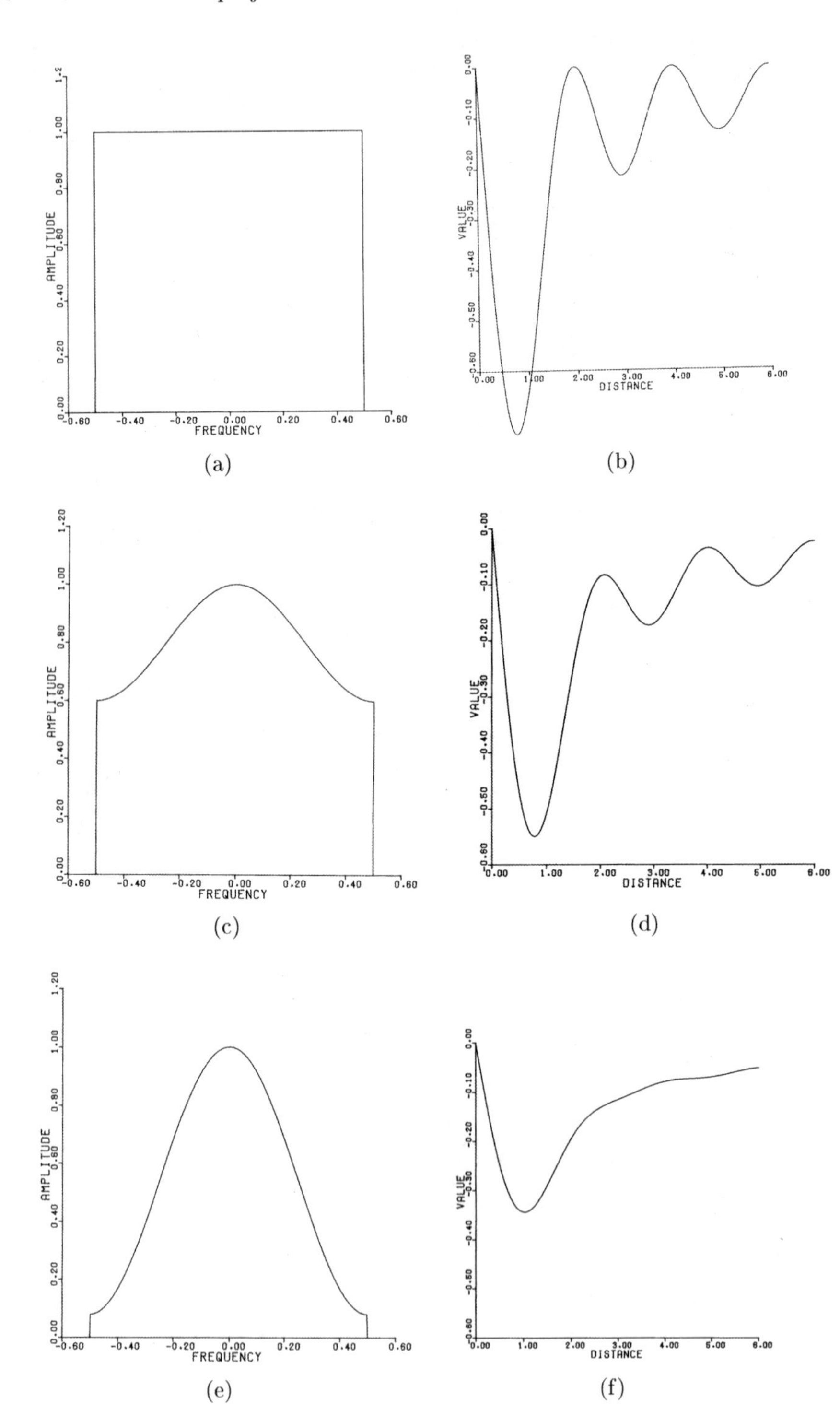

(a) (b)

(c) (d)

(e) (f)

8.2 Derivation of the FBP Method

We are now going to show that the first two stages of evaluating the inverse Radon transform, namely differentiation of the data and taking the Hilbert transform, see (6.16), can be approximated by a simple convolution of the data with a fixed convolving function.

As in Section 6.2, let p be the function of two variables whose inverse Radon transform we wish to find. For now, let us consider θ fixed and define

$$p_\theta(\ell) = p(\ell, \theta). \tag{8.11}$$

Then, for any ℓ',

$$[\mathscr{H}_Y \mathscr{D}_Y p](\ell', \theta) = [\mathscr{H} p'_\theta](\ell'), \tag{8.12}$$

where p'_θ is the derivative of p_θ. In view of (8.9), the right-hand side of (8.12) can be approximated by

$$[p'_\theta * \rho_A](\ell') = \int_{-\infty}^{\infty} p'_\theta(\ell)\rho_A(\ell' - \ell)\, d\ell. \tag{8.13}$$

Observe that $p'_\theta(\ell) = 0$ if $|\ell| \geq E$. If ρ_A is defined by (8.10) and F_A satisfies conditions (i)–(iii) in Section 8.1, then the derivative ρ'_A of ρ_A exists and

$$\rho'_A(u) = -4\pi \int_0^{A/2} U F_A(U) \cos(2\pi U u)\, dU. \tag{8.14}$$

(Here we made use of the standard technique which in mathematical analysis is usually referred to as "differentiation under the integral sign.") Using these facts, we can integrate the right-hand side of (8.13) by parts and obtain

$$[p'_\theta * \rho_A](\ell') = \int_{-\infty}^{\infty} p_\theta(\ell)\rho'_A(\ell' - \ell)\, d\ell. \tag{8.15}$$

Let us define p_A by

$$p_A(\ell', \theta) = [p_\theta * \rho'_A](\ell'). \tag{8.16}$$

Combining the facts just stated, we can say that $[\mathscr{H}_Y \mathscr{D}_Y p](\ell', \theta)$ is approximated by $p_A(\ell', \theta)$. We define the estimate produced by FBP as

$$f^* = -(1/2\pi)\mathscr{B} p_A, \tag{8.17}$$

see (6.16) and (6.10).

Fig. 8.1: Shapes of the generalized Hamming window for (a) $\alpha = 1.0$, (c) $\alpha = 0.8$, (e) $\alpha = 0.54$. Plots of the corresponding ρ_A for (b) $\alpha = 1.0$, (d) $\alpha = 0.8$, (f) $\alpha = 0.54$.

We now introduce notation that allows us to describe concisely the FBP method. We define a new operator $*_Y$, which we call *convolution with respect to the first variable*. It associates with a function p of two variables and a function q of one variable a new function $p *_Y q$ of two variables, defined by

$$[p *_Y q](\ell, \theta) = [p_\theta * q](\ell), \tag{8.18}$$

where p_θ is defined by (8.11). The mathematical idealization of the FBP method of reconstruction (with *convolving function* q) is the estimate

$$f^* = \mathscr{B}(p *_Y q). \tag{8.19}$$

The functions defined by (8.17) and (8.19) are the same provided that

$$q(u) = -(1/2\pi)\rho_A'(u). \tag{8.20}$$

Substitution into (8.14) gives

$$q(u) = 2\int_0^{A/2} UF_A(U)\cos(2\pi Uu)\,dU. \tag{8.21}$$

In Fig. 8.2 we show plots of q determined by different choices of F_A.

To summarize, the FBP method of reconstruction approximates the inverse Radon transform in two steps:

(i) a convolution with respect to the first variable; followed by
(ii) a backprojection.

The convolving function in the first step is usually chosen by (8.21), where F_A is one of a family of windows satisfying (i)–(iii) of Section 8.1. How this window is to be chosen is discussed in Section 8.6.

8.3 Implementation of the FBP Method

In Section 7.2 we have discussed how the backprojection operator is implemented. That discussion assumed that the function p to be backprojected is known at points $(nd, m\Delta)$, $-N \le n \le N$, $0 \le m \le M-1$ and $M\Delta = \pi$. In order to apply the techniques developed there we need to calculate the values of $p *_Y q$ at these points from the values of p at the same points.

Combining (8.18) with (8.11) and (8.1) we get

$$[p *_Y q](n'd, m\Delta) = \int_{-\infty}^{\infty} p(\ell, m\Delta) q(n'd - \ell)\,d\ell. \tag{8.22}$$

Recall that $p(\ell, \theta)$ is projection data (and hence we can assume that $p(\ell, \theta) = 0$ if $|\ell| \ge E$) and our assumption in Section 7.2 that $Nd \ge E$. Then a Riemann sum approximation to the integral on the right-hand side of (8.22) is

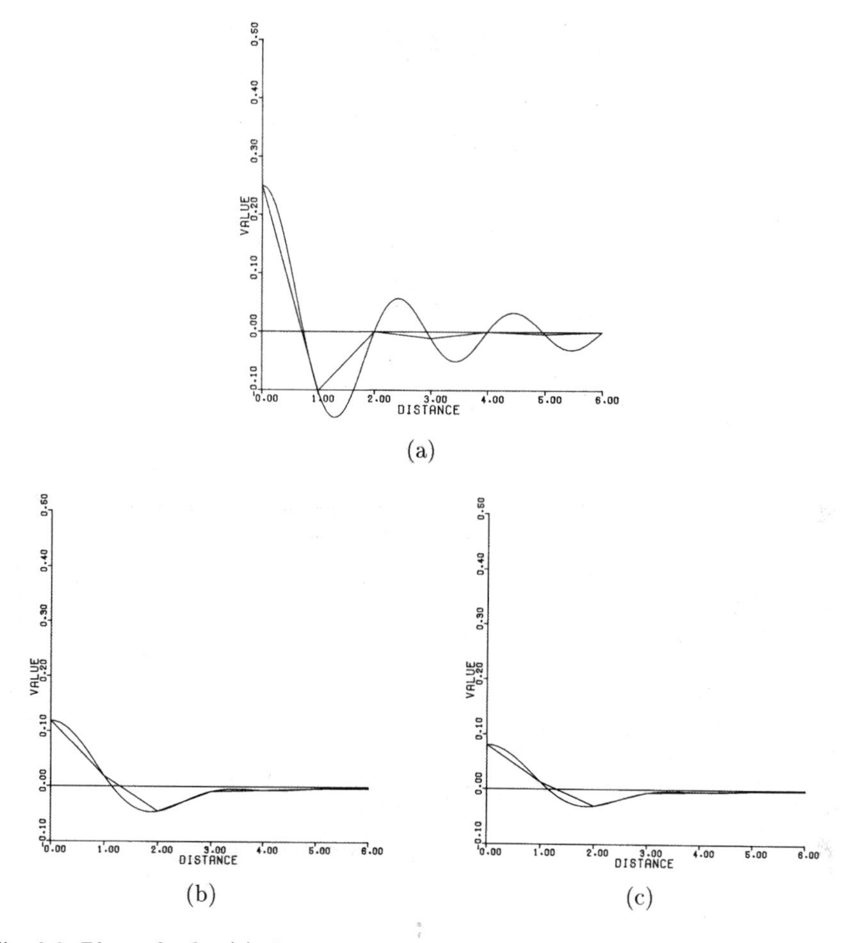

Fig. 8.2: Plots of q for (a) the window in Fig. 8.1(a), (b) the window in Fig. 8.1(c), (c) the window in Fig. 8.1(e). The straight line segments connect the sample points of Section 8.3.

$$p_c(n'd, m\Delta) = d \sum_{n=-N}^{N} p(nd, m\Delta) q((n'-n)d). \tag{8.23}$$

The sum in (8.23) is referred to as a *discrete convolution.*

We now bring together the whole process of calculating $f^*(r, \phi)$ for projection data collected along equally-spaced parallel lines at equal angular increments. More precisely, we assume that we have estimates $p(nd, m\Delta)$ of $[\mathscr{R}f](nd, m\Delta)$ for integers n and m with $-N \le n \le N$ and $0 \le m \le M-1$.

(i) For each m, $0 \le m \le M-1$, we evaluate $p_c(n'd, m\Delta)$ for $-N \le n' \le N$ using (8.23). Thus, p_c is evaluated at $I = (2N+1)M$ points; the associated

I-dimensional vector y_c is often referred to as the *convolved projection data*.

(ii) $f^*(r,\phi)$ is calculated using (7.2), but with p_c in place of p. This involves interpolation for estimating $p_c(r\cos(m\Delta - \phi), m\Delta)$ from values of $p_c(n'd, m\Delta)$.

There are a number of computational points that need to be emphasized.

Since $-N \le n \le N$ and $-N \le n' \le N$, the values of q need to be known for at most $4N+1$ points. For a fixed geometry of data collection, these values can be precalculated and used with the different sets of measured projection data. In fact, usually $q(-v) = q(v)$, as can be seen from (8.21), and in such a case q needs to be calculated for only $2N+1$ points. See Fig. 8.2 for some of these points for the windows shown in Fig. 8.1.

For any fixed m, the values of $p_c(n'd, m\Delta)$, $-N \le n' \le N$, are obtained from the values of $p(nd, m\Delta)$, $-N \le n \le N$. Hence the projection data in one view (i.e., in one set of parallel lines) completely determines the convolved projection data in that view. Evaluation of (8.23) for a particular view can begin as soon as all data for that view are collected, and does not need any data from the other views. Similarly, the contribution to $f^*(r,\phi)$ of the convolved projection data $p_c(nd, m\Delta)$, for any one view (i.e., m fixed, n varies), can be calculated from that view alone, since the interpolations described in Section 7.2 estimate $p_c(r\cos(m\Delta - \phi), m\Delta)$ from values of $p_c(nd, m\Delta)$ with $-N \le n \le N$.

Hence, in practice, the process of convolution followed by backprojection need not be repeated for every (r,ϕ) at which $f^*(r,\phi)$ is evaluated. Instead, the computer algorithm operates as follows.

A sequence $f_0, \ldots, f_{M-1}, f_M$ of digitized pictures is produced, by assigning to the jth pixel the value at its center (r_j, ϕ_j). These values are calculated as follows. The process is initialized by setting

$$f_0(r_j, \phi_j) = 0, \tag{8.24}$$

for $1 \le j \le J$. For each value of m, $0 \le m \le M-1$, we produce from the mth picture the $(m+1)$st picture by a two-step process.

(i) Calculate $p_c(n'd, m\Delta)$ for $-N \le n' \le N$, from $p_c(nd, m\Delta)$ for $-N \le n \le N$, using (8.23) and the precalculated values of $q((n'-n)d)$.

(ii) Let, for $1 \le j \le J$,

$$f_{m+1}(r_j, \phi_j) = f_m(r_j, \phi_j) + \Delta p_c(r_j \cos(m\Delta - \phi_j), m\Delta). \tag{8.25}$$

Interpolation may have to be used in evaluating (8.25).

The digitized picture f_M produced by this process is our estimate f^*. Note that once we have calculated $f_{m+1}(r_j, \phi_j)$ we no longer need $f_m(r_j, \phi_j)$, and the computer can reuse the same memory location repeatedly for $f_0(r_j, \phi_j)$, $\ldots$, $f_M(r_j, \phi_j) = f^*(r_j, \phi_j)$.

The reader should note that the implementation, as just described, is more efficient than brute force implementation of the convolution and backprojection formulas repeatedly for all points $(r_1, \phi_1), \ldots, (r_j, \phi_j)$. The efficiency comes from the observation that we do not have to calculate the convolution step described by (8.23) JM times (once for each pixel and each view), but only $(2N+1)M$ times (once for each line in each view). Since typically J is of the same order as $(2N+1)^2$, this is a significant saving.

The only thing we have left vague in our discussion of the implementation of the FBP method is the choice of the convolving function. In order to discuss this choice, we need to know something about Fourier transforms and sampling.

8.4 Fourier Transforms

Fourier transforms are operators that act on functions whose arguments are real, but whose values are *complex numbers*, i.e., numbers of the form $a + ib$, where a and b are real numbers and i denotes $\sqrt{-1}$. In particular, we use the notation $\exp(i\alpha)$ to denote the complex number $\cos\alpha + i(\sin\alpha)$. In fact, any complex number $a + ib$ can be written in the form $r\exp(i\alpha)$, by choosing r to be the nonnegative square root of $a^2 + b^2$ and α so that $a\tan\alpha = b$. In such a case r is called the *modulus* and α is called an *argument* of $a + ib$. The modulus of $a + ib$ is often denoted by $|a + ib|$. Note that this is consistent with the notation $|a|$ for the absolute value of a real number a. If ϕ is a complex-valued function of a real variable, we define

$$\int_s^t \phi(u)\,du = \left(\int_s^t a(u)\,du\right) + i\left(\int_s^t b(u)\,du\right), \tag{8.26}$$

where a and b are the real-valued functions such that $a(u) + ib(u) = \phi(u)$.

The (*one-dimensional*) *Fourier transform* is an operator that associates with a complex-valued function ϕ of a real variable another complex-valued function $\mathscr{F}\phi$ of a real variable, defined by

$$[\mathscr{F}\phi](U) = \int_{-\infty}^{\infty} \phi(u)\exp(-2\pi i U u)\,du. \tag{8.27}$$

The (*one-dimensional*) *inverse Fourier transform* is an operator that associates with a complex-valued function ϕ of a real variable another complex-valued function $\mathscr{F}^{-1}\phi$ of a real variable, defined by

$$\left[\mathscr{F}^{-1}\phi\right](u) = \int_{-\infty}^{\infty} \phi(U)\exp(2\pi i U u)\,dU. \tag{8.28}$$

The fundamental relationship between these operators is that for many functions ϕ (and we assume that the functions we use fall into this category)

$$\mathscr{F}^{-1}\mathscr{F}\phi = \mathscr{F}\mathscr{F}^{-1}\phi = \phi. \tag{8.29}$$

This is why $\mathscr{F}^{-1}$ is called the inverse Fourier transform.

In order to give an intuitive explanation of the relationship between a function and its Fourier transform we need to digress a little. A *harmonic function* is a function of one of the types $R\cos(2\pi Uu+\alpha)$ or $R\sin(2\pi Uu+\alpha)$, where R, U, and α are constants and u is the variable. The *amplitude* of such a function is $|R|$ (i.e., its value lies between $-R$ and $+R$) and the function is *periodic* with *period* $1/|U|$ (for example, $R\cos\left(2\pi U\left(u+(1/|U|)\right)+\alpha\right) = R\cos\left(2\pi Uu+\alpha\right)$, for all u). The shape of just over a period of a harmonic function can be seen in Fig. 7.2. Since such a function has $|U|$ complete periods in a unit interval, U is called the *frequency* of the function. The number α is called the *initial phase* of the function.

To get an intuitive feeling for the relationship between a function ϕ and its Fourier transform Φ consider the following.

$$\begin{aligned}\phi(u) = &\int_{-\infty}^{\infty} |\Phi(U)| \cos\left(2\pi Uu + \alpha(U)\right) dU \\ &+ i\int_{-\infty}^{\infty} |\Phi(U)| \sin\left(2\pi Uu + \alpha(U)\right) dU,\end{aligned} \tag{8.30}$$

where $\alpha(U)$ is an argument of $\Phi(U)$. This is easily proved from (8.29), (8.28), and (8.26). Note that, for any fixed value of U, both the integrands on the right-hand side of (8.30) are harmonic functions of u with frequency U, with amplitude equal to the modulus of $\Phi(U)$ and with initial phase equal to an argument of $\Phi(U)$. Roughly speaking (8.30) says that both the real and the imaginary part of the function ϕ can be "decomposed" into harmonic functions of different frequencies, and that the amplitude and initial phase of the harmonic function with frequency U in this decomposition are determined by the value of the Fourier transform of ϕ at the point U.

It appears reasonable that the smoother the function ϕ is, the less important are the contributions of high frequency harmonic functions, i.e., for a smooth function ϕ we expect $[\mathscr{F}\phi](U)$ to be small for large $|U|$. This statement can be made mathematically precise, but this book is not the place for that. We are, however, very interested in functions ϕ that are *bandlimited*; i.e., which are such that $[\mathscr{F}\phi](U) = 0$ if $|U| \geq A/2$. In such a case A is said to be the *bandwidth* of ϕ. A function we are likely to come across in image reconstruction is probably not bandlimited, but usually there exists a bandlimited function that is practically indistinguishable from it.

We have, however, already introduced some bandlimited functions: in fact the convolving functions q as defined by (8.21) are bandlimited. In order to see this, we define

$$\Phi(U) = |U|\, F_A\left(|U|\right). \tag{8.31}$$

Note that $\Phi(U) = 0$ if $|U| \geq A/2$ and $\Phi(-U) = \Phi(U)$. Using these facts, substitution into (8.28) yields

$$\left[\mathscr{F}^{-1}\Phi\right](u) = 2\int_0^{A/2} \Phi(U)\cos(2\pi U u)\, dU. \tag{8.32}$$

Comparison with (8.21) shows that $q(u) = \left[\mathscr{F}^{-1}\Phi\right](u)$, and so $\mathscr{F}q$ is the function Φ defined by (8.31). This shows that a convolving function based on a window of bandwidth A is a bandlimited function of the same bandwidth.

The following argument now appears quite natural. The functions F_A were introduced in Section 8.1, since they gave rise using (8.10) to a family $\{\rho_A \mid A > 0\}$ of regularizing functions. The purpose of such a family is to approximate the Hilbert transform; see (8.9). The approximation at any point can be made as accurate as we wish by choosing A large enough. The value of the functions F_A at any fixed point tends to 1 as A increases. So why not use instead of (8.31) its limit as A increases; namely, why not define $\Phi(U) = |U|$? If we did this, it appears reasonable that we would get

$$\mathscr{R}^{-1}p = \mathscr{B}\left(p *_Y \mathscr{F}^{-1}\Phi\right); \tag{8.33}$$

i.e., we would have replaced the approximating formula (8.19) by one that gives $\mathscr{R}^{-1}p$ exactly. There is a major flaw in this argument: if Φ is defined by $\Phi(U) = |U|$, then $\mathscr{F}^{-1}\Phi$ is not defined, in the sense that the infinite integral on the right-hand side of the definition of the inverse Fourier transform (8.28) does not exist.

Hence this limiting argument fails, and we still need to choose an F_A. The desire to approximate the Hilbert transform accurately seems to imply that A should be chosen large, but as we shall see, the nature of the data may dictate otherwise.

Let us now recall the notation of Section 8.2. The function of two variables whose inverse Radon transform we wish to estimate is denoted by p. For any angle θ, we define p_θ by (8.11). The convolution step consists of convolving p_θ with q, for each θ; see (8.18). One way towards understanding how q should be chosen is to look at what convolving p_θ with q does to the Fourier transform of p_θ.

The important relevant result here is the well-known *convolution theorem*. It states that the Fourier transform of the convolution of two functions is the product of their Fourier transforms, or in symbols

$$\left[\mathscr{F}\left[\phi * \psi\right]\right](U) = \left[\mathscr{F}\phi\right](U)\left[\mathscr{F}\psi\right](U). \tag{8.34}$$

Applying this theorem to our case yields

$$\left[\mathscr{F}\left[p_\theta * q\right]\right](U) = |U|\, F_A(|U|)\left[\mathscr{F}p_\theta\right](U), \tag{8.35}$$

which means that the value of the Fourier transform of $p_\theta * q$ at the point U is $|U|\, F_A(|U|)$ times the value of the Fourier transform of p_θ at the point U. This has many interesting consequences; for example, $p_\theta * q$ is a bandlimited function with bandwidth A. However, our real interest lies not in the approximate formula to the inverse Radon transform given in (8.19), but in the actual implementation described in Section 8.3. Hence, we need to look at the discrete versions of the convolution and Fourier transform operators.

8.5 Sampling and Interpolation

In (8.19) we have defined the estimate f^* produced by the mathematical idealization of the FBP method as the backprojection of $p *_Y q$, where p is the function of two variables whose inverse Radon transform we wish to find and q is the convolving function. In Section 8.3 we have pointed out that in practice the backprojection is applied not to $p * q$, but to an approximation of it, which we have denoted by p_c. In order to apply our approximation (7.2) of the backprojection operator, $p_c(\ell, \theta)$ needs to be known for those values of ℓ and θ that are of the form $\ell = r\cos(m\Delta - \phi)$ and $\theta = m\Delta$. Since the point (r, θ) at which we wish to estimate the picture can be anywhere in the picture region, p_c needs to be defined at all points (ℓ, θ), where $-E \leq \ell \leq E$ and $\theta = m\Delta$ with m an integer in the range $0 \leq m \leq M - 1$. Defining p_c at these points has been done in two stages. First, in (8.23), we have defined p_c explicitly at points $(n'd, m\Delta)$, where n' is an integer in the range $-N \leq n' \leq N$, and then we have stated that $p_c\left(r\cos(m\Delta - \phi), m\Delta\right)$ is obtained by interpolation from the values of $p_c(n'd, m\Delta)$. In this section we discuss the relationship between $p * q$ and its approximation p_c.

Note, first of all, that the discussion here is concerned with functions that are essentially functions of one variable only. This is so because, for any fixed $m\Delta$, $p_c(\ell, m\Delta)$ is defined based on the values of $p(\ell, m\Delta)$, i.e., on the values of $p_{m\Delta}(\ell)$, see (8.11). Hence we can rephrase our problem as follows.

Assume that p_θ is a function of one real variable such that $p_\theta(\ell) = 0$ if $|\ell| \geq E$ (where E is a positive real number) and that q is another function of one variable. Let d be a real number and N be an integer such that $Nd > E$. Define a new function t as follows. For integer values of n',

$$t(n'd) = d \sum_{n=-N}^{N} p_\theta(nd)q\left((n' - n)\,d\right). \tag{8.36}$$

For all values of the real variable ℓ, $t(\ell)$ is defined by interpolation from the values of $t(n'd)$. *Problem*: Investigate how the choices of q and the method of interpolation influence the relationship between p_θ and t.

We have stated the problem in this particular form, since p_θ represents the projection data, which are obtained by our physical device. On the other hand, the choices of the convolving function and of the interpolation method are ours to make; it is the effect of these choices that is our current interest.

To solve our problem, we need to discuss the nature of interpolation more precisely. For every positive real number d (called the *sampling interval*) and every function on the real numbers ψ (called the *interpolating function*) we define an operator $\mathscr{I}_d^\psi$ (called the *interpolation operator* with sampling interval d and interpolating function ψ), which associates with any function ϕ of one real variable another function $\mathscr{I}_d^\psi \phi$ of one real variable defined by

$$\left[\mathscr{I}_d^\psi \phi\right](v) = \sum_{n=-\infty}^{\infty} \phi(nd)\psi(v - nd). \tag{8.37}$$

In practice the sum in (8.37) is usually finite, since in most applications the interpolating function assumes zero value outside a small interval. For example, for the nearest neighbor interpolation we can use the function ψ_n, defined by

$$\psi_n(u) = \begin{cases} 1, & \text{if } -d/2 < u < d/2, \\ 0.5, & \text{if } \mid u \mid = d/2, \\ 0, & \text{if } \mid u \mid > d/2 \end{cases} \tag{8.38}$$

(we assume that the average is desired at a point exactly half-way between two sample points), and for linear interpolation we can use the function ψ_ℓ, defined by

$$\psi_\ell(u) = \begin{cases} 1 - |u/d|, & \text{if } |u| < d, \\ 0, & \text{if } |u| \geq d. \end{cases} \tag{8.39}$$

Note that for both these interpolating functions

$$[\mathscr{I}_d^\psi \phi](nd) = \phi(nd), \tag{8.40}$$

for any function ϕ and any integer n. We call interpolating functions satisfying this property *proper interpolating functions*.

Let us assume that the function t of our problem is to be defined using a proper interpolating function ψ. The precise method of definition is the following. Define t at points $n'd$ (for all integers n') using (8.36). Then, using (8.37) with t in place of ϕ, we define t $(= \mathscr{I}_d^\psi t)$ at all real numbers u. Under these circumstances, we can characterize the Fourier transform of t as follows.

Let

$$F_1(U) = \sum_{k=-\infty}^{\infty} [\mathscr{F} p_\theta] (U + k/d), \tag{8.41}$$

$$F_2(U) = \sum_{k=-\infty}^{\infty} [\mathscr{F} q] (U + k/d), \tag{8.42}$$

and

$$F_3(U) = [\mathscr{F} \psi] (U)/d. \tag{8.43}$$

Then

$$[\mathscr{F} t] (U) = F_1(U) F_2(U) F_3(U). \tag{8.44}$$

The proof of this claim requires a deeper mathematical background than what we have assumed in writing this book. The claim has important implications for the FBP method, in the next section we discuss the choice of convolving and interpolating functions based entirely on (8.41)–(8.44).

8.6 The Choice of Convolving and Interpolating Functions

Equations (8.41)–(8.44) provide a handle on how to choose the convolving function q and the interpolating function ψ. The function t is supposed to be an approximation to $p_\theta * q$. By the convolution theorem (Section 8.4), the Fourier transform of $p_\theta * q$ is the product of the Fourier transforms of p_θ and of q. On the other hand, the Fourier transform of t is expressed as the product of three terms in (8.44): $F_1(U)$, which depends on the projection data p_θ; $F_2(U)$, which depends on the convolving function q; and $F_3(U)$, which depends on the interpolating function ψ. Roughly speaking, we aim to identify F_1 with $\mathscr{F} p_\theta$, F_2 with $\mathscr{F} q$, and F_3 with a function whose value is always 1. However, the interrelations between the three functions are also important, especially since our previously stated aim turns out to be unachievable in practice. We deal with the functions F_1, F_2 and F_3 one by one.

The function F_1, in (8.41) is a periodic function with period $1/d$. (Recall that d is the sampling interval in the ℓ variable; in other words, d is the spacing between the parallel lines along which ray sums are collected.) If the projection data are reasonably smooth compared with the sampling distance, one finds that the value of $|[\mathscr{F} p_\theta](U)|$ is very small for $|U| > 1/2d$. (In other words, the amplitudes of high frequency harmonic functions in the Fourier decomposition of p_θ are small.) In such a case, for $|U| < 1/2d$,

$$F_1(U) \simeq [\mathscr{F} p_\theta](U), \tag{8.45}$$

which is desirable, since we wish to identify F_1 with $\mathscr{F} p_\theta$. However, (8.45) is clearly violated for $|U| > 1/2d$, since the values of F_1 outside the range $-1/2d \leq U \leq 1/2d$ are just periodic repeats of the values inside that range, while the values of $\mathscr{F} p_\theta$, for projection functions p_θ, do not have this property. It follows that while we may use $F_1(U)$ to be an approximation to $[\mathscr{F} p_\theta](U)$ in the range $-1/2d < U < 1/2d$, we must not do this outside this range. If we can assume that the function p_θ is smooth relative to the sampling distance, then a reasonable approximation to $[\mathscr{F} p_\theta](U)$ for $|U| \geq 1/2d$ is zero.

An important point to consider is the following. If the values of $[\mathscr{F} p_\theta](U)$ are not insignificant for $|U| \geq 1/2d$, then we are in a serious difficulty because we have no idea how to approximate $\mathscr{F} p_\theta$ for large values of $|U|$. Even worse, (8.45) is no longer valid even in the range $-1/2d < U < 1/2d$ as can be seen by comparing (8.41), which defines $F_1(U)$, with (8.45), since the values $[\mathscr{F} p_\theta](U + k/d)$ cannot be ignored for $k \neq 0$. Thus, the amplitudes of high frequency components of p_θ influence the values of $F_1(U)$ for small values of $|U|$. This phenomenon, called *aliasing*, is demonstrated in Fig. 8.3.

What is happening here is the following. If we do not sample p_θ finely enough, not only do we lose information about the high-frequency components of our data, but we also contaminate the low-frequency components. Prior knowledge (see Section 6.4) may be helpful for recovering from such a situation, but the FBP method does not make use of such knowledge. If a finer sampling is not available (machine design usually limits the sampling rate), we just have to accept that in those cases in which the projection data have significant high-frequency components we obtain low-quality reconstructions.

Of course, the change in amplitude is unlikely to be abrupt at the frequency $1/2d$. It is to be expected that the amplitudes slightly over $1/2d$ are small but

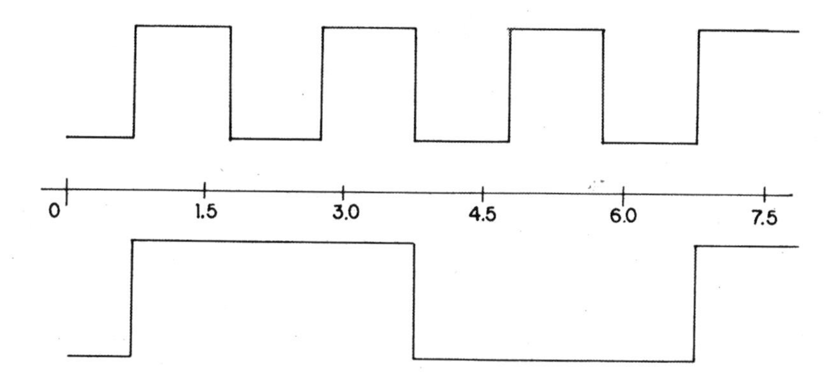

Fig. 8.3: Illustration of aliasing. The periodic function (shown on the top) with period 2 (frequency 1/2) is sampled at the sampling interval 1.5. Nearest neighbor interpolation gives a function (shown at the bottom) with period 6 (frequency 1/6).

not totally insignificant. In this case aliasing does not affect the amplitudes at significantly smaller frequencies than $1/2d$, see Fig. 8.4. We thus have a fairly typical intermediate situation between the ideal (but unobtainable) case of bandlimited projection data (with bandwidth $1/d$) and the totally hopeless case where frequencies up to $3/2d$ have large amplitudes. In this intermediate situation $F_1(U)$ approximates $[\mathscr{F}p_\theta](U)$ well for small values of $|U|$, but the approximation deteriorates as U approaches $\pm 1/2d$, becoming useless beyond these points.

One other point needs to be mentioned in our consideration of F_1 as an approximation to $\mathscr{F}p_\theta$. Since we are discussing data obtained from physical experiments, the values of p_θ only approximate the values of the Radon transform of the picture f that we wish to reconstruct. We may write p_θ as

$$p_\theta = \mathscr{R}_\theta f + n_\theta \tag{8.46}$$

where $\mathscr{R}_\theta f$ represents the projection data for angle θ without any photon statistics (i.e., in the limiting case in which the number of photons used to collect the data approaches infinity, see Section 3.1), but with all other sources of error in estimating the line integrals, such as those discussed in Chapter 3. Under this assumption, n_θ is the additional *noise* due to photon statistics. From the definition of Fourier transform (8.27) we see that, for all U,

$$[\mathscr{F}p_\theta](U) = [\mathscr{F}\mathscr{R}_\theta f](U) + [\mathscr{F}n_\theta](U). \tag{8.47}$$

For the statistical noise n_θ, the value of $|[\mathscr{F}n_\theta](U)|$ (amplitude in the noise at frequency U) can be considered as a sample from a random variable. The expected value of this random variable is approximately the same for all values of U. On the other hand, for sufficiently smooth $\mathscr{R}_\theta f$, $|[\mathscr{F}\mathscr{R}_\theta f](U)|$, becomes small as $|U|$ approaches $1/2d$. Hence, when $|U|$ is near $1/2d$, the values

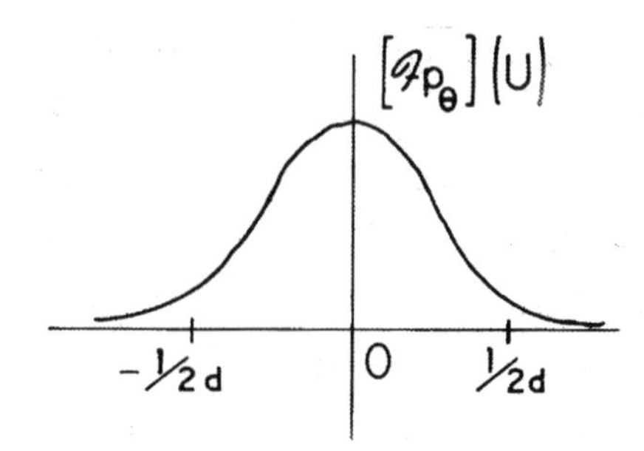

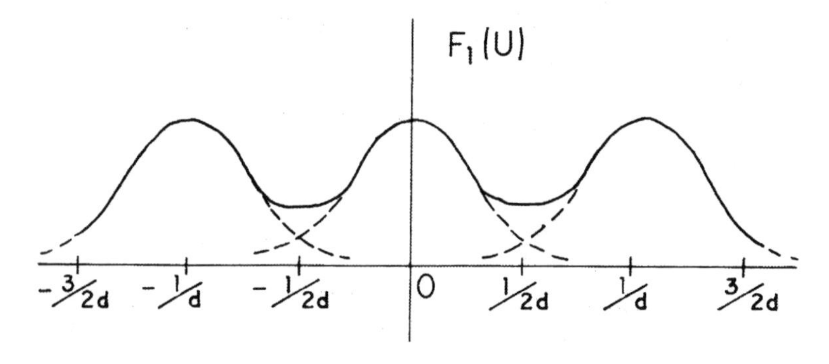

Fig. 8.4: The amplitudes at frequencies near $\pm\frac{1}{2d}$ in $[\mathscr{F}p_\theta](U)$ affect the values of $F_1(U)$ only near $\pm\frac{1}{2d}$. In the illustration both $\mathscr{F}p_\theta$ and F_1 are shown (on the top and the bottom, respectively) as if they were real valued. In practice they will be complex valued, but the moduli of their values have the indicated behavior.

$[\mathscr{F}p_\theta](U)$ are often determined more by the noise in the data than by the Radon transform of the function that we wish to reconstruct. This observation also influences our selection of the convolving and interpolating functions.

We illustrate the nature of the function F_1 by plotting, in Fig. 8.5, $|F_1(U)|$ for some noisy parallel projection data of the piecewise homogeneous head phantom of Fig. 4.4 for the angle $\theta = 0$.

The function F_2 defined by (8.42) appears to have the same relationship to q as F_1 has to p_θ. However, the situation here is much simpler, since the choice of q is under our control.

In the first place, we can select q so that it is bandlimited with bandwidth no greater than $1/d$. If we do that, then, for $|U| < 1/2d$,

$$F_2(U) = [\mathscr{F}q](U), \tag{8.48}$$

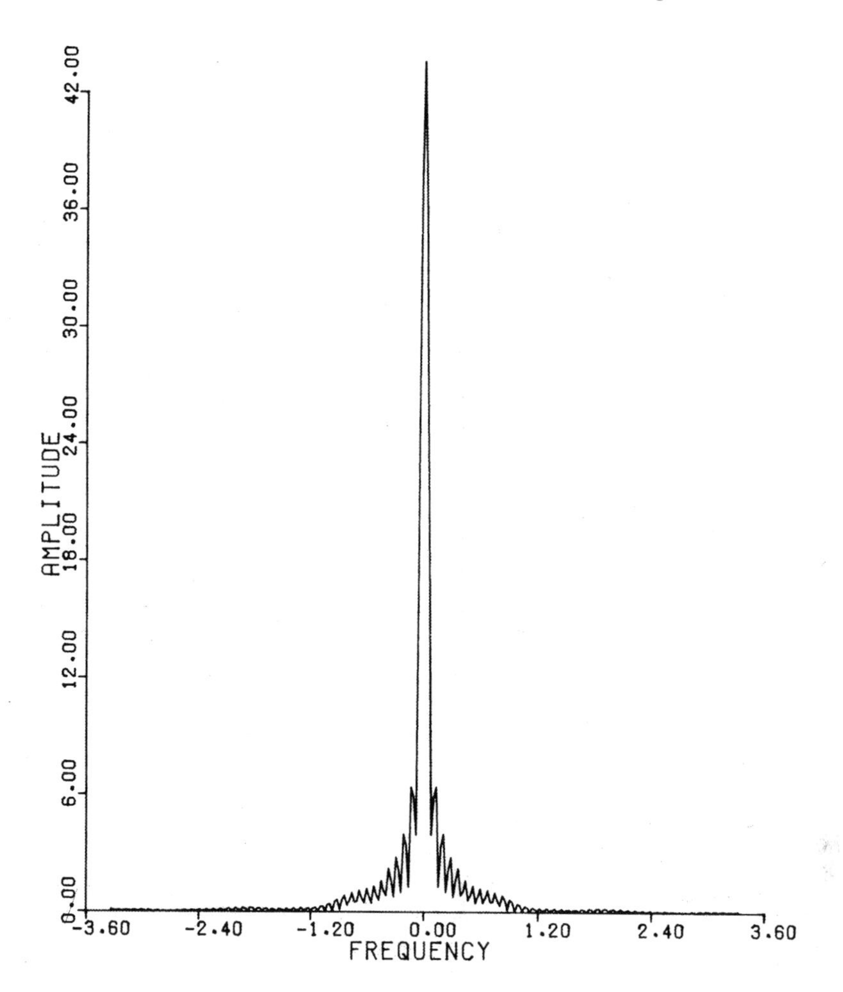

Fig. 8.5: The function $|F_1(U)|$ for noisy parallel projection data of the piecewise homogeneous head phantom of Fig. 4.4 for the angle $\theta = 0$ sampled with sampling interval $d = 0.1504$, and hence with $\frac{1}{2d}$ slightly smaller than 3.33. Past $\pm\frac{1}{2d}$ the values of the function are periodic repeats of the values between $-\frac{1}{2d}$ and $+\frac{1}{2d}$.

where we now have a precise equality, rather than an approximation as in (8.45).

The discussion in Section 8.4 shows that the convolving functions that arise out of the regularization arguments of Sections 8.1 and 8.2 are indeed bandlimited. In fact, $\mathscr{F}q$ is the function Φ defined by (8.31). If we choose A to be no greater than $1/d$, then (8.48) is satisfied.

We now have to resolve a dilemma: the regularization argument suggests that A should be as large as possible, but now we are talking about restricting it to $1/d$. The resolution of the dilemma comes from the recognition that we are working in two different contexts. In the mathematical idealization a high value of A appears desirable. In the practical implementation there appears to be just about no point in having A higher than $1/d$. $F_2(U)$ is used as one term in a product where another term is $F_1(U)$. This term is already known to be totally unreliable for $|U| > 1/2d$; we may as well give up making $F_2(U)$ reliable for such values of U. On the other hand, by making $F_2(U)$ equal to $[\mathscr{F}q](U)$ within the range $-1/2d < U < 1/2d$, we make our second approximation as precise as possible in the range where it matters.

It also appears that there is no reason to choose A anything but $1/d$. This is the highest possible value within the constraints just discussed, hence it is desirable based on the regularization argument. Often the values of q at multiples of d become easy to calculate when q is defined as $[\mathscr{F}^{-1}\Phi]$, with $\Phi(U) = |U| F_{1/d}(|U|)$; see (8.31), (8.32) and Fig. 8.2, especially for the bandlimiting window. Finally, if for some family of windows $\{F_A\}$ a choice of A which is $A_0 < 1/d$ appears ideal, then there is very likely to be another family of windows $\{G_A\}$, such that $G_{1/d} = F_{A_0}$. From now on, therefore, we assume that $A = 1/d$, i.e., that the bandwidth of our window is the inverse of our sampling interval.

Assuming that we remain with the formulation that q is $\mathscr{F}^{-1}\Phi$, where Φ is defined by (8.31), the question still remains: how do we choose the window $F_A(U)$? The regularization argument in Section 8.4 indicates that for the families of windows under discussion the ideal limiting value of Φ is given by $\Phi(U) = |U|$. One may therefore argue that the bandlimiting window, which sets Φ to this ideal value in the range up to $A/2$, may be the best. However, the regularization argument is based on the assumption of perfect data. As we have seen in our discussion on the nature of F_1, the values of $F_1(U)$ for U near $1/2d$ may be far from the ideal assumed in the regularization argument. Furthermore, since in this case we would have $F_2(U) = |U|$, F_2 would multiply F_1 by the largest values where F_1 is least reliable.

From all this we may conclude the following. If the data collection is very reliable and if $\mathscr{F}p_\theta$ is very nearly bandlimited with bandwidth $1/d$, then it is appropriate to choose q so that $[\mathscr{F}q](U) = F_2(U) = |U|$ for $-1/2d \leq U \leq 1/2d$. However, if there is considerable noise in the data or if there are aliasing errors near $1/2d$, then a choice of an $F_A(U)$ that is small for U near $1/2d$ is more likely to produce good results, since it avoids multiplication of the erroneous amplitudes at frequencies near $1/2d$ by the relatively large value of $|U|$. The exact choice of the filter must be dependent on the data collection method and the type of object that is to be reconstructed.

Finally, we come to the discussion of F_3. Under ideal circumstances $F_3(U)$ should have the value 1 everywhere. In real life a very different objective occurs. We have assumed that $[\mathscr{F}p_\theta](U)$; and hence the product $[\mathscr{F}p_\theta](U)\,[\mathscr{F}q](U)$, is nearly zero if $|U| > 1/2d$. However, both F_1 and F_2 are periodic with period $1/d$. Thus, for $|U| > 1/2d$, the product $F_1(U)F_2(U)$ is unlikely to be near zero. We can use $F_3(U)$ to remedy this situation. Thus,

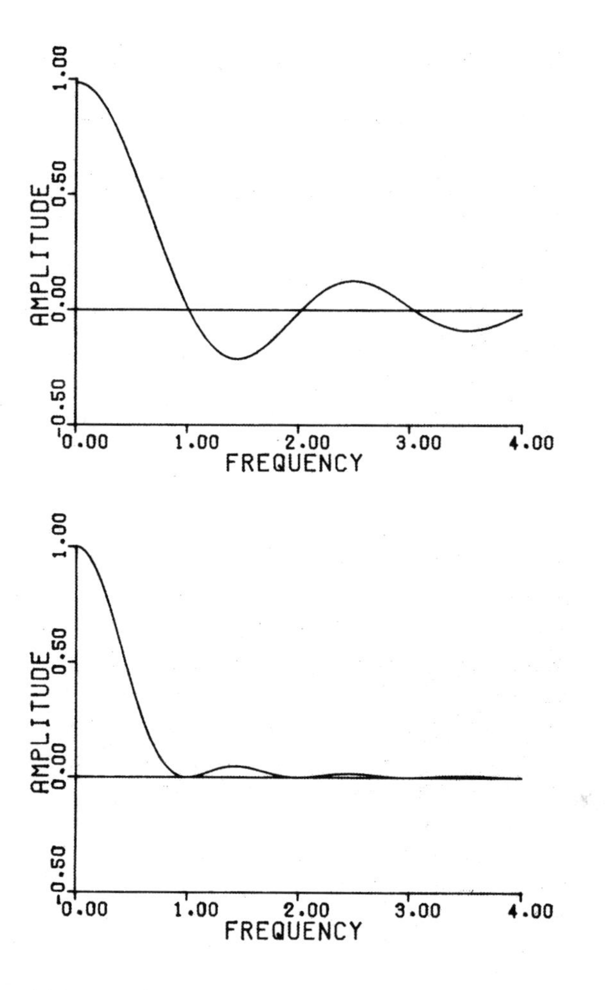

Fig. 8.6: Plots of F_3 assuming interpolation interval $d = 1$ for nearest neighbor interpolation (top) and linear interpolation (bottom).

it is desirable to have $|F_3(U)|$ small if $|U| > 1/2d$. Even for $|U| < 1/2d$ we may not wish $F_3(U)$ to have the value 1 because $F_3(U)$ can be used, in conjunction with $F_2(U)$, to suppress the erroneous values in $F_1(U)$ when $|U|$ is near $1/2d$. Hence, a desirable F_3 is one which has value 1 at the origin, but dies away as it nears $1/2d$ and remains near zero past $1/2d$. In Fig. 8.6 we plot the values of $F_3(U)$ for the nearest neighbor and the linear interpolation. In view of the comments just made, it is not surprising that linear interpolation usually leads to better reconstructions than the nearest neighbor interpolation.

We illustrate this discussion using a number of experiments all involving the standard parallel projection data. (Further relevant discussion is given in Chapter 10.)

In Fig. 8.7(a), (b) and (c) we show reconstructions using linear interpolation and the generalized Hamming window with three different values of the parameter α. The case $\alpha = 1$ is the same as the bandlimiting window; there is no suppression of frequencies near $U = 1/2d$. The case $\alpha = 0.54$ is near the other extreme; it is the Hamming window. The case $\alpha = 0.8$ is in-between these extremes. Note that smaller values of α give smoother looking pictures (suppression of high-frequency harmonics), but this may eliminate small tumors as well as the noise; see the discussion in Section 5.3. The first three rows of Table 8.2 report on the picture distance measures and the computer times for these three reconstructions.

In Figs. 8.7(b) and (d) and in Fig. 8.8(a) and (b) we compare the linear and nearest neighbor methods of interpolation, for the generalized Hamming filter with $\alpha = 0.8$. These figures indicate that linear interpolation is superior to nearest neighbor interpolation. Nevertheless, the picture distance measure d (but not r) in Table 8.2 indicates that nearest neighbor interpolation is superior to linear interpolation. The reason for this is that this measure is highly influenced by the accuracy of the reconstruction of the skull. Linear interpolation is less accurate than nearest neighbor interpolation for the region of the picture occupied by the skull, but is more accurate than nearest neighbor interpolation for the interior of the skull. This is a prime example of a general principle in CT: the appropriate choices of the free parameters in a reconstruction algorithm are dependent on the information we wish to obtain about the picture to be reconstructed. In view of the discussion in Section 5.3, we investigated whether the visual superiority of linear interpolation over nearest neighbor interpolation is contradicted by an evaluation of task-oriented performance. We found that there is no such contradiction for our task of detecting small low-contrast tumors. The null-hypothesis that linear interpolation and nearest neighbor interpolation (within FBP for parallel data with generalized Hamming window with $\alpha = 0.8$) are equally efficacious can be rejected in favor of the alternative hypothesis that linear interpolation is better with P-value less than 10^{-11} for both the IROI and HITR figures of merit. The average values are given in Table 8.2.

It is also interesting to note that the reported time for nearest neighbor interpolation is greater than that for linear interpolation. There is no inherent reason for this. It is a consequence of the programmers of SNARK09 recog-

Table 8.2: Picture distance measures and timings (in seconds) for the reconstructions in Fig. 8.7 and average FOMs for comparing interpolation methods.

reconstruction in	interpolation	α	d	r	t	IROI	HITR
Fig. 8.7(a)	linear	1.00	0.0655	0.0325	1.0		
Fig. 8.7(b)	linear	0.80	0.0814	0.0340	1.0	0.2348	0.9499
Fig. 8.7(c)	linear	0.54	0.1071	0.0369	1.0		
Fig. 8.7(d)	nearest neighbor	0.80	0.0797	0.0435	1.5	0.2150	0.9136

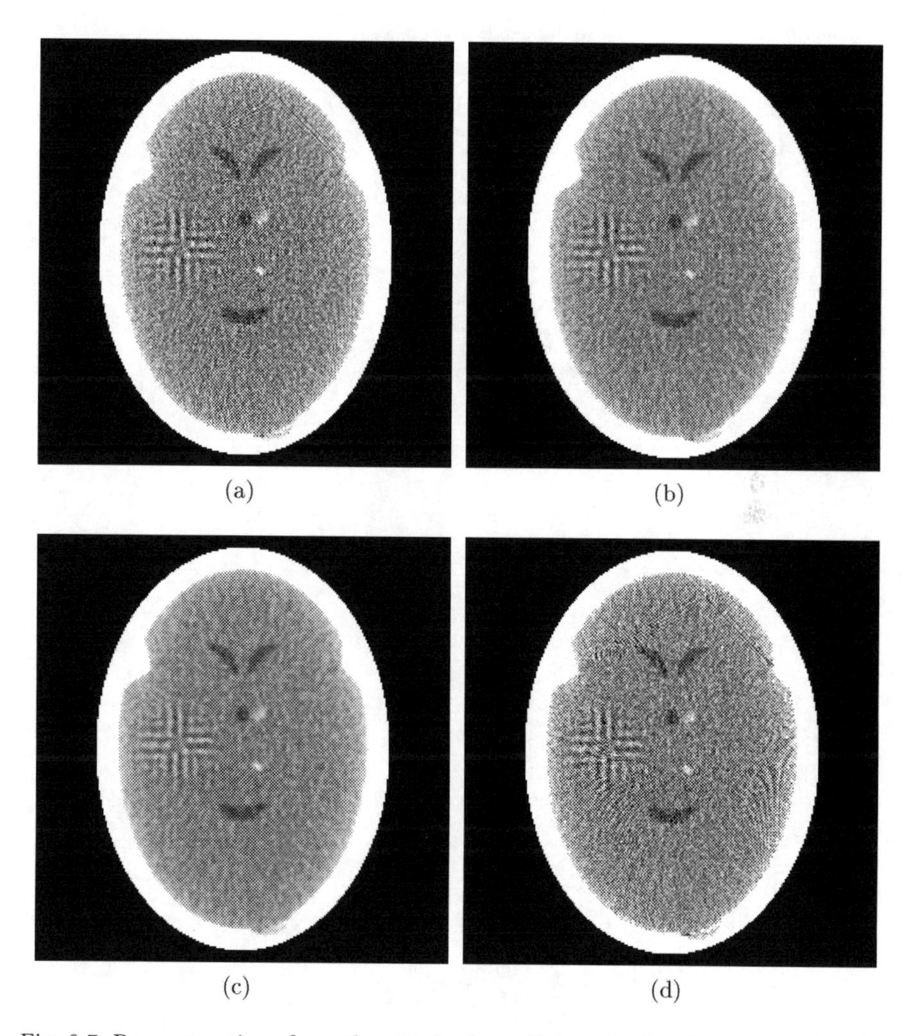

Fig. 8.7: Reconstructions from the standard parallel projection data using FBP for parallel beams with linear interpolation and generalized Hamming window with (a) $\alpha = 1.0$, (b) $\alpha = 0.8$, (c) $\alpha = 0.54$ and (d) nearest neighbor interpolation and generalized Hamming window with $\alpha = 0.8$.

nizing that linear interpolation is more efficacious and hence investing extra effort in making its code particularly efficient; see Section 6.6.

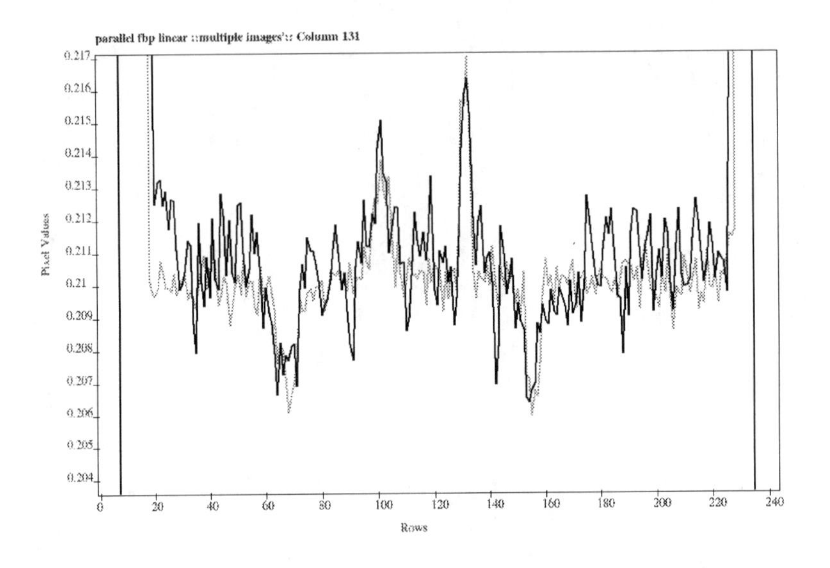
standard head phantom
standard par_linear alpha_CONV_0001_r_a
parallel fbp linear ::multiple images':: Column 131
Pixel Values
0.217
0.216
0.215
0.214
0.213
0.212
0.211
0.21
0.209
0.208
0.207
0.206
0.205
0.204
0
20
40
60
80
100
120
140
160
180
200
220
240
Rows

(a)

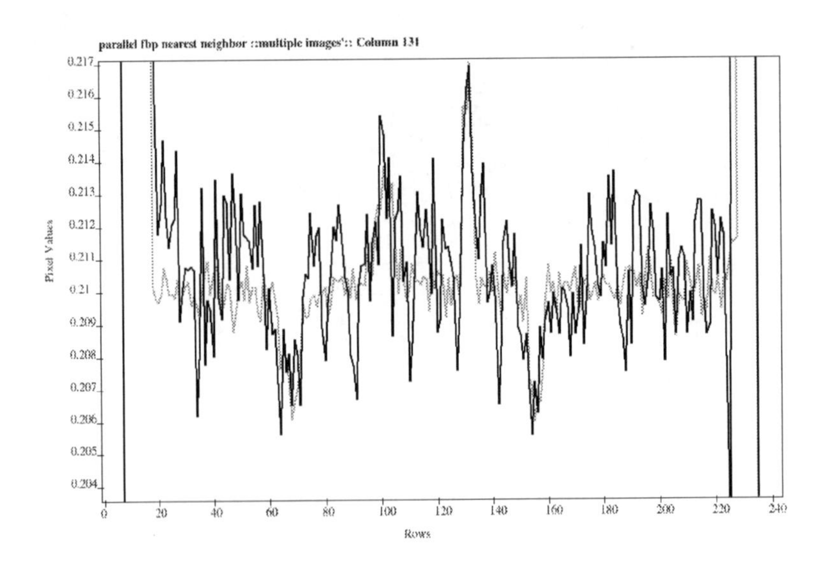
standard head phantom
standard par_nearest neig_CONV_0001_r_a
parallel fbp nearest neighbor ::multiple images':: Column 131
Pixel Values
0.217
0.216
0.215
0.214
0.213
0.212
0.211
0.21
0.209
0.208
0.207
0.206
0.205
0.204
0
20
40
60
80
100
120
140
160
180
200
220
240
Rows

(b)

8.7 Why So Popular?

The FBP method is a widely-used method for reconstruction from data obtained by the parallel modes of data collection. There are many reasons for this.

A major reason is its computational simplicity. As discussed in Section 8.3, the demands of the FBP method on computer time and storage are surprisingly small, even when implemented on a general-purpose computer. Examination of the method reveals that it is relatively easy to build special-purpose computing hardware that implements the FBP method very efficiently. The data from each view can be convolved and backprojected independently of the other views; the final outcome is simply a sum of such convolved and backprojected views. In state-of-the-art devices, large digitized pictures (e.g., 1000×1000) are reconstructed from many views (over 1000) in the order of a second.

The quality of the reconstructions produced by the FBP method is generally competitive with, and is often better than, the quality of those produced by other methods. There are situations in which other reconstruction techniques produce more efficacious images than the FBP method; but when accurate data are available in abundance (x-ray reconstruction appears to fall in this category, but positron emission tomography and electron microscopy do not), then the FBP method seems to be as efficacious as any other.

The electrical engineering and physics background of many people involved in scanner design also makes the FBP method popular. The type of analysis that we have carried out in the last section, using the Fourier transforms of the functions involved to explain the effects of our choices, is very familiar to scientists and engineers. In fact, this familiarity leads to statements of the type "the FBP method is preferable to series expansion techniques, because the underlying mathematics is well understood." This particular reason for the popularity of the FBP method appears weak; the theory that we develop in this book for the series expansion methods is every bit as rigorous as the theory underlying the FBP and other transform methods. Different aspects of the problem are more easily explained in the different theories: while it is difficult to explain the behavior of some of the series expansion techniques using Fourier analysis, it is easier to incorporate prior knowledge into the series expansion techniques than into a transform method; see Section 6.4. We return to this point later.

Fig. 8.8: Plots of the head phantom of Fig. 4.6(a), shown light, and its reconstructions, shown dark, from the standard parallel projection data using FBP for parallel data with generalized Hamming window with $\alpha = 0.8$ and (a) linear interpolation (cf., Fig. 8.7(b)) and (b) nearest neighbor interpolation (cf., Fig. 8.7(d)).

In conclusion, the FBP method produces efficacious reconstructions at a small cost. Unless evidence is available to the contrary in a particular application area, it is as or more likely to be an appropriate method to use than any other method designed for the parallel mode of data collection.

Notes and References

The mathematical form of the FBP method was first proposed for image reconstruction from data collected along parallel lines in [29], while [227] described an implementation that took care of the discrete nature of the data. Both these approaches used the bandlimiting window, as it was made explicit in the derivation provided in [138]. L. A. Shepp and B. F. Logan [241] introduced the idea of using windows other than the bandlimiting window; they suggested the use of the sinc window, combined with linear interpolation. The use of the Hamming window was proposed in [52]. It was shown, for example in [234], that the use of the generalized Hamming window is equivalent to applying the bandlimiting window to data that have been smoothed by a three-point averaging process of the type discussed, for example, in [241]. An exhaustive study of these windows was carried out by S.W. Rowland [234], who was the first to carefully separate the convolving function and the interpolating function. Our presentation is highly influenced by that work.

The notion of a regularizing family was introduced into the image reconstruction literature in [136]. We followed the approach of [49].

A precise statement of the theorem used to differentiate under the integral sign can be found in most standard books on mathematical analysis; see, e.g., [10], Theorem 9-37.

The general context of our approach to Fourier transforms, sampling and interpolation can be easily obtained from a basic text on these topics, such as [28]. Discussion of different windows can be found in standard texts on signal processing, such as [223].

Examples of difficulties with the FBP method when the data have high frequency components were given in [126].

There have been a number of publications comparing the performance of the FBP method with series expansion techniques, examples are [138, 198, 241].

An interesting variant of FBP that is particularly popular in reconstruction in electron microscopy is weighted backprojection (WBP); see [224]. Comparisons of this approach with a series expansion method are presented in [38, 195].

9

Other Transform Methods for Parallel Beams

In this chapter we discuss three alternative transform methods for image reconstruction from data collected along parallel lines: the Fourier method, the linogram method and the method of rho-filtered layergrams. All these methods make use of the concept of the two-dimensional Fourier transform.

9.1 Two-Dimensional Fourier Transforms

The *two-dimensional Fourier transform* $\mathscr{F}_2$ is an operator that associates with a complex-valued function f of two polar variables another complex-valued function $\mathscr{F}_2 f$ of two polar variables defined by

$$[\mathscr{F}_2 f](R,\Phi) = \int_0^{\pi}\int_{-\infty}^{\infty} |r|\, f(r,\phi) \exp\left(-2\pi i r R \cos(\Phi-\phi)\right) dr d\phi. \tag{9.1}$$

The *inverse two-dimensional Fourier transform* is an operator that associates with a complex-valued function F of two polar variables another complex-valued function $\mathscr{F}_2^{-1} F$ of two polar variables defined by

$$\left[\mathscr{F}_2^{-1} F\right](r,\phi) = \int_0^{\pi}\int_{-\infty}^{\infty} |R|\, F(R,\Phi) \exp\left(2\pi i R r \cos(\Phi-\phi)\right) dR d\Phi. \tag{9.2}$$

For many functions f and F (including all in this book, except where otherwise stated),

$$\mathscr{F}_2^{-1}\mathscr{F}_2 f = f \quad \text{and} \quad \mathscr{F}_2\mathscr{F}_2^{-1} F = F. \tag{9.3}$$

Similarly to the one-dimensional case, (8.30), a function f of two polar variables can be "decomposed" into harmonic functions of two variables, and the two-dimensional Fourier transform indicates the nature of these harmonic components. We now explain this in more detail.

Let f be a function of two polar variables and F be its two-dimensional Fourier transform. Let $\alpha(R,\Phi)$ denote an argument of $F(R,\Phi)$. Then it follows from (9.2) and (9.3) that

$$f(r,\phi) = \int_0^\pi \int_{-\infty}^\infty |R|\,|F(R,\Phi)| \cos(2\pi Rr\cos(\phi-\Phi)+\alpha(R,\Phi))\,dRd\Phi \\ + i\int_0^\pi \int_{-\infty}^\infty |R|\,|F(R,\Phi)| \sin(2\pi Rr\cos(\phi-\Phi)+\alpha(R,\Phi))\,dRd\Phi. \tag{9.4}$$

For any fixed R and Φ, the functions

$$|F(R,\Phi)|\cos(2\pi Rr\cos(\phi-\Phi)+\alpha(R,\Phi)) \tag{9.5}$$

and

$$|F(R,\Phi)|\sin(2\pi Rr\sin(\phi-\Phi)+\alpha(R,\Phi)) \tag{9.6}$$

are *harmonic functions of two polar variables* (r,ϕ) with *frequency* $|R|$, *direction* Φ, *amplitude* $|F(R,\Phi)|$, and *initial phase* $\alpha(R,\Phi)$.

What do harmonic functions of two polar variables look like? Note first of all that if we fix ϕ, then the resulting function of r is a harmonic function with amplitude $|F(R,\Phi)|$, initial phase $\alpha(R,\Phi)$, and frequency $|R\cos(\phi-\Phi)|$. In particular, on the line L through the origin that makes an angle Φ with the x axis (the line $\phi=\Phi$), the resulting harmonic function has frequency $|R|$. On any line perpendicular to L (i.e., on any line with equation $r\cos(\phi-\Phi)=r_0$, where r_0 is constant), the harmonic function of two polar variables is constant (see Fig. 9.1).

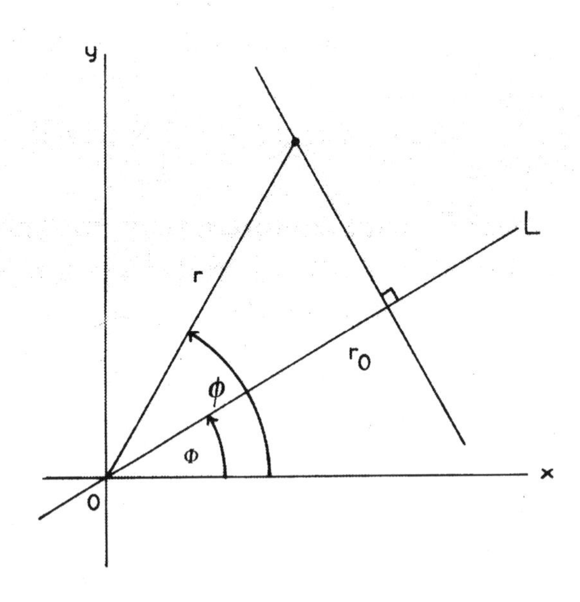

Fig. 9.1: A harmonic function of two polar variables (r,ϕ) with frequency R and direction Φ is, when restricted to the line L for which $\phi=\Phi$, a harmonic function of the variable r with frequency R. On any line perpendicular to L (such as the line determined by $r\cos(\phi-\Phi)=r_0$), the value of the harmonic function of two polar variables is constant.

If a function f is smooth, we expect a small amplitude $|F(R, \Phi)|$ for components with large $|R|$ in the decomposition (9.4). A function f is said to be *bandlimited* if $[\mathscr{F}_2 f](R, \Phi) = 0$ for $|R| \geq A/2$, where A is a positive real number, called the *bandwidth* of f. (See similar definitions for functions of one variable in Section 8.4.)

Of the many interesting and useful properties of the two-dimensional Fourier transform, the most important one for image reconstruction is the so-called projection theorem. It gives a basic relationship between the Radon transform, the two-dimensional Fourier transform, and an operator $\mathscr{F}_Y$, which is a two-dimensional version of the one-dimensional Fourier transform, defined as follows.

Let p be a function of two variables, and let p_θ be defined, as in (8.11), by $p_\theta(\ell) = p(\ell, \theta)$. Then $\mathscr{F}_Y p$ is another function of two variables defined by

$$[\mathscr{F}_Y p]\,(R, \theta) = [\mathscr{F} p_\theta]\,(R). \tag{9.7}$$

In other words, $\mathscr{F}_Y$ is a *Fourier transform with respect to the first variable.*

The *projection theorem* can now be stated as the operator equation:

$$\mathscr{F}_2 = \mathscr{F}_Y \mathscr{R}. \tag{9.8}$$

In words, taking the two-dimensional Fourier transform is the same as taking the Radon transform and then applying the Fourier transform with respect to the first variable. The proof of the projection theorem follows easily from the definitions of the Radon and Fourier transforms; we omit the details.

9.2 The Fourier Method of Reconstruction

From (9.3) and (9.8) we see that for a function f of two polar variables

$$f = \mathscr{F}_2^{-1} \mathscr{F}_Y \mathscr{R} f. \tag{9.9}$$

This leads to the mathematical idealization of the *Fourier method* of reconstruction. For any function p, representing projection data of an image, we estimate the image by

$$\mathscr{R}^{-1} p = \mathscr{F}_2^{-1} \mathscr{F}_Y p. \tag{9.10}$$

The major difficulty with the Fourier method lies in its implementation on real data. We look at what is involved step by step.

Let us recall our assumption that in the parallel mode of data collection p is known at points $(nd, m\Delta)$, where $-N \leq n \leq N$ and $0 \leq m \leq M-1$, see Fig. 6.2. For any value of R, we may calculate $[\mathscr{F}_Y p](R, m\Delta)$ using (9.7) in conjunction with (8.11) and (8.27) as

$$[\mathscr{F}_Y p](R, m\Delta) = \int_{-E}^{E} p(\ell, m\Delta) \exp(-2\pi i R\ell)\, d\ell. \tag{9.11}$$

We have made use of the fact that $p_\theta(\ell) = 0$ if $|\ \ell\ | \geq E$.

The right-hand side of (9.11) has to be numerically evaluated for some selected values of R. A Riemann sum approximation using the sample points gives:

$$[\mathscr{F}_Y p](R, m\Delta) \simeq d \sum_{n=-N}^{N} p(nd, m\Delta) \exp\left(-2\pi i R n d\right). \tag{9.12}$$

This approximation is accurate for at most a limited range of values of R. In fact, the right-hand side of (9.12) is equal to

$$F_1(R) = \sum_{k=-\infty}^{\infty} [\mathscr{F}_Y p](R + k/d, m\Delta). \tag{9.13}$$

The use of the same function name, F_1, that has been defined in (8.41) and discussed in detail in Section 8.6 is not accidental; as simple observation shows, the function defined in (9.13) is the same function that was called F_1 in Chapter 8. As discussed in Section 8.6, $F_1(R)$ can only be an accurate approximation of $[\mathscr{F}_Y p](R, m\Delta)$ $(= [\mathscr{F} p_{m\Delta}](R))$ if $|\ R\ | < 1/2d$, and it may be inaccurate even within that interval, especially near its two ends. For $|R| > 1/2d$, it is probably better to approximate $[\mathscr{F}_Y p](R, m\Delta)$ by zero than by the use of (9.12).

Also, we have to select the points R in the interval $-1/2d \leq R \leq 1/2d$ at which we wish to evaluate $[\mathscr{F}_Y p](R, m\Delta)$. It is computationally desirable, for reasons that are now given, to select values of R that are multiples of $1/(2N+1)d$. Note that this is not a real restriction on how finely these sample points are spaced, since the evaluation in (9.12) would not change if we decided to use a larger value for N. (Recall that $p(nd, m\Delta) = 0$ if $nd \geq E$.) Combining these statements we see that the first step of the Fourier method is to estimate, for $0 \leq m \leq M - 1$, $-N \leq n' \leq N$, $[\mathscr{F}_Y p]\left(n'/(2N + 1)d, m\Delta\right)$ by

$$[\mathscr{F}_Y p]\left(\frac{n'}{(2N+1)d}, m\Delta\right) \simeq d \sum_{n=-N}^{N} p(nd, m\Delta) \exp\left(\frac{-2\pi i n n'}{2N+1}\right). \tag{9.14}$$

The right-hand side of (9.14) is d multiplied by what is called the *discrete Fourier transform* in the first variable of the sampled version of p. We introduce the abbreviation

$$[\mathscr{D}\mathscr{F}_Y p](n', m) = \sum_{n=-N}^{N} p(nd, m\Delta) \exp\left(\frac{-2\pi i n n'}{2N+1}\right). \tag{9.15}$$

The evaluation of $\mathscr{D}\mathscr{F}_Y p$ at the $M(2N+1)$ points $(0 \leq m \leq M-1, -N \leq n' \leq N)$ is much less expensive than it would appear at first sight. Note first of all that, just as in FBP, we deal with each view separately. The $2N + 1$ different values of $[\mathscr{D}\mathscr{F}_Y p](n', m)$ for a fixed m but varying n', are evaluated from the $2N + 1$ values of $p(nd, m\Delta)$, for the same fixed m and varying n. Since the values of $\exp(-2\pi inn'/(2N+1))$ can be precalculated and stored (they do not depend on the data), it appears that the evaluation of (9.15), for a fixed m but varying n', requires $2(2N+1)^2$ multiplications. (The factor 2 in the front comes from the fact that in each term of the sum a real number is multiplied by a complex number, which requires two real multiplications.) However, there is a much more efficient way of evaluating (9.15) for $-N \leq n' \leq N$ than the method that evaluates the expression for each value of n' separately. This method is called the *fast Fourier transform* (FFT). Its description is beyond the scope of this book, but we must comment on its performance, since this is essential in appreciating the computational efficiency of the Fourier reconstruction method.

Using FFT, the calculation of (9.15), for a fixed m but for all the $2N+1$ values of n' between $-N$ and N, requires approximately $N(3 + \lceil \log_2 N \rceil)$ multiplications, where $\lceil \log_2 N \rceil$ is the smallest integer not smaller than the base 2 logarithm of N.

Consider the standard parallel projection data. In this case $M = 360$ and $N = 172$, and the straightforward evaluation of (9.15) requires $2M(2N+1)^2 = 85{,}698{,}800$ multiplications. Using the FFT, we need $MN(3 + \lceil \log_2 N \rceil) = 681{,}120$. This is a reduction by over two orders of magnitude, a very considerable saving. In commercial scanners, where N may be several times larger than in our example, the saving is even more substantial. Thus, by using the FFT, the first step of the Fourier method consisting of the evaluation of (9.15), for $0 \leq m \leq M-1$, $-N \leq n' \leq N$, can be done at a relatively low cost.

We are now faced with the problem of numerically evaluating $\mathscr{F}_2^{-1}\mathscr{F}_Y p$ of (9.10) based on the estimated values of $\mathscr{F}_Y p$ at the points $(n/(2N+1)d, m\Delta)$. One possible way of doing this is to combine our claim that $[\mathscr{F}_Y p](R, m\Delta)$ is best approximated by zero for $|R| \geq E$ with the Riemann sum approximation of (9.2) and obtain the estimated picture

$$f^*(r,\phi) = \frac{\Delta}{2N+1} \sum_{m=0}^{M-1} \sum_{n=-N}^{N} \left| \frac{n}{(2N+1)d} \right| [\mathscr{D}\mathscr{F}_Y p](n,m) \times \exp\left(\frac{2\pi in}{(2N+1)d} r \cos(\phi - m\Delta) \right). \tag{9.16}$$

In fact, the Fourier reconstruction method is usually not implemented in this way. The reason for this is computational. Getting back to our example of the head phantom and the standard parallel projection data, we see that f^* has to be evaluated at $J = 243 \times 243 = 59{,}049$ points. If (9.16) is used separately for each point, then the total number of the required multiplications is

$$2JM(2N+1) > 10^{10}, \tag{9.17}$$

even if we assume that the values

$$\frac{\Delta}{2N+1}\left|\frac{n}{(2N+1)d}\right| \exp\left(\frac{2\pi i n}{(2N+1)d} r\cos(\phi - m\Delta)\right) \tag{9.18}$$

are precalculated and stored. This is quite a sizable computational requirement, especially since our example is actually small as compared with a commercial scanner, for which the number of calculations would be at least an order of magnitude larger. Another way of indicating the unreasonableness of implementing the Fourier method using (9.16) is to consider the total number of multiplications needed for FBP for the head phantom and standard parallel projection data. As the reader can easily work out, it is less than 10^8, which is more than two orders of magnitude less than what was calculated for evaluating (9.16). Clearly, a better alternative method has to be found for numerically evaluating $\mathscr{F}_2^{-1}\mathscr{F}_Y p$ based on the estimated values of $\mathscr{F}_Y p$ at the points $(n/(2N+1)d, m\Delta)$.

One way is to break up the evaluation of (9.16) into a two-stage process:

(i) For each m, $0 \le m \le M-1$, we evaluate $p_c(n'd, m\Delta)$, for $-N \le n' \le N$, using

$$p_c(n'd, m\Delta) = \frac{1}{(2N+1)^2 d} \sum_{n=-N}^{N} \mid n \mid [\mathscr{D}\mathscr{F}_Y p](n', m) \exp\left(\frac{2\pi i n n'}{2N+1}\right). \tag{9.19}$$

(ii) $f^*(r, \phi)$ is then calculated by

$$f^*(r, \phi) = \Delta \sum_{m=0}^{M-1} p_c(r\cos(\phi - m\Delta), m\Delta). \tag{9.20}$$

This involves interpolation for approximating $p_c(r\cos(\phi - m\Delta), m\Delta)$ from values of $p_c(n'd, m\Delta)$.

This approach is just about identical to FBP, except that p_c is defined by (9.19) rather than by (8.23). In fact, (9.19) can be rewritten as a discrete convolution of p with a convolving function q, and so the approach just described is essentially identical to FBP. We therefore say no more about it in this chapter.

An alternative efficient implementation, and this is the alternative that we refer to as the *Fourier method*, makes use of the availability of a two-dimensional fast Fourier transform. There is a version of the FFT that can be used to estimate the values of the two-dimensional inverse Fourier transform $\mathscr{F}_2^{-1}F$ at J points from the values of F at J points, and the number of multiplications required for this process is of the order $J\log_2 J$. (The point-by-point Riemann sum evaluation discussed previously requires order J^2 multiplications.)

The difficulty with this process is that the points at which $\mathscr{F}_2^{-1}$ are to be calculated and the points at which the values of F have to be given must lie in a regular rectangular arrangement (such as the centers of pixels provided by

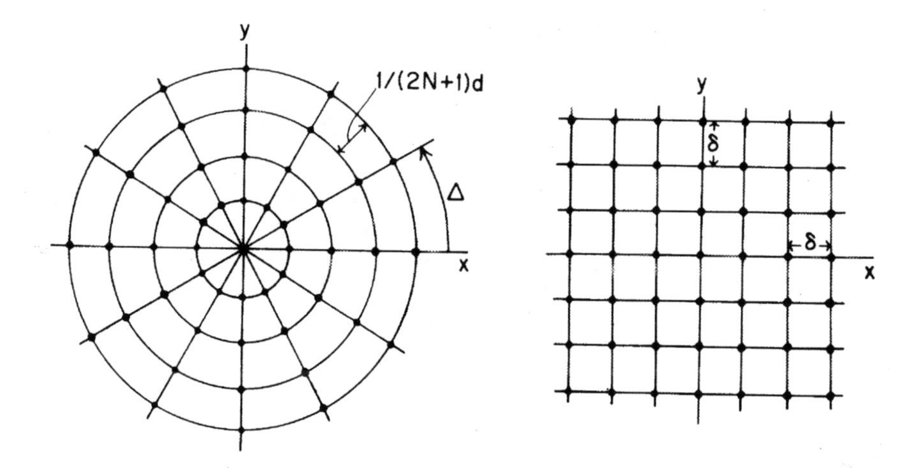

Fig. 9.2: Left: The arrangement of points at which we have estimates of $\mathscr{F}_Y p$. Right: The arrangement of points at which we need to know the values of a function before the inverse two-dimensional fast Fourier transform can be applied.

an n-element grid, see Section 4.1). For our application this is not a restriction as far as the output is concerned, since we desire to estimate $f^* = \mathscr{F}_2^{-1}\mathscr{F}_Y p$ at points that are centers of pixels. The input is a different matter. The first stage of the Fourier method provides us with values at points with polar coordinates $(n/(2N+1)d, m\Delta)$. These points lie in a radial arrangement, rather than in a rectangular one (see Fig. 9.2).

Hence, the Fourier method of reconstruction has two further stages beyond the already described first stage. The second stage is the approximation of the values of $\mathscr{F}_Y p$ at points on a rectangular grid from the values of $\mathscr{F}_Y p$ produced by the first stage (on a radial grid). The third stage is the use of the fast Fourier transform to obtain f^* at the centers of pixels. It is beyond the scope of this book to give a detailed description of these two stages, but we mention some considerations that go into the design of a Fourier method to ensure that it provides acceptable reconstructions.

A major difficulty comes from the fact that the FFT algorithm only provides an estimate of the two-dimensional inverse Fourier transform. The relationship between the output of the FFT and the true inverse Fourier transform is similar to the one between the function F_1 of (9.13) and $\mathscr{F} p_{m\Delta}$. In particular, if the spacing between the points at which values of $\mathscr{F}_Y p$ are interpolated is δ (see Fig. 9.2), then the output of the FFT can only be accurate in the rectangular region defined by $\mid r\cos\phi \mid < 1/2\delta$ and $\mid r\sin\phi \mid < 1/2\delta$. Furthermore, near the edges of this region it is likely to be contaminated with aliasing errors (see Section 8.6). Hence, to get an accurate reconstruction, we have to select δ small enough so that $1/\delta$ is considerably larger than E. This has two computationally undesirable consequences.

First, the FFT has to be calculated for a number of points that is much larger than J (the number of pixels in the final display), corresponding to additional pixels that are introduced to make the picture region $1/\delta \times 1/\delta$ instead of $E \times E$. The necessary increase may be as large as a factor of 9 (if $1/\delta = 3E$), removing much of the computational advantage of the FFT.

Second, in order to have accurate estimates of $\mathscr{F}_Y p$ at the rectangular grid with spacing δ, we may have to evaluate during the first stage of the process $\mathscr{F}_Y p$ at points $(n'/(2N'+1)d, m\Delta)$ with an N' that is greater than N, where $2N+1$ is the number of lines in a view. Doing this for all points n' such that $-N \leq n' \leq N$ results in a further increase in computational cost.

The calculated values of $[\mathscr{F}_Y p](n'/(2N'+1)d, m\Delta)$ for $\mid n' \mid$ near N' may be inaccurate (see (9.13) and the discussion in Section 8.6). It sometimes improves the result if, prior to interpolation, $F_Y p$ is multiplied pointwise by a window function $F_{1/d}$ of the type defined in Table 8.1. That is, instead of $[\mathscr{F}_Y p](n/(2N+1)d, m\Delta)$, one uses $[\mathscr{F}_Y p](n/(2N+1)d, m\Delta)F_{1/d}(\mid n \mid /(2N+1)d)$.

So far we have not discussed the interpolation from the polar to the rectangular grid. There are a number of ways of doing this. A relatively inexpensive method is *bilinear interpolation*, which approximates the value of $\mathscr{F}_Y p$ at a point P of the rectangular grid from its already-approximated values at four points A, B, C, and D of the polar grid. These four points are chosen so that the region between the lines AB and CD and the arcs AC and BD contains P and that this region is the smallest possible such region. In this case the interpolation is done by first linearly interpolating along the radial lines and then linearly interpolating along a circular arc. Unfortunately, this inexpensive interpolation is not good enough; when incorporated into the Fourier method, the resulting reconstructions are of much worse quality than what is provided by FBP. The underlying reason for this is that even for reasonably smooth functions, their Fourier transforms may be quite oscillatory, as can be seen for example in Fig. 8.5. Linear interpolation reduces the amplitudes of such oscillations and thereby destroys essential information regarding the object to be reconstructed.

There are alternative methods of interpolation that overcome this problem, but we do not discuss them in this book. We turn instead to a different approach that does away altogether with the need of performing explicit interpolations to approximate the values of a Fourier transform at new points from its already-approximated values at other points.

9.3 Linograms

Just as in the Fourier method of reconstruction, the method using linograms is based on the projection theorem (9.8). We first explain the reason for the terminology.

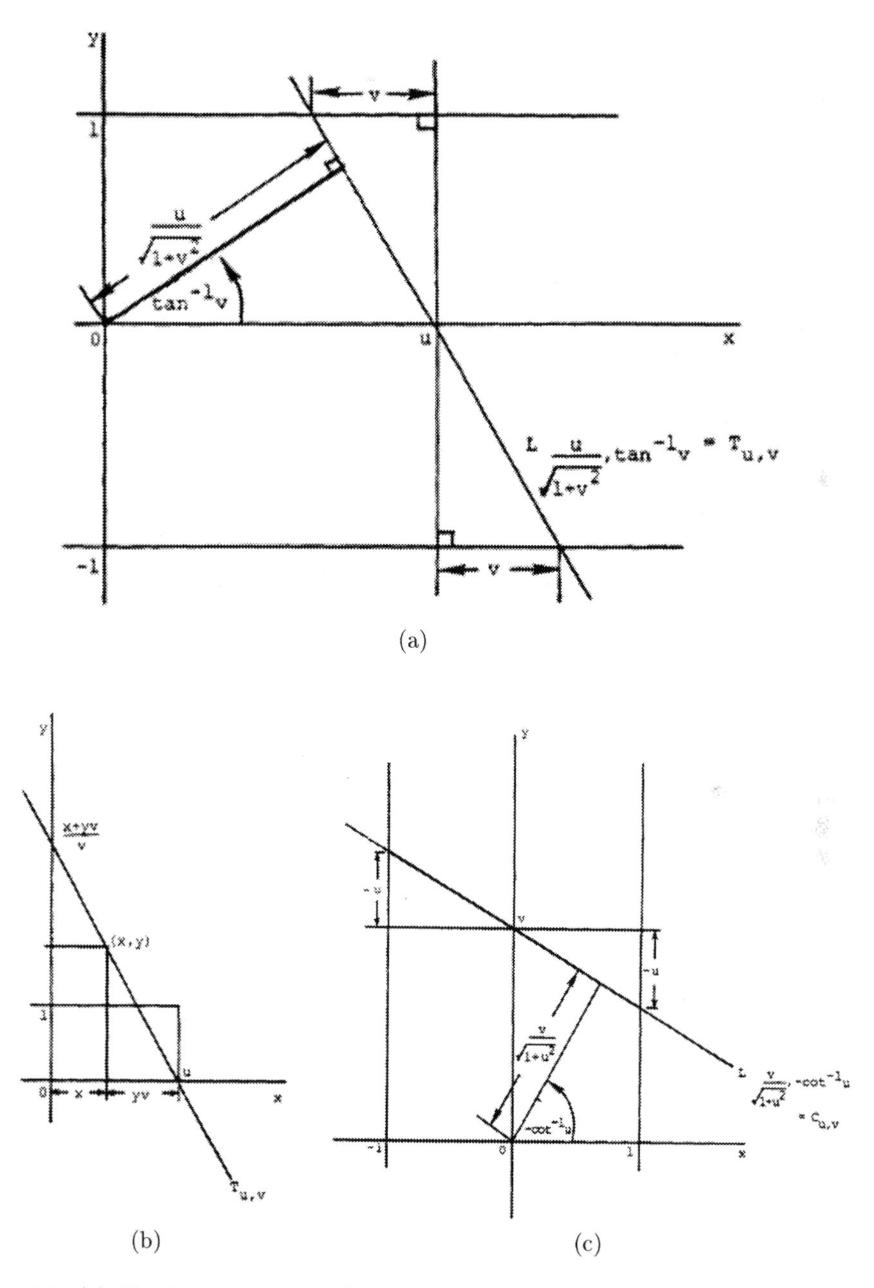

Fig. 9.3: (a) The location in the (x, y) space of the line $T_{u,v}$. (b) A geometrical illustration that for each line $T_{u,v}$ that goes through a fixed point (x, y) the parameters (u, v) must satisfy (9.22). (c) The location in the (x, y) space of the line $C_{u,v}$. (Reproduced from [72] with permission, © 1987 IEEE.)

As can be seen in Fig. 6.1, when lines are parametrized by (ℓ, θ), as defined in Fig. 2.4, then the locus of the points in (ℓ, θ) space that corresponds to the set of lines going through a fixed point in the (r, ϕ) space is a sinusoid. Consequently, when the projection data are displayed as an image in which the gray level at a point with rectangular coordinates (ℓ, θ) is proportional to the estimated line integral $p(\ell, \theta)$, we see a superposition of sinusoids, as in Fig. 1.5(b), and that is why such an image is referred to as a *sinogram*. Consider now an alternate parametrization (u, v) of lines, which has the property that the locus of the points in (u, v) space that corresponds to the set of lines going through a fixed point in the (r, ϕ) space is a line. Consequently, when the projection data are displayed as an image in which the gray level at a point with rectangular coordinates (u, v) is proportional to the estimated integral along the line parametrized by (u, v), we see a superposition of lines and such an image can be referred to as a *linogram*.

Using $L_{\ell,\theta}$ to denote the line parametrized by (ℓ, θ), we define the line parametrized by (u, v) as

$$T_{u,v} = L_{\frac{u}{\sqrt{1+v^2}}, \tan^{-1} v}, \tag{9.21}$$

see Fig. 9.3(a). All lines $L_{\ell,\theta}$ can be parametrized in this way, with the exception of those for which $\theta = \frac{\pi}{2}$ (since there is no real number v for which $\tan^{-1} v = \frac{\pi}{2}$). Using the rectangular coordinates (x, y), rather than the polar coordinates (r, ϕ), it is easy to show that $T_{u,v}$ goes through (x, y) if, and only if,

$$yv - u + x = 0; \tag{9.22}$$

a geometrical illustration of this fact is given in Fig. 9.3(b). This proves that, for every fixed (x, y), the locus of those points in the (u, v) space for which $T_{u,v}$ goes through (x, y) is a line.

To overcome the problem of not being able to represent lines $L_{\ell,\theta}$ for which $\theta = \frac{\pi}{2}$ as a $T_{u,v}$ (as well as for some other reasons that are soon to become obvious), we introduce the alternative (u, v) parametrization of lines

$$C_{u,v} = L_{\frac{v}{\sqrt{1+u^2}}, -\cot^{-1} u}, \tag{9.23}$$

see Fig. 9.3(c). Note that lines $L_{\ell,\theta}$ for which $\theta = 0$ cannot be parametrized this way. Clearly, the $C_{u,v}$ representation also leads to linograms. In what follows we use the $T_{u,v}$ representation for those lines $L_{\ell,\theta}$ for which $-\pi/4 \leq \theta < \pi/4$ and the $C_{u,v}$ representation for those lines $L_{\ell,\theta}$ for which $\pi/4 \leq \theta < 3\pi/4$.

The linogram property has some very interesting mathematical consequences that lead to very efficient reconstruction algorithms. The essential idea is that since in the linogram representation backprojection corresponds to integration along straight lines, it is possible to express the backprojection operator $\mathscr{B}$ defined in (6.14) in terms of the Radon transform $\mathscr{R}$ defined in (6.4) and simple changes of variables. In this book we do not go into the details of the mathematical theory, but concentrate instead on specifying the reconstruction algorithm that is based on it.

For such a specification, it is easiest to assume that the data were collected in a particular way. It is possible to adapt the method to more general modes of data collection, but we will not go into that here. To define the data collection, let us assume that an estimate f^* produced by the method is to be evaluated at points of a $(2W+1) \times (2W+1)$ regular rectangular grid that covers the picture region. Let d denote the distance between nearest neighbor grid points, both horizontally and vertically. Then the linogram reconstruction method that we explain in the rest of this section assumes that the complete projection data set available to us consists of the two subsets:

$$\{p(nd_m, \theta_m) \mid -2W-1 \le n \le 2W+1,\ -2W-1 \le m \le 2W+1\} \quad (9.24)$$

and

$$\{p(nd_m, \theta_m + {\pi}/{2}) \mid -2W-1 \le n \le 2W+1,\ -2W-1 \le m \le 2W+1\}, \quad (9.25)$$

$$\theta_m = \tan^{-1}\frac{2m}{4W+3} \quad \text{and} \quad d_m = d\cos\theta_m. \quad (9.26)$$

For $-2W-1 \le m \le 2W+1$, we have that $-{\pi}/{4} \le \theta_m < {\pi}/{4}$ in (9.24) and ${\pi}/{4} \le \theta_m < {3\pi}/{4}$ in (9.25). In fact, the samplings described in these equations come from uniform samplings in u and v of the lines $T_{u,v}$ and $C_{u,v}$, respectively. This is of course different from our standard parallel mode of data collection, which samples ℓ and θ uniformly, see Fig. 6.2.

The linogram reconstruction method consists of five steps:

(i) Fourier transforming the data.
(ii) Windowing.
(ii) Separating into two functions.
(iv) Chirp z-transforming in one of the variables.
(v) Inverse transforming in the other variable.

In the first step, for each value of the second variable in (9.24) and (9.25), we estimate the Fourier transform in the first variable using the FFT. By the projection theorem, the nature of the FFT and (9.26), this provides us with estimates of the two-dimensional Fourier transform of the object to be reconstructed at the points (in the rectangular coordinate system)

$$\left\{\left(\frac{k}{(4W+3)d}, \frac{2km}{(4W+3)^2 d}\right) \middle| -2W-1 \le k,\ m \le 2W+1\right\} \quad (9.27)$$

and

$$\left\{\left(\frac{2km}{(4W+3)^2 d}, \frac{k}{(4W+3)d}\right) \middle| -2W-1 \le k,\ m \le 2W+1\right\}. \quad (9.28)$$

The intuition behind the windowing in the linogram method is the following. Consider the formulation of FBP in (8.19). Where the linogram method diverges from FBP is in its implementational details, which are based on a theorem (not stated in this book) giving an alternate mathematical expression for the f^* of (8.19). Just as in (8.19), this expression also depends on a window function F_A, see (8.21). The role of the window function is made explicit in (8.44), in which the Fourier transform of the processed projection data is expressed as the product of three terms. The first term is F_1, which is the Fourier transform of the unprocessed projection data; one can think of the first step described in the previous paragraph as the evaluation of F_1 for the linogram data. The third term is F_3, which has to do with the interpolation needed for backprojection; it is one of the advantages of the linogram method that it does not use any explicit interpolations and so we do not have to worry about F_3 at all. On the other hand, F_2 comes from the window function; in order to produce a linogram result that matches the idealized FBP result, we need to multiply the values obtained as described in the previous paragraphs by $|U|\, F_{1/d}\,(|U|)$. Since $U = 0$ when $k = 0$ in (9.27) and (9.28), the information regarding the value of the Fourier transform at the origin is lost. This is equivalent to losing the information regarding the total density of the picture; we discuss this in greater detail in the next section.

The two steps described so far give us, for the points specified by (9.27) and (9.28), values that can be roughly interpreted as samples of a function F from which our reconstruction should be estimated by some kind of Fourier inversion. An essential trick of the linogram method is to write $F = G + H$, where G has the same values as F at the points specified by (9.27) and is zero-valued elsewhere, while H has the same values as F at the points specified by (9.28) and is zero-valued elsewhere. As we soon explain, Fourier inversion of both G and H can be carried out accurately and efficiently. Summing the results of these inversions and adding a constant to bring the average value of the reconstructed picture to that of the accurately estimated average value (see Section 6.4, especially the discussion following (6.44)), provides us with the output of the linogram method. The next two steps are described for the inversion of G only; the treatment of H is strictly analogous.

Looking carefully at the set of (9.27), we see uniform sampling in the first variable. Also, for any fixed value of its first variable, sampling is uniform in the second variable, although the sampling rate varies with the value of the first variable. Taking the inverse two-dimensional Fourier transform using rectangular coordinates can be done by taking sequentially the one-dimensional inverse Fourier transform in the second variable and then taking a one-dimensional inverse Fourier transform in the first variable. The problem with the data as presented by (9.27) is that if we use the FFT for the second variable, we end up after inversion with values at points whose spacing depends on the first variable and these values do not line up suitably for taking the inverse Fourier transform in the first variable using the FFT. This is where our separation into two functions comes into play. For any fixed value of the first variable, the sampling of G in the second variable that is provided by (9.27) is uniform and we know that the value of G is zero outside the sampled region. Under these circumstances there is an alternative fast way of inverting the Fourier transform, called the *chirp z-transform,* that can be used to estimate the inverse Fourier transform at any user-specified sampling distance (and not just at the one that would be automatically provided by the FFT). The chirp z-transform can be implemented using three FFTs. We use it to estimate, for each value of the first variable, the one-dimensional inverse Fourier transform in the second variable at $2W + 1$ points with sampling distance d.

In the final step, we perform, for each value of the second variable, an inverse one-dimensional FFT in the first variable to obtain the estimated reconstruction at all the points of our specified regular rectangular grid.

In order to compare the performance of FBP with that of the linogram method, we need to apply FBP to data collected in the linogram mode. This is easy to do, since the Riemann sum approximations used to evaluate the convolution and the backprojection in (8.19) do not actually require that the sampling distances in angles and between lines be uniform all through the data collection, a slight alteration to the previously presented discrete formulas provides the needed more general implementation. For our experiments we used all the parameters for the standard parallel projection data except for the sampling: using the linogram mode for a 243×243 image (i.e., $W = 121$), we needed to generate 974 projection directions with data collected for 487 parallel lines in each. The resulting reconstructions are illustrated in Fig. 9.4. The picture distance measures and timings are given in Table 9.1.

Note that FBP needed nearly five times as much computer time as the linogram method. While the exact timings are implementation dependent, the basic tendency is that the linogram method is faster than FBP, since it uses only FFTs, while FBP needs to perform a backprojection, which requires a considerably larger number of computer operations.

Regarding the relative accuracy of the two reconstructions we note, especially in Fig. 9.4(c), that the reconstructed values in the linogram method are slightly elevated. Since, as discussed in the third step of the linogram method, we made sure that the average density in the reconstruction region is correct, this seems curious. In fact, the average densities of the two reconstructions of Fig. 9.4 are exactly the same. The linogram reconstruction has slightly lower values in the corners of the picture region (these cannot be seen in our displays due to the selected display window) and this is compensated for by slightly elevated values in the rest of the picture region.

Table 9.1: Picture distance measures and timings (in seconds) for the reconstructions from linogram data in Fig. 9.4, as well as the average FOMs.

reconstruction method	d	r	t	IROI	HITR
FBP	0.0625	0.0262	3.7	0.2885	0.9921
linogram	0.0647	0.0281	0.8	0.3092	0.9945

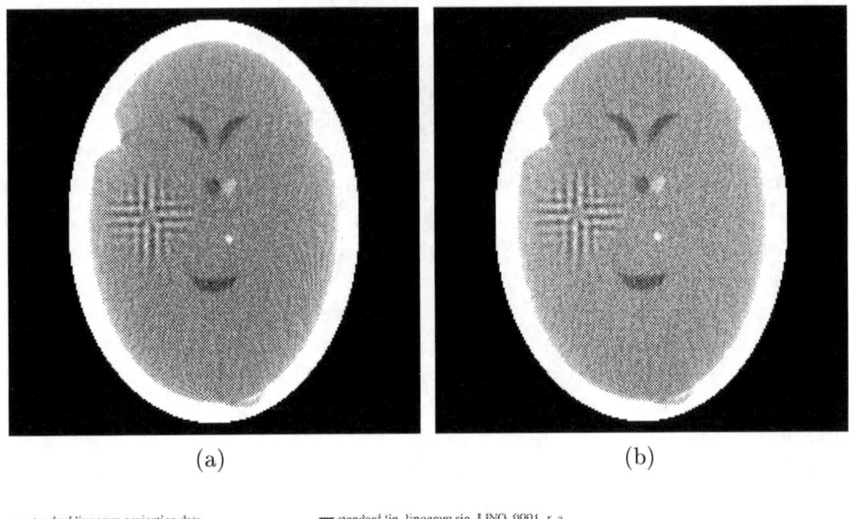

(a) (b)

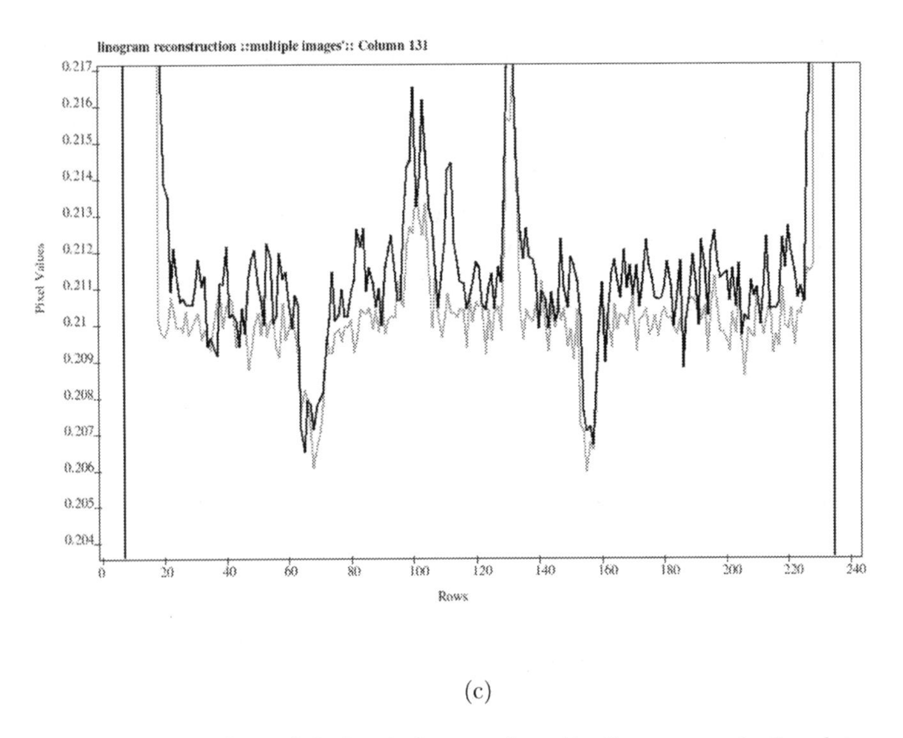

(c)

Fig. 9.4: Reconstructions of the head phantom from the linogram projection data. (a) Using FBP with the sinc window and linear interpolation. (b) Using the linogram method with the sinc window. (c) Plots of the 131st column of the phantom (light) and the linogram reconstruction (dark).

As far as tumor detectability is concerned, a uniform elevation of values within the skull should make no difference; tumors are detected by the contrast to their backgrounds. In fact, examining the IROI figure of merit (5.3), we see that if we add the same density to all pixels in the reconstruction, it will make no difference to the value of IROI. The same is clearly true for HITR. So, while the inaccuracies in the reconstructed densities in the linogram method that are mentioned in the previous paragraph adversely affect the picture distance measures, they may have no effect on a task-oriented measure of algorithm performance. This is indeed the case for our task of detecting small low-contrast tumors. Using either of our two FOMs, the null-hypothesis that the linogram method and FBP, both using the sinc window, are equally efficacious can be rejected in favor of the alternative hypothesis that the linogram method is better with P-value less than 10^{-5}. (The average values of the FOMs are given in Table 9.1.) This, combined with the superior speed of the linogram method, implies that, in spite of all that has been said in Section 8.7, FBP is not necessarily the reconstruction algorithm of choice!

It is worth emphasizing the reasons for the superior performance of the linogram method. The speed comes from having to do only FFTs in steps (i), (iv) and (v), and even less time-consuming operations in the other two steps. The accuracy comes from not having to do interpolations at all; the way the data collection is determined by (9.24) and (9.25) ensures that the points at which values are needed for any of the five steps are points at which those values were calculated in the previous step. If the data are collected according to a different scheme, one can estimate what the data would have been if it were collected as for linograms. This can be done by interpolation of the measured projections, which is a less challenging task than the interpolation of the Fourier transforms of the projection data, since the original data tends to be locally much smoother than its Fourier transform (compare the sinogram in Fig. 1.5(b) with the Fourier transform of a single projection in Fig. 8.5).

9.4 Rho-Filtered Layergram

In our discussion of the continuous backprojection method we have pointed out that the method produces a blurred version of the original picture, where the contribution of the original density at a point A to the reconstructed density at a point B is inversely proportional to the distance between the two points. The *rho-filtered layergram* is a method that attempts to deblur the picture that is obtained by backprojection alone.

The method of deblurring is based on a relationship between the two-dimensional Fourier transform of a picture and the two-dimensional Fourier transform of the backprojected Radon transform of the picture. This relationship is given by

$$[\mathscr{F}_2 f](R, \Phi) = | R | \times [\mathscr{F}_2 \mathscr{B} \mathscr{R} f](R, \Phi), \tag{9.29}$$

for any point (R, Φ) with $R \neq 0$.

Equation (9.29) gives rise to a four-stage process for estimating a picture f from projection data p:

(i) Backproject p, to obtain $\mathscr{B}p$.
(ii) Calculate the two-dimensional Fourier transform $\mathscr{F}_2\mathscr{B}p$.
(iii) Obtain a new function F of two polar variables by

$$F(R, \Phi) = \mid R \mid \times [\mathscr{F}_2\mathscr{B}p](R, \Phi). \tag{9.30}$$

(iv) Estimate the picture by

$$f^* = \mathscr{F}_2^{-1} F. \tag{9.31}$$

The reason for the name of the method is the following. The result of the process of backprojection has sometimes been called in the literature a *layergram*. In the articles that introduced the concept of the rho-filtered layergram, the first polar variable of the two-dimensional Fourier transform was denoted by the Greek letter ρ (rho), and hence the operations described in (ii)–(iv) were given the name rho-filtering.

The difficulty with the rho-filtered layergram is its implementation. We discuss the implementation of the four steps just described one by one.

It is easy to estimate the value of $\mathscr{B}p$ at any point (r,ϕ) using a Riemann sum approximation combined with an interpolation (see Section 7.2). However, even though $p(\ell, \theta) = 0$ for $\mid \ell \mid \geq E$, there is no value of E' such that $[\mathscr{B}p](r,\phi) = 0$ for $r \geq E'$. In other words, the set of points at which $\mathscr{B}p$ is not zero is unbounded. On the other hand, as the reader can easily prove, it is the case that

$$\lim_{r \to \infty} \sup_{0 \leq \phi \leq 2\pi} [\mathscr{B}p](r, \phi) = 0, \tag{9.32}$$

i.e., $[\mathscr{B}p](r,\phi)$ is guaranteed to be arbitrarily small provided r is large enough.

In practice, we can evaluate $\mathscr{B}p$ only at finitely many points. In view of the fact that the next thing to be done is to apply the two-dimensional Fourier transform to $\mathscr{B}p$, it makes sense to evaluate $\mathscr{B}p$ at equally-spaced points of a rectangular grid. (Recall our discussion of the FFT for two-dimensional Fourier transforms in Section 9.2.) The central part of this grid should form the picture region, with the pixel centers being points on a regular rectangular grid. The rest of the grid should form a frame around the picture region. The frame should be big enough so that the values of $\mathscr{B}p$ outside it can be ignored with relative safety.

For the second stage of the rho-filtered layergram, we apply the FFT to estimate $\mathscr{F}_2\mathscr{B}p$ from values of $\mathscr{B}p$. As discussed before, the number of points at which the FFT provides us with estimates of $\mathscr{F}_2\mathscr{B}p$ is the same as the number of points at which we had estimates for $\mathscr{B}p$. The spacing (parallel to the rectangular axis) between the points at which we have estimates of $\mathscr{F}_2\mathscr{B}p$ is the inverse of the size of the backprojection region (i.e, the picture region plus the frame around it that is discussed in the previous paragraph).

Estimates of $\mathscr{F}_2\mathscr{B}p$ at points near the edge of the rectangular grid on which it is estimated are usually unreliable, because of aliasing and noise in the data. (This statement is not supported by anything we have said in this section. However, the reader should be able to argue this out, similarly to what we have presented on this matter for FBP and the Fourier method.)

Implementation of the third stage is a trivial matter. However, for reasons that are similar to those given in previous sections, rather than multiplying by $\mid R \mid$, we multiply by $\mid R \mid \times F_{1/d}(\mid R \mid)$, where $F_{1/d}$ is a window function whose bandwidth is the inverse of the sampling distance.

An important fact trivially follows from (9.30): $F(0, \Phi) = 0$. Looking at (9.31), (9.3), and (9.1), we see that this means that

$$\int_0^\pi \int_{-\infty}^\infty \mid r \mid f^*(r, \phi)\, dr\, d\phi = 0, \tag{9.33}$$

which says that the total density of the estimate f^* is zero, irrespective of the nature of the picture f that we are estimating. This appears at first sight to be very undesirable, but two comments are in order.

First, (9.33) is somewhat misleading. The function f^* defined by it may (and usually does) have nonzero values everywhere in the plane. Knowing that we are estimating a picture, we can set all values outside the picture region to zero. The resulting picture function may very well have a total density that is nearly the same as that of the picture we are attempting to reconstruct.

Second, the problem is not new, but it has never been so obvious before. In FBP, the convolved projection data $p_{m\Delta} * \mathscr{F}^{-1}\Phi$ has zero total density, see (8.31). Nevertheless, in the reconstructions produced by FBP, the total density (inside the picture region) is quite accurate; see Figs. 8.7 and 8.8. Similarly, in the implementation of the Fourier method that is indicated by (9.16), $[\mathscr{D}\mathscr{F}_Y p](0,m)$ is always multiplied by zero, and the value of the total density of $p_{m\Delta}$ is irrelevant, but nevertheless the reported reconstructions with that method also tend to have accurate average density inside the reconstruction region.

However, in the case of the rho-filtered layergram (somewhat similarly to the linogram method) this problem does not resolve itself as nicely as with the two methods mentioned in the previous paragraph. The reason for this is that since the fourth stage is implemented by the use of the FFT, we end up with values of f^* on a rectangular grid that is identical in size and location with the grid onto which we backprojected in the first stage. The sum of the values of f^* on this grid is zero. Unless this grid is very much bigger than the grid associated with the digitized picture region, the total density even in the picture region will be noticeably inaccurate. Fortunately, this can be easily corrected by additive normalization (see Sections 7.2 and 9.3). Note that, in this case, multiplicative normalization is not appropriate.

We do not report in this book on reconstructions using the rho-filtered layergram method.

Notes and References

The relationship between the Radon transform and the Fourier transforms has been studied in a number of mathematical texts; see, for example, [188] and its references. The first mention (and proof) of the projection theorem in application oriented image reconstruction is in [25]. A useful practical text on Fourier transforms is [28].

The equivalence of (9.19) to (8.23) follows from the convolution theorem for the discrete Fourier transform; see, e.g., [28]. Some researchers, e.g., [241], refer to all transform methods, in particular FBP, as "Fourier reconstruction." Since neither the derivation nor the implementation of FBP requires the use of Fourier transforms (although both can be done that way), this name seems inappropriate, especially in view of the fact that the implementational differences between what we called FBP and what we called the Fourier method are sufficiently significant to require separate names to distinguish them. A good overview of early work on the Fourier method can be obtained by reading [201] and its references, especially [60]. The claim of [227] that FBP is superior to the Fourier method is valid for certain implementations, for example if bilinear interpolation is used with the Fourier method. However, recent work involving alternative ways of interpolating indicates otherwise. One particularly efficacious interpolation method is called gridding; this is discussed in the book [211] and also in [82]. An interesting aspect of that line of work is that the recommended interpolation makes use of the blobs that we have introduced in Section 6.5 for a very different reason.

The FFT, very important for the implementation of the methods in this chapter, is of sufficient general importance that there have been whole books devoted to the topic, such as [31].

Linograms were introduced in [72], with details of the implementation of the reconstruction algorithm based on them in [71]. This approach has generated quite a large follow-up literature, a recent example of which is [88]. The linogram mode of data collection can be used with various kinds of instrumentation discussed in Section 1.1, including PET [24, 214, 265] and MRI [15]. Rather interestingly, linograms were reported [16] to be also useful for designing efficient algorithms for truly three-dimensional reconstruction from cone-beam data (see Section 3.4).

The phrase rho-filtered layergram was introduced in [247]. Our development is based on the more detailed study of [234], which also contains reports on experiments with this technique using different windows and interpolating functions. The reader should consult these works for other relevant literature. The method has been extended to the divergent beam data collection techniques in [104]. The WBP method mentioned in the Notes and References of the previous chapter has a variant that is very similar in flavor to the rho-filtered layergram [224].

For implementational details of the reconstruction methods in this chapter the reader should consult [61].

10

Filtered Backprojection for Divergent Beams

An alternative to the parallel mode of data collection is when data are collected so that they naturally divide into subsets containing estimated ray sums for lines diverging from a single point. Our standard projection data are of this type. There are two basic approaches to designing an FBP-type algorithm for such data. The first is to find an FBP-type implementation of the Radon inversion formula that is appropriate for the divergent mode of data collection. The second is to use interpolation in the (ℓ, θ) space to estimate ray sums for sets of parallel lines from the measured ray sums for sets of divergent lines (this process is called *rebinning*) and then apply the parallel beam FBP method. In this chapter we concentrate on the first of these methods. We also return to the topic of window selection in the context of the divergent beam FBP method.

10.1 The Divergent Beam FBP Algorithm

The data collection geometry we deal with is described in Fig. 10.1. The x-ray source is always on a circle of radius D around the origin. The detector strip is an arc centered at the source. Each line can be considered as one of a set of divergent lines (σ, β), where β determines the source position and σ determines which of the lines diverging from this source position we are considering. This is an alternative way of specifying lines to the (ℓ, θ) notation used previously (in particular in Fig. 2.4). Of course, each (σ, β) line is also an (ℓ, θ) line, for some values of ℓ and θ that depend on σ and β. In fact, as is easily seen from Fig. 10.1, the line (σ, β) corresponds to the point $(D \sin \sigma,\ \beta + \sigma)$ in (ℓ, θ) space.

As usual in this book, we use f to denote the function of two polar variables r and ϕ that we wish to reconstruct. Recall that $f(r, \phi) = 0$ if $r \geq E$. We assume that $D > E$ and use δ to denote the inverse sine of E/D. Note that

$$0 < \delta = \sin^{-1}(E/D) < \pi/2. \tag{10.1}$$

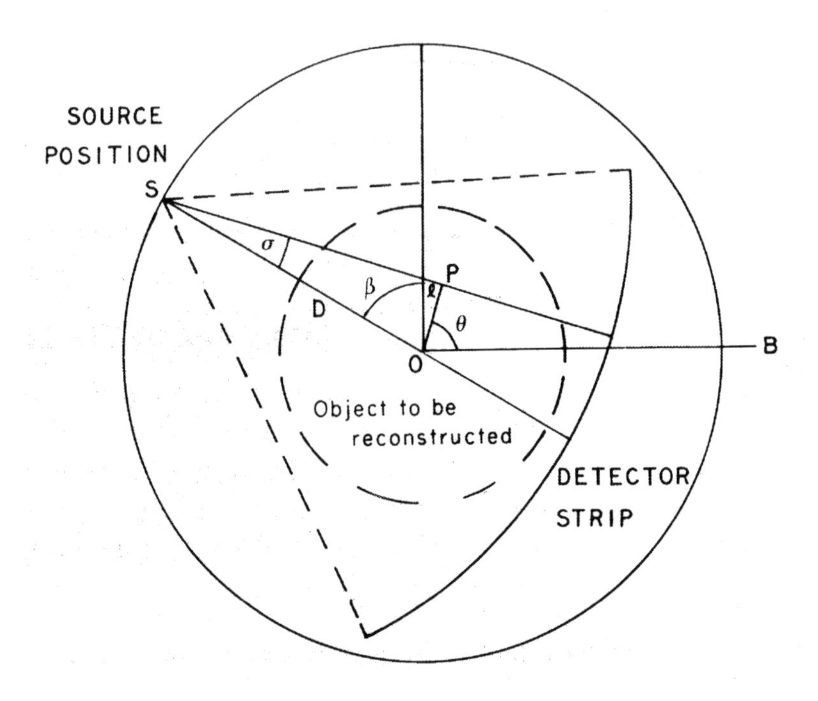

Fig. 10.1: Geometry of divergent beam data collection. Every one of the diverging lines is determined by two parameters β and σ. Let O be the origin and S be the position of the source, which always lies on a circle of radius D around O. Then $\beta + {}^{\pi}/2$ is the angle the line OS makes with the baseline B and σ is the angle the divergent line makes with SO. The divergent line is also one of a set of parallel lines. As such it is determined by the parameters ℓ and θ. Let P be the point at which the divergent line meets the line through O that is perpendicular to it. Then ℓ is the distance from O to P and θ is the angle that OP makes with the baseline. (Reproduced from [115], Copyright 1981.)

We use $g(\sigma, \beta)$ to denote the line integral of f along the line (σ, β). That is,

$$g(\sigma, \beta) = [\mathscr{R} f] (D \sin \sigma,\ \beta + \sigma). \tag{10.2}$$

It follows from (10.1) that $g(\sigma, \beta) = 0$ if $|\sigma| > \delta$.

Suppose we have all possible projection data $g(\sigma, \beta)$ for $0 \leq \beta < 2\pi$ and $|\sigma| \leq \delta$. It can be shown that the Radon inversion formula gives rise to the following. If the derivatives of $g(\sigma, \beta)$ with respect to σ and β both exist and are denoted by $g_1(\sigma, \beta)$ and $g_2(\sigma, \beta)$, then

$$f(r, \phi) = \frac{1}{4\pi^2} \int_0^{2\pi} \int_{-\infty}^{\infty} \frac{1}{\sigma' - \sigma} G(\sigma, \beta, \sigma')\, d\sigma\, d\beta, \tag{10.3}$$

with

$$G(\sigma,\beta,\sigma') = \begin{cases} \dfrac{\sigma'-\sigma}{W\sin(\sigma'-\sigma)}\left(g_1(\sigma,\beta)-g_2(\sigma,\beta)\right), & \text{if } |\sigma|\le\delta, \\ 0, & \text{if } |\sigma|>\delta, \end{cases} \tag{10.4}$$

where

$$\sigma' = \tan^{-1}\frac{r\cos(\beta-\phi)}{D+r\sin(\beta-\phi)}, \qquad -\frac{\pi}{2}\le\sigma'\le\frac{\pi}{2}, \tag{10.5}$$

and

$$W = \left((r\cos(\beta-\phi))^2+(D+r\sin(\beta-\phi))^2\right)^{1/2}, \quad W>0. \tag{10.6}$$

Note that σ' and W depend on β, r, and ϕ, but not on σ. The meanings of σ' and W are that when the source is at angle β, the line that goes through (r,ϕ) is (σ',β) and the distance between the source and (r,ϕ) is W.

We see that (10.3), called the *Radon inversion formula for divergent rays*, is in the form of a singular integral. The inner integral is essentially a Hilbert transform of the function $G(\sigma,\beta,\sigma')$ considered as a function of σ alone. Hence our discussion of regularization in Section 8.1 applies here as well.

Let us assume that the function $G(\sigma,\beta,\sigma')$, as a function of σ, is reasonable at the point σ. Then, for any choice of $\{F_A \mid A>0\}$ that satisfies the conditions stated prior to (8.10), we get a family of regularizing functions $\{\rho_A \mid A>0\}$ such that (10.3) can be rewritten in the form

$$f(r,\phi) = \lim_{A\to\infty}\frac{1}{4\pi^2}\int_0^{2\pi}\int_{-\infty}^{\infty}\rho_A(\sigma'-\sigma)G(\sigma,\beta,\sigma')\,d\sigma\,d\beta, \tag{10.7}$$

see (8.9) and (8.10). The advantage of rewriting (10.3) as (10.7) is that for any fixed A the inner integral in (10.7) is easy to handle, since one can evaluate it using integration by parts. We denote the approximation to f provided by a fixed A by $\tilde{f}$, that is

$$\tilde{f}(r,\phi) = \frac{1}{4\pi^2}\int_0^{2\pi}\int_{-\infty}^{\infty}\rho_A(\sigma'-\sigma)G(\sigma,\beta,\sigma')\,d\sigma\,d\beta. \tag{10.8}$$

Having chosen a particular function ρ_A as the regularizing function, substitution of the value of $G(\sigma,\beta,\sigma')$ into (10.8) and integration by parts (note that, according to (8.14), ρ_A is differentiable) leads to

$$\begin{aligned}\tilde{f}(r,\phi) = \frac{D}{4\pi^2}\int_0^{2\pi}\frac{1}{W^2}\int_{-\delta}^{\delta}\Big(&q^{(1)}(\sigma'-\sigma)\cos\sigma \\ &+ q^{(2)}(\sigma'-\sigma)\cos\sigma'\Big)\,g(\sigma,\beta)\,d\sigma\,d\beta,\end{aligned} \tag{10.9}$$

where

$$q^{(1)}(u) = -u\rho_A(u)/\sin^2 u, \tag{10.10}$$

and

$$q^{(2)}(u) = \left(\rho_A(u) + u\rho_A'(u)\right) / \sin u, \tag{10.11}$$

for $u \neq 0$, and (10.10) and (10.11) are assigned their limit values for $u = 0$. (We omit the somewhat cumbersome details.) Equation (10.9) gives the FBP reconstruction formula for the divergent beam geometry.

We have thus far presented an easy way to generate FBP-type reconstruction formulas for divergent beam x-ray data. There are two choices to be made: a family of windows F_A has to be selected and a value has to be assigned to A. Once they are made, we find the *convolving functions* $q^{(1)}$ and $q^{(2)}$ from (10.10) and (10.11) and get the formula for approximating $f(r, \phi)$ from (10.9).

Up to this point, we have assumed for the simplicity of mathematical analysis that the projection data are available for all possible σ and β. In practice, we can have only finitely many source positions, and for each source position we can have only finitely many detector readings. As shown in Fig. 5.5, we assume that projections are taken for M equally-spaced values of β with angular spacing Δ, and that for each view the projected values are sampled at $2N + 1$ equally-spaced angles with angular spacing λ. Thus g is known at points $(n\lambda, m\Delta)$, $-N \leq n \leq N$, $0 \leq m \leq M - 1$, and $M\Delta = 2\pi$. Our standard projection data are collected in this way (see Section 5.8). Even though the projection data consist of estimates (based on measurements) of $g(n\lambda, m\Delta)$, we use the same notation $g(n\lambda, m\Delta)$ for these estimates for the rest of this chapter. Similarly to the parallel beam FBP method, the numerical implementation of (10.9) is carried out in two stages.

First, the inner integral in (10.9) is evaluated using a Riemann sum approximation for values of σ' that are multiples of λ. We obtain

$$\begin{aligned} g_c(n'\lambda, m\Delta) &= \lambda \sum_{n=-N}^{N} \cos(n\lambda) g(n\lambda, m\Delta) q^{(1)}\left((n' - n)\lambda\right) \\ &\quad + \lambda \cos(n'\lambda) \sum_{n=-N}^{N} g(n\lambda, m\Delta) q^{(2)}\left((n' - n)\lambda\right). \end{aligned} \tag{10.12}$$

This corresponds to (8.23). Note that the first sum is a discrete convolution of $q^{(1)}$ and the projection data weighted by a cosine function, and the second sum is a discrete convolution of $q^{(2)}$ and the projection data.

Second, the outer integral in (10.9) is evaluated using a Riemann sum approximation. We obtain

$$f^*(r, \phi) = \frac{D\Delta}{4\pi^2} \sum_{m=0}^{M-1} \frac{1}{W^2} g_c\left(\sigma', m\Delta\right), \tag{10.13}$$

where σ' and W are defined by (10.5) and (10.6), but with $m\Delta$ in place of β. Implementation of (10.13) involves interpolation for approximating $g_c(\sigma', m\Delta)$ from values of $g_c(n'\lambda, m\Delta)$. The nature of such an interpolation has been discussed in some detail in Section 8.5. Note that (10.13) can be described as a "weighted backprojection." Given a point (r, ϕ) and a source position $m\Delta$, the line $(\sigma', m\Delta)$ is exactly the line from the source position $m\Delta$ through the point (r, ϕ). The contribution of the convolved ray sum $g_c(\sigma', m\Delta)$ to the value of f^* at points (r, ϕ) that the line goes through is inversely proportional to the square of the distance of the point (r, ϕ) from the source position $m\Delta$.

The actual computer implementation of this process is nearly identical to the computer implementation of the parallel FBP method, as described by (8.24) and (8.25). We do not repeat this discussion for the divergent case, but turn our attention instead to the choice of the window F_A.

10.2 Choice of the Window Function

In Section 8.6 we have given a general discussion of some of the principles involved in choosing the convolving and interpolating functions for the parallel beam FBP method. Linear interpolation was found to be clearly superior to nearest neighbor interpolation; for the divergent method we adopt linear interpolation without further discussion in this book.

The purpose of this section is to answer the question: How does the selection of the window F_A influence the quality of the reconstruction? Three approaches may be taken to answer this question.

(i) Specify some criteria for measuring the quality of reconstructions and find windows that are "optimal" by these criteria.
(ii) Take a representative selection of window functions and investigate these according to some "physical" criteria that measure such things as how well an isolated signal is reconstructed and how resistant is the method to noise.
(iii) Investigate the consequences of the selection on test cases typical of the intended application area, as discussed in detail in Sections 5.1–5.3.

While the first approach is mathematically attractive, it may not lead to efficacious windows because it is hard to translate the desirable properties of a window for a particular application into mathematical terms. (How does one translate into mathematics: "I want a window that produces diagnostically informative head cross sections from x-ray projections"?) More easily expressed general properties are likely to have some arbitrary parameters in them, and the "optimal" window may be strongly dependent on the values assigned to these parameters. Once the criterion for the optimality of the window is fixed, it may still be very difficult to find the optimal window. Usually, simplifying assumptions are made in its derivation (such as the availability of views from all directions, or that the noise in the measurement is independent of the signal) making it doubtful that the derived window is really optimal for the actual method of data collection. Even with simplifying assumptions, it is often hard to find a closed-form solution for the optimal window.

For the reasons just listed, we use only the second and third approaches in investigating the influence of the window selection on reconstruction quality. In choosing our windows we take the following considerations into account.

Under ideal circumstances, we should use a window whose value is 1 within its bandwidth and whose bandwidth is as large as possible. The purpose of using any other window is to reduce the effect of errors introduced by using finite numbers of views, by discretizing the projection data, and by various kinds of noise. Generally, the Fourier transform of the projection data dies away rapidly at higher frequencies, and so the effects of aliasing due to sampling of the projection data and the effects of noise are usually more significant at high frequencies than at low frequencies. In trying to find a "good" window, we may wish to de-emphasize these effects.

According to the conditions for F_A together with the consideration of de-emphasizing the errors without too much loss of information, windows of interest should be nonincreasing functions of U with $F_A(U) \leq 1$ over the interval $[0, A/2]$. In order to investigate a range of possibilities, we look at the generalized Hamming window with three different values of the parameter α, namely 1.0, 0.8, and 0.54, and also at the sinc window (see Table 8.1 and Section 8.6). The last of these when combined with linear interpolation, as we do here, is also referred to in the literature as the *Shepp–Logan window*. In all cases the bandwidth A was chosen to be $1/\lambda$, for reasons that are clear from the discussion in Section 8.6.

For each of the four windows mentioned in the previous paragraph we carried out experiments to test the ability of the method to reconstruct signal in the absence of noise, to evaluate the noise resistance of the method, and to test the efficacy of the method for reconstructing from x-ray data cross sections of the human head. In all experiments we used the standard geometry of data collection (see Section 5.4), and the function to be reconstructed was estimated at the pixel centers of a 243-element grid (see Section 4.1) with spacing between the grid points being 0.0752 cm. The experiments are discussed in separate sections below.

10.3 Point Response Function

Since the projection process and the divergent beam FBP reconstruction process are both linear (see Section 6.3, especially (6.20)), a reasonable choice of the reconstruction algorithm is the one that gives the most desirable reconstruction when the original picture to be reconstructed is a single point. Unfortunately, looking at the discrete reconstruction formula (10.13) it is clear that the reconstruction of a point is not *translation invariant*, meaning that the reconstruction of a point at a new location cannot be obtained by shifting the reconstruction at an old location. We now demonstrate this with a simple experiment.

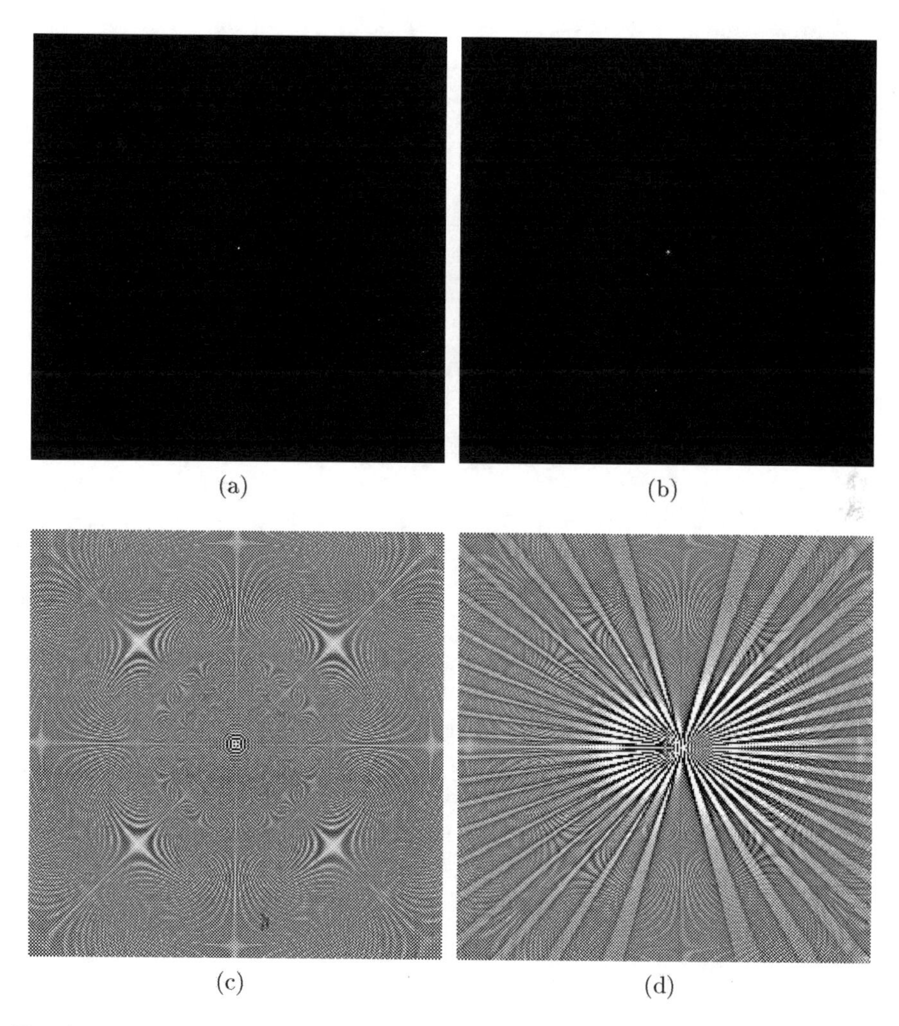

Fig. 10.2: Point response functions. (a) A "centrally located point" phantom displayed with value −0.1 shown as black and value 10.1 shown as white. (b) Reconstruction of this phantom by FBP (linear interpolation, bandlimiting window) for divergent beams from perfect data collected according to the standard geometry, displayed using the same display range. (c) The same reconstruction displayed with value −0.01 shown as black and value 0.01 shown as white. (d) Reconstruction of an "off-center point" phantom by FBP (linear interpolation, bandlimiting window) for divergent beams from perfect data collected according to the standard geometry, displayed using the same display range.

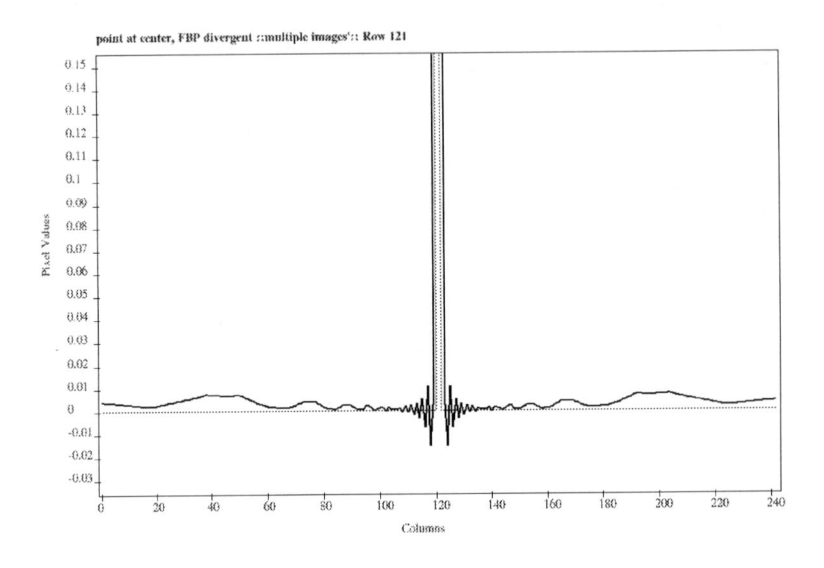
point center, standard geometry
point center_POINT WITH b_DCON_0001_r_a
point at center, FBP divergent ::multiple images'':: Row 121
Pixel Values
0.15
0.14
0.13
0.12
0.11
0.1
0.09
0.08
0.07
0.06
0.05
0.04
0.03
0.02
0.01
0
-0.01
-0.02
-0.03
0
20
40
60
80
100
120
140
160
180
200
220
240
Columns

(a)

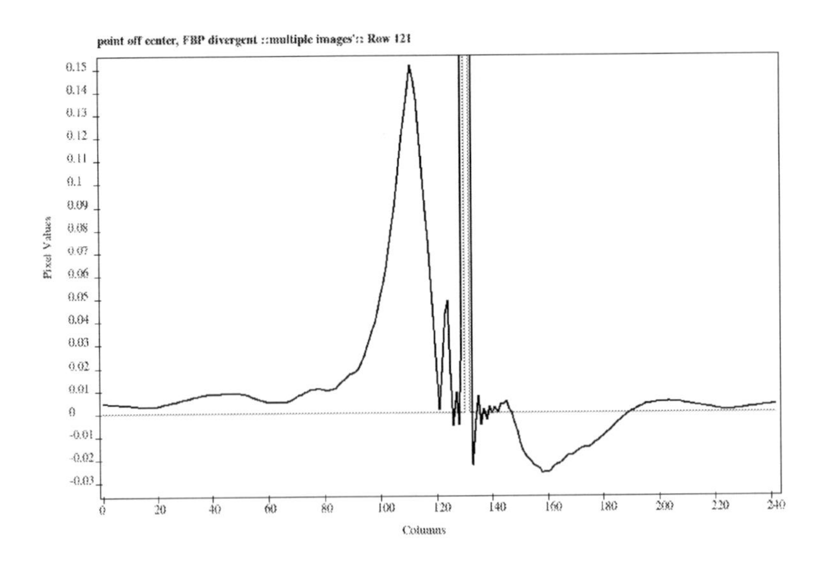
point 0ff center, standard geometry
point 0ff ce_POINT WITH b_DCON_0001_r_a
point off center, FBP divergent ::multiple images'':: Row 121
Pixel Values
0.15
0.14
0.13
0.12
0.11
0.1
0.09
0.08
0.07
0.06
0.05
0.04
0.03
0.02
0.01
0
-0.01
-0.02
-0.03
0
20
40
60
80
100
120
140
160
180
200
220
240
Columns

(b)

Consider a "point" phantom that is specified to have linear attenuation 10 cm^{-1} inside a circle of diameter 0.1 cm. If we center this circle at the origin, as in Fig. 10.2(a), then in our standard geometry the perfect ray sum is 1 for the center line in each view and is 0 for other lines. We reconstructed from these data using FBP for divergent beams with linear interpolation and the bandlimiting window and obtained the reconstruction shown in Fig. 10.2(b); it appears to be perfect. However it is not, by narrowing the display range as in Fig. 10.2(c), we see that the reconstructed values are not zero away from our "point." Worse than that, when the "point" is shifted by ten pixels to the right, the reconstructed pattern changes substantially. Plots of these reconstructions along the central row are shown in Fig. 10.3. We see that the structure of the response to projection taking and reconstruction of a point is complicated and is dependent on where the point is located.

In view of this, it is unlikely that something insightful can be gained for the choice of the window function by looking at just a few parameters that can be obtained from an associated point response function. For the sake of completeness we discuss the kind of point response function parameters that are commonly used to indicate the quality of an imaging procedure.

We use $P_{(r^*,\phi^*)}(r,\phi)$ to denote the reconstructed value at (r,ϕ) for a point at (r^*,ϕ^*). This value is provided by substitution of the discrete projection data into (10.12) and (10.13). Ideally, $P^*(r,\phi)$ should have value zero at $(r,\phi) \neq (r^*,\phi^*)$. In practice this is not the case, as can be seen in Figs. 10.2 and 10.3. We now discuss two aspects of the point response function that translate in a straightforward way into the quality of the reconstruction in general. The associated parameters depend both on the location of the point (r^*,ϕ^*) and on a chosen direction ψ. Let us fix both of these for now and use, for any nonnegative real number s, the notation $P(s)$ to denote the value of $P_{(r^*,\phi^*)}(r,\phi)$ at the point (r,ϕ) that is at a distance s in direction ψ from (r^*,ϕ^*) divided by $P_{(r^*,\phi^*)}(r^*,\phi^*)$. Consequently, $P(0) = 1$. Then we define:

(i) *Half-width at half-maximum* (HWHM) is the smallest positive s such that $P(s) = 0.5$.
(ii) Size of the *first overshoot* is the value of $|P(s)|$ at the smallest positive real number s such that $\frac{dP}{ds}(s) = 0$.

Roughly speaking the first of these measures the blurring in direction ψ, while the second measures the size of the locally maximal fake value that is nearest to the point in the direction ψ. If the values of $P(s)$ were independent of both (r^*,ϕ^*) and ψ, then for each window function we would have only one

---

Fig. 10.3: Plots of the "points" (shown light) and their reconstructions (shown dark) from perfect data collected according to the standard geometry using FBP for divergent data with linear interpolation and bandlimiting window for a "point" (a) at the center and (b) off center.

Table 10.1: Values of $P(s)$ when the "point" to be reconstructed is at the origin, $\psi = \pi/2$, and $s = 0.0752n$, where 0.0752 cm is the distance between adjacent pixel centers.

window	$n = 0$	$n = 1$	$n = 2$	$n = 3$	$n = 4$
generalized Hamming, α =1.00	1.0000	0.1049	0.0002	-0.0014	0.0011
generalized Hamming, α =0.54	1.0000	0.3871	0.0474	-0.0012	0.0003

HWHM and only one size of the first overshoot and so the window function would have these two parameters associated with it, both of which should be as small as possible. The dependence of $P(s)$ on both (r^*, ϕ^*) and ψ makes this approach to window function selection of questionable usefulness. There are additional practical problems that we now discuss.

While the blurring in the point response function (as compared with the original "point") is observable in Fig. 10.3, this blurring is quite small as compared with the distance between pixel centers. So while HWHM gets smaller as α increases when we use the generalized Hamming window, the differences are hardly noticeable in a practical reconstruction.

Another practical point is that the first overshoot may not be the largest overshoot, see Fig. 10.3(b), and so its use may result in an incorrect choice as far as the overall quality of the resulting reconstructions are concerned. A further difficulty with these physical measures is their inconsistency, which we now illustrate on a simple example.

Consider the case when the point is at the center, that is $r^* = 0$. We reconstructed it from perfect data collected according to the standard geometry by FBP for divergent beams using linear interpolation and the generalized Hamming window with $\alpha = 1.0$ (this is the same as the bandlimiting window, the resulting reconstruction is shown in Figs. 10.2(b) and (c)) and with $\alpha = 0.54$. In Table 10.1 we report on the values of $P(s)$ when $\psi = \pi/2$ and the values of s are selected at consecutive pixel centers. As far as HWHM is concerned $\alpha = 1.0$ is better than $\alpha = 0.54$, but the size of the first overshoot seems to indicate otherwise. Other experiments lead to the same conclusion. So the two parameters provided by the point response function give contradictory indications as to the better value of α. All these considerations make us conclude that the physical parameters associated with the point response function are not particularly useful for window selection for the divergent beam FBP.

10.4 Noise Reconstruction

In addition to the point response, the efficacy of a reconstruction algorithm is affected by its resistance to noise in the data. Let us assume that the projection data are corrupted by additive noise. Due to the linearity of the FBP method, the reconstruction is the sum of the reconstruction provided by the true signal and the reconstruction of the noise. Hence we concentrate on the behavior of the algorithm on pure noise.

In order to get a rough feeling for the relationship between the noise in the reconstruction and the noise in the data, we investigate the nature of the reconstruction of a very simple (and for our application, unrealistic) type of noise. We assume that each measurement of $g(n\lambda, m\Delta)$ is an independent sample of the same random variable R such that $\mu_R = 0$ (see Section 1.2). Then the reconstructed value at the point (r, ϕ), as determined by (10.13), is also a random variable, which we denote by $F^*(r, \phi)$. It is easy to show that $\mu_{F^*(r,\phi)} = 0$. In words, if the data are zero mean noise, then the reconstructed value at a point has also zero mean. The variance $V_{F^*(r,\phi)}$ depends on several things: the variance of the data V_R, the convolving functions $q^{(1)}$ and $q^{(2)}$ used in the reconstruction, the interpolating function ψ for the interpolation used in (10.13), the number of views M, the sampling angle λ, and the location of the point (r, ϕ). The precise formula can be obtained by using (10.12) and (10.13) in conjunction with (8.37) and (1.14). Evaluating this formula for a number of points, one finds that a window that suppresses more the higher frequency components (such as the Hamming window, which is the generalized Hamming window with $\alpha = 0.54$) is more resistant to noise in the data than a window that suppresses less the higher frequency components (such as the bandlimiting window, which is the generalized Hamming window with $\alpha = 1.0$). We now illustrate this with an example.

In our example we used the standard Gaussian random variable N to take the place of R in the previous paragraph. We generated the noise data for the standard geometry and reconstructed from it using FBP for divergent beams with linear interpolation, both with the bandlimiting window and the Hamming window. The results are shown in Fig. 10.4. The variance of the values in the image that is produced by the bandlimiting window is six times that in the image produced by the Hamming window. However, this overall variance is only part of the story, it says nothing about the way noise in the reconstruction is correlated. A window with a low value of α may be considered undesirable for noisy data because it produces *structured noise*, meaning noise that influences reconstructed values at neighboring points in a sufficiently similar way so as to introduce false features spreading over relatively large areas. This possibility is demonstrated in Figs. 10.4(c) and (d) and in Fig. 10.5. Thus again we find that investigating a physical property, in this case resistance to noise, provides some general insight, but does not really help in deciding on a window function. We therefore return to using the methodologies introduced in Sections 5.1–5.3.

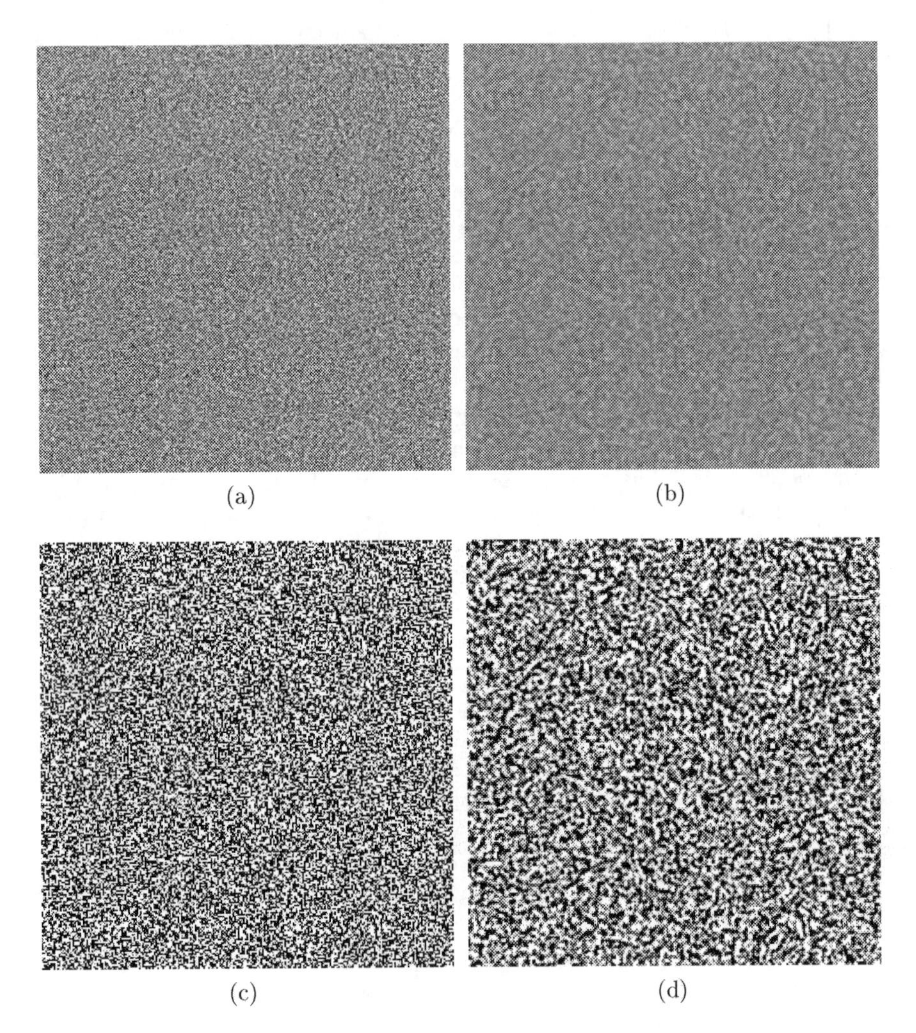

Fig. 10.4: Reconstructions from pure noise, collected according to the standard geometry, using FBP for divergent beams with linear interpolation and (a) generalized Hamming window with $\alpha = 1.0$ (same as the bandlimiting window), (b) generalized Hamming window with $\alpha = 0.54$ (same as the Hamming window). For these images the display range was adjusted so that -1.2 is black and 1.2 is white. (c) and (d) are the same as (a) and (b), respectively, but the display range was adjusted so that -0.12 is black and 0.12 is white.

10.5 Comparison of Algorithms Based on Reconstructions

We applied variants of the reconstruction method discussed in this chapter to the standard projection data. We used linear interpolation and investigated

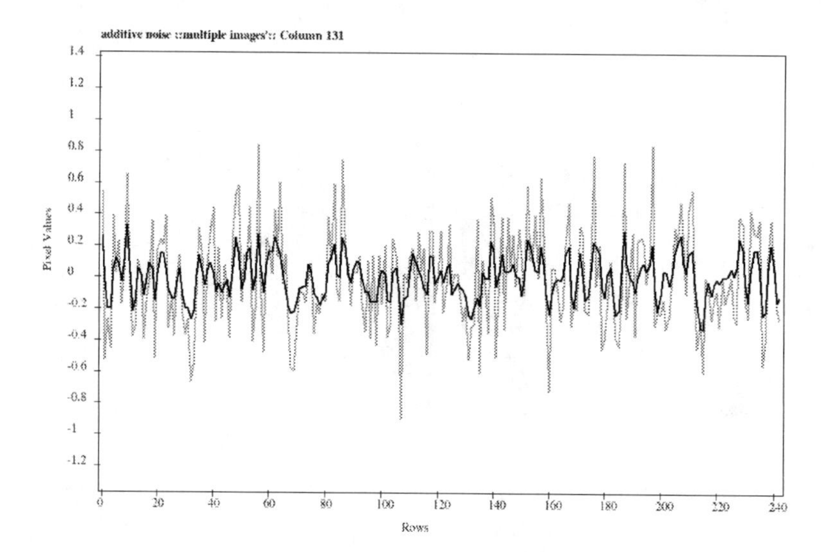

Fig. 10.5: Plots of reconstructions from pure noise using FBP for divergent data with linear interpolation and the generalized Hamming window with $\alpha = 1.0$ (light) and $\alpha = 0.54$ (dark).

four windows: the generalized Hamming window with $\alpha = 1.0$, $\alpha = 0.8$, $\alpha = 0.54$, and the sinc window. The reconstructions are reported in Figs. 10.6 and 10.7, and in Table 10.2.

When we applied our task-oriented comparison methodology we found that the average values of our two FOMs, as reported in the last two columns of Table 10.2, indicate opposite tendencies. This occurs in spite of the fact that for both FOMs the observed differences between any pair of windows are extremely significant, with P-values always less than 10^{-12} with the exception of HITR when comparing generalized Hamming with α =0.54 with sinc, in which case the P-value is 0.0053. Thus we see, yet again, that the smoother looking reconstructions are not better for the task of detecting small low-contrast tumors as measured by IROI, but they are better as measured by HITR. Judgment on the medical efficacy of the choice of the window cannot be made without a better understanding of how the images are used by the radiologist: we need to know which of the two numerical observers IROI and HITR correspond more closely to the actual diagnostic process. This is beyond the scope of this book.

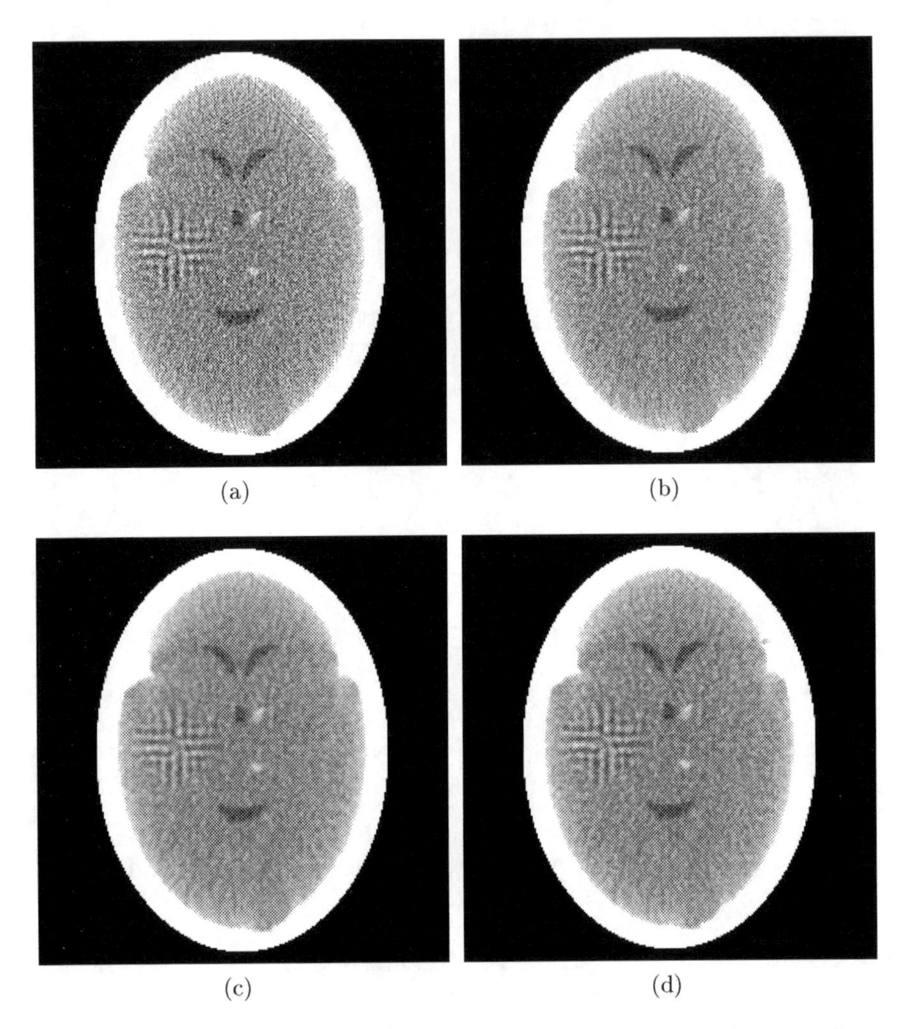

Fig. 10.6: Reconstructions from the standard projection data using FBP for divergent beams with linear interpolation and (a) generalized Hamming window with $\alpha = 1.0$ (same as the bandlimiting window), (b) generalized Hamming window with $\alpha = 0.8$, (c) generalized Hamming window with $\alpha = 0.54$ and (d) sinc window.

Fig. 10.7: Plots of the head phantom of Fig. 4.6(a), shown light, and its reconstructions, shown dark, from the standard projection data using FBP for divergent data with linear interpolation and the generalized Hamming window with (a) $\alpha = 1.0$ (which is the same as the bandlimiting window) and (b) $\alpha = 0.54$.

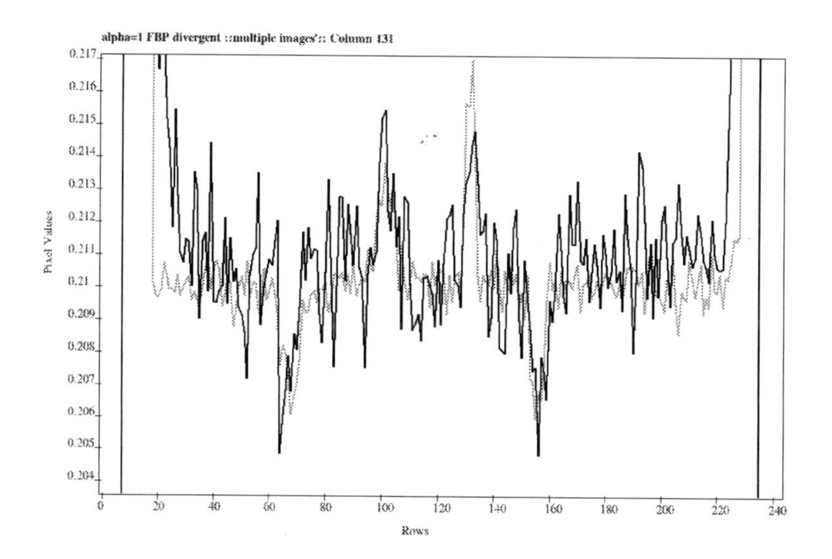
standard head phantom
standard pro_ALPHA=1 FBP_DCON_0001_r_s
alpha=1 FBP divergent ::multiple images':: Column 131
0.217
0.216
0.215
0.214
0.213
0.212
0.211
0.21
0.209
0.208
0.207
0.206
0.205
0.204
Pixel Values
0
20
40
60
80
100
120
140
160
180
200
220
240
Rows

(a)

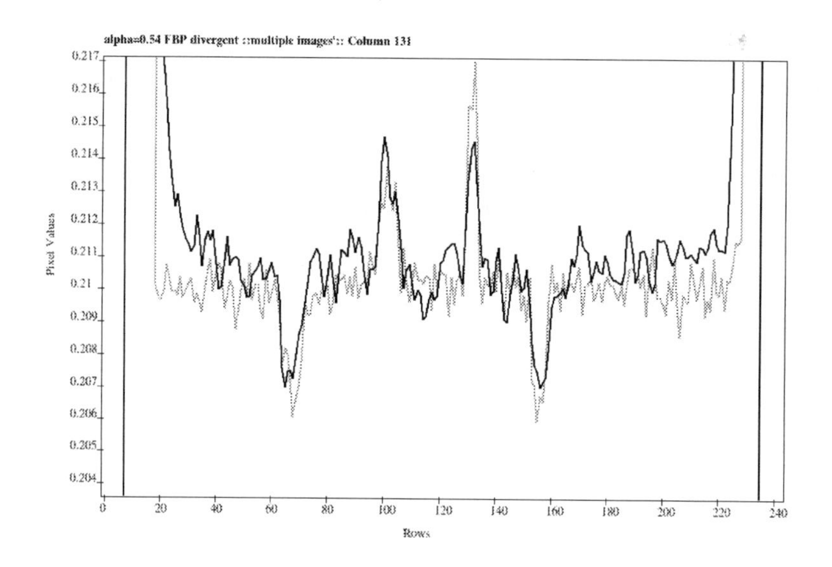
standard head phantom
standard pro_ALPHA=0.54 F_DCON_0001_r_s
alpha=0.54 FBP divergent ::multiple images':: Column 131
0.217
0.216
0.215
0.214
0.213
0.212
0.211
0.21
0.209
0.208
0.207
0.206
0.205
0.204
Pixel Values
0
20
40
60
80
100
120
140
160
180
200
220
240
Rows

(b)

Table 10.2: Picture distance measures and timings (in seconds) for the reconstructions in Fig. 10.6. The last two columns report on the average values of the FOMs for the various algorithms that were produced by a task-oriented evaluation experiment.

window	d	r	t	IROI	HITR
generalized Hamming, $\alpha = 1.00$	0.0764	0.0400	8.7	0.1813	0.9197
generalized Hamming, $\alpha = 0.80$	0.0901	0.0413	8.7	0.1741	0.9356
generalized Hamming, $\alpha = 0.54$	0.1138	0.0443	8.7	0.1601	0.9517
sinc	0.1060	0.0423	8.7	0.1667	0.9496

An overall conclusion that can be reached based on the material presented in this and the previous three sections is that while the choice of the window function has an effect on the appearance of the reconstruction, this effect is not such that we can say based on it how the window function should be chosen from the point of view of diagnostic efficacy. Compare this with our more definitive conclusion regarding interpolation in Table 8.2: all measures with the exception of the picture distance measure d indicate superiority of linear interpolation over the nearest neighbor interpolation.

Notes and References

To learn about rebinning, read for example [134], which gives references to earlier work on which it is based; see, in particular, [69].

The earliest development of an FBP reconstruction method for divergent beams without rebinning seems to be due to J. Pavkovich [218]. Detailed derivations of the Radon inversion formula for divergent rays (10.3), as well as of (10.9), are given in [136], together with an illustration of the superiority of linear interpolation to nearest neighbor interpolation in conjunction with the divergent beam FBP algorithm.

Our presentation of the FBP method for divergent beams and our discussion of the choice of the convolving function is based on [49, 136]. Those papers reference earlier literature on related approaches and also contain some details, for example on finding an "optimal" window, which were not included in this book. The approach described in those papers is in current use; see, for example, [228]. The mathematical theory underlying the inversion of the transform that corresponds to the divergent beam method of data collection is reported in [245]. The study of FBP-like algorithms for divergent beams is still of active interest; for a recent study see [79]. Modifications that provide satisfactory reconstructions even from truncated projections, which do not cover the whole object to be reconstructed, have long been known [131, 182].

The ability of designing devices capable of implementing a divergent beam reconstruction algorithm so that each reconstruction takes less than one hundredth of a second (1/100 sec) was already in evidence in the late 1970s [92].

11

Algebraic Reconstruction Techniques

In this and the next chapter we discuss series expansion methods for image reconstruction. The *algebraic reconstruction techniques* (*ART*) form a large family of reconstruction algorithms. The name is a historical accident; there is nothing more "algebraic" about these techniques than about the techniques that are discussed in the next chapter. The distinguishing feature of ART needs careful discussion, which is given in the following section.

11.1 What Is ART?

All series expansion methods are procedures for the solution of the discrete reconstruction problem. As discussed in Section 6.3, this is the problem of estimating an image vector x such that $y = Rx + e$, given a measurement vector y. The estimation is done by requiring x, and the error vector e, to satisfy some specified optimization criterion of the type discussed in Section 6.4. We use x^* to denote the required estimate.

All ART methods of image reconstruction are iterative procedures: they produce a sequence of vectors $x^{(0)}$, $x^{(1)}, \ldots$ that is supposed to *converge* to x^*. This means that, for $1 \leq j \leq J$, $x_j^{(k)}$ (the jth component of the kth iterate) should be arbitrarily near to x_j^*, provided that k is chosen large enough. The process of producing $x^{(k+1)}$ from $x^{(k)}$ is referred to as an *iterative step*.

In ART, $x^{(k+1)}$ is obtained from $x^{(k)}$ by considering a single one of the I approximate equations, see (6.23). In fact, the equations are used in a *cyclic order*. We use i_k to denote $k(\text{mod } I) + 1$; i.e., $i_0 = 1$, $i_1 = 2, \ldots, i_{I-1} = I$, $i_I = 1$, $i_{I+1} = 2, \ldots$, and we use r_i to denote the J-dimensional column vector whose jth component is $r_{i,j}$. In other words, r_i is the transpose of the ith row of R. An important point here is that this specification is incomplete because it depends on how we index the lines for which the integrals are estimated. It is stated in Section 6.1 that we assume that estimates of $[\mathscr{R}f](\ell, \theta)$ are known for I pairs: $(\ell_1, \theta_1), \ldots, (\ell_I, \theta_I)$. However, until now we have not specified the geometrical locations of the lines that are parametrized by these pairs. Since the order in which we do things in ART depends on the indexing i for the set of lines for which data are collected, the specification of ART as a reconstruction algorithm is complete only if it includes the indexing method for the lines, which we refer to as the *data access ordering*. We return to this point later on in this chapter.

The kth iterative step in ART can be described by a function α_k, whose arguments are two J-dimensional vectors and one real number and whose value is a J-dimensional vector. (In mathematical jargon, $\alpha_k : \mathbb{R}^J \times \mathbb{R}^J \times \mathbb{R} \to \mathbb{R}^J$, where $\mathbb{R}$ denotes the set of real numbers.) Then,

$$x^{(k+1)} = \alpha_k \left(x^{(k)}, r_{i_k}, y_{i_k} \right). \tag{11.1}$$

In words, a particular algebraic reconstruction technique is defined by a sequence of functions $\alpha_0, \alpha_1, \alpha_2, \ldots$. In order to get the $(k+1)$st iterate we apply α_k to the kth iterate, the i_kth row of the projection matrix R, and the i_kth component of the measurement vector y. Such algorithms have been referred to as *storage efficient*, because the J-dimensional vector $x^{(k+1)}$ can be stored in the same part of computer memory where $x^{(k)}$ has been kept, since $x^{(k)}$ is not needed by the algorithm after the kth step. (Note that the implementation of the FBP described near the end of Section 8.3 is also storage efficient. The same cannot be said for the iterative procedures that are discussed in the next chapter.) Various ART methods differ from each other in the way the sequence of α_ks is chosen. We now illustrate the previous discussion on a particularly simple example.

One way of choosing the α_ks is the following. For any J-dimensional vectors x and t and for any real number z, let

$$\alpha_k (x, t, z) = \begin{cases} x + \frac{z - \langle t, x \rangle}{\langle t, t \rangle} t, & \text{if} \quad \langle t, t \rangle \neq 0, \\ x, & \text{if} \quad \langle t, t \rangle = 0, \end{cases} \tag{11.2}$$

where $\langle \bullet, \bullet \rangle$ denotes the *inner product* of two J-dimensional vectors; i.e.,

$$\langle t, x \rangle = \sum_{j=1}^{J} t_j x_j. \tag{11.3}$$

Note that, in this case, the α_ks have the same functional form for all k. Defining α_k in this way has a number of attractive properties.

One is that, if $\langle r_{i_k}, r_{i_k} \rangle \neq 0$, then

$$y_{i_k} = \sum_{j=1}^{J} r_{i_k,j} x_j^{(k+1)}, \tag{11.4}$$

i.e., the i_kth approximate equality is exactly satisfied after the kth step. To see this, combine (11.1) and (11.2) and use the notation of (11.3) to get

$$\begin{aligned}\left\langle r_{i_k}, x^{(k+1)}\right\rangle &= \left\langle r_{i_k}, \alpha_k\left(x^{(k)}, r_{i_k}, y_{i_k}\right)\right\rangle \\ &= \left\langle r_{i_k}, x^{(k)}\right\rangle + \frac{y_{i_k} - \left\langle r_{i_k}, x^{(k)}\right\rangle}{\left\langle r_{i_k}, r_{i_k}\right\rangle}\left\langle r_{i_k}, r_{i_k}\right\rangle \\ &= y_{i_k}.\end{aligned} \tag{11.5}$$

Another attractive property of defining α_k by (11.2) is that the updating of $x^{(k)}$ becomes very simple: we just add to $x^{(k)}$ a multiple of the vector r_{i_k}. In practice, this updating of $x^{(k)}$ can be computationally very inexpensive.

Consider, for example, the basis functions associated with a digitization into pixels (6.17). Then $r_{i,j}$ is just the length of intersection of the ith line with the jth pixel. This has two consequences. First, most of the components of the vector r_{i_k} are zero. At most $2\ell - 1$ pixels can be intersected by a straight line in an $\ell \times \ell$ digitization of a picture. Thus, of the ℓ^2 components of r_{i_k}, at most $2\ell - 1$ (and typically only about ℓ) are nonzero. Second, the location and size of the nonzero components of r_{i_k} can be rapidly calculated using a DDA from the geometrical location of the i_kth line relative to the $\ell \times \ell$ grid, as discussed in Section 4.6. Thus, the projection matrix R does not need to be stored in the computer. Only one row of the matrix is needed at a time, and all essential information about this row is easily calculable. For this reason such methods are also referred to as *row-action methods*.

We investigate this point further, since it is basic to the understanding of the computational efficacy of ART. Suppose that we have a list $j_1, \ldots, j_U$ of indices such that $t_j = 0$ unless j is one of the $j_1, \ldots, j_U$. Then evaluation of (11.3) requires only U multiplications, which in our application is much smaller than J, as discussed above. Similarly, $\langle t, t\rangle$ can be evaluated using U multiplications. Having evaluated $(z - \langle t, x\rangle) / \langle t, t\rangle$ using $2U$ multiplications (and one division), the updating of x can be achieved by a further U multiplications. This is because only those x_j need to be altered for which $j = j_u$ for some u, $1 \le u \le U$, and the alteration requires adding to x_j a fixed multiple of t_j. This shows that a single step of the algorithm, as described by (11.2), is very simple to implement in a computationally efficient way.

Apart from its computational efficiency, (11.2) is an intuitively reasonable way of producing $x^{(k+1)}$ from $x^{(k)}$. Suppose that, in addition to requiring the satisfaction of (11.4) after the kth iterative step, we impose the following conditions on the way the kth step should be carried out.

(i) Only those pixels that are intersected by the i_kth line should have their densities changed.
(ii) The density change of a pixel should be proportional to $y_{i_k} - \left\langle r_{i_k}, x^{(k)}\right\rangle$ (the "error" in the i_kth approximate equality prior to the kth step).
(iii) The change in the jth pixel should be proportional to $r_{i_k,j}$.

These conditions, nearly identical to the conditions for discrete backprojection stated in Section 7.3, uniquely determine how the α_ks are defined; and they lead to (11.2). The early literature on ART relied on justifying the algorithms by showing that they are derived from such reasonable conditions.

Before we get into the details of specific ART methods, two comments are in order. First, for (11.1) to specify the sequence $x^{(0)}, x^{(1)}, x^{(2)}, \ldots$ precisely, we need to select the *initial vector* $x^{(0)}$. The choice of $x^{(0)}$ is quite important in the practical behavior of these algorithms. More is said about this below. Second, if the version of the discrete reconstruction problem that is represented by the system of inequalities $Nx \leq q$ (see Section 6.4) is used, then the general description of ART given by (11.1) is not always adequate. In such a case, a slightly more complicated general framework may be required, but one that has essentially similar computational requirements. We discuss a similar situation in Section 11.3 in some detail.

11.2 Relaxation Methods for Solving Systems of Inequalities and Equalities

In this section we give the mathematical background to ART. We do this in the framework of the mathematical problem "find a vector that satisfies all of a given set of linear inequalities." In other words, we are interested in finding a J-dimensional vector x such that

$$\langle n_i, x \rangle \leq q_i, \quad \text{for } 1 \leq i \leq P, \tag{11.6}$$

where the n_i are given J-dimensional vectors and the q_i are given real numbers. Equation (11.6) is a rewrite of (6.42).

In what follows we assume that each n_i has at least one nonzero component. A physical interpretation of this assumption is that we do not make use of a measurement if none of the basis functions contributed to it. The reason for making this assumption is to avoid having to make special cases all the time when $\langle n_i, n_i \rangle = 0$, like we had to do in (11.2).

We introduce some sets of vectors N_i ($1 \leq i \leq P$) and N. For $1 \leq i \leq P$,

$$N_i = \{x \mid \langle n_i, x \rangle \leq q_i\} \tag{11.7}$$

and

$$N = \bigcap_{i=1}^{P} N_i. \tag{11.8}$$

In words, N_i is the set of vectors that satisfies the ith of the P inequalities in (11.6), and N is the set of vectors that satisfies all P inequalities. Our aim, for now, is to find an element of N.

More precisely, we need an algorithm that, for given $n_1, \ldots, n_P, q_1, \ldots, q_P$, finds an x in N. We propose an ART-type method using functions

$$\alpha_k(x, t, z) = \begin{cases} x, & \text{if } \langle t, x \rangle \leq z, \\ x + \lambda^{(k)} \frac{z - \langle t, x \rangle}{\langle t, t \rangle} t, & \text{otherwise}, \end{cases} \tag{11.9}$$

where $\lambda^{(k)}$ is a real number, referred to as the *relaxation parameter.*

Consider the following procedure, which we refer to as the *relaxation method for inequalities.*

$$\begin{aligned} &x^{(0)} \text{ is arbitrary,} \\ &x^{(k+1)} = \alpha_k(x^{(k)}, n_{i_k}, q_{i_k}), \end{aligned} \tag{11.10}$$

where α_k is defined by (11.9) and $i_k = k(\text{mod } P) + 1$. If the relaxation parameters satisfy the weak condition that, for some ε_1 and ε_2 and for all k,

$$0 < \varepsilon_1 \leq \lambda^{(k)} \leq \varepsilon_2 < 2, \tag{11.11}$$

then the relaxation method for inequalities produces a sequence $x^{(0)}, x^{(1)}, x^{(2)}$, ... that converges to a vector in N, provided only that N is not empty. Proof of this result appears in Section 15.8.

Next we discuss the geometrical nature of the relaxation method for inequalities and, in particular, the role of the relaxation parameters. Let

$$H_i = \{x \mid \langle n_i, x \rangle = q_i\}. \tag{11.12}$$

In words, H_i is the set of vectors x for which the ith inequality is satisfied by the two sides of the inequality being actually equal. Note that H_i is a subset of N_i. Each H_i is what mathematicians call a *hyperplane*. If the dimension J of x is three, then a hyperplane is a plane in three-dimensional space. If the dimension J of x is two, then a hyperplane is a straight line in two-dimensional space (i.e., in a plane).

The two-dimensional case is illustrated in Fig. 11.1. There are two hyperplanes H_1 and H_2. For these hyperplanes

$$n_1 = \begin{pmatrix} 4 \\ 1 \end{pmatrix}, \quad n_2 = \begin{pmatrix} 2 \\ 5 \end{pmatrix}, \tag{11.13}$$

$$q_1 = 24, \quad q_2 = 30. \tag{11.14}$$

Observe the following simple geometrical fact: The vector n_i (think of it as the line drawn from the origin to the point n_i in the plane) is perpendicular to the line H_i. This statement generalizes to any dimensions, as a reader acquainted with analytic geometry can easily see from (11.12).

Since in the relaxation method for inequalities, (11.10), the role of t in (11.9) is taken by n_{i_k}, we see that if $x^{(k+1)}$ differs from $x^{(k)}$ at all, then $x^{(k+1)} - x^{(k)}$ (which is a multiple of n_{i_k}) is perpendicular to H_{i_k}.

The geometrical interpretation in the two-dimensional case is that N_i is a set of points lying on one side of the line H_i (including the line H_i). For example, in Fig. 11.1, both N_1 and N_2 are those half-planes that include the origin. Their intersection N, is shown dark in Fig. 11.1. This notion also generalizes, and we say that N_i is a *half-space* that is the set of points lying on one side of the hyperplane H_i (including the hyperplane H_i). The set N, as defined by (11.8), is an intersection of such half-spaces.

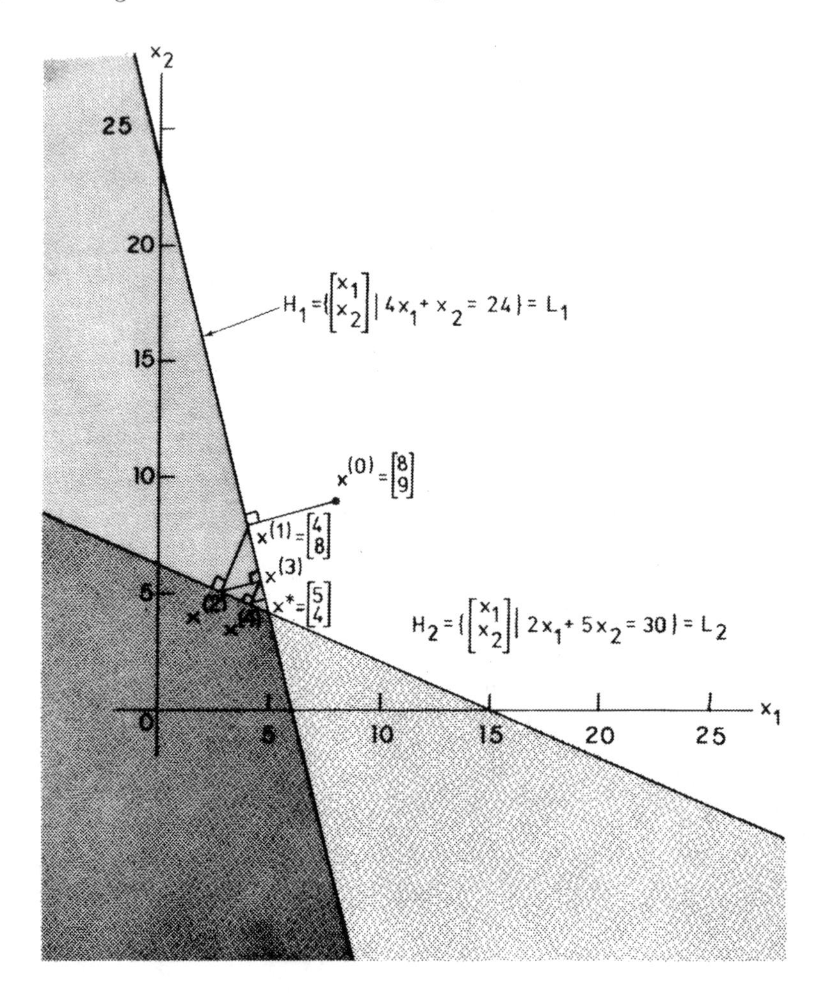

Fig. 11.1: Demonstration of the relaxation method (with $\lambda^{(k)} = 1$, for all k) for the simple case when $I = J = 2$. In the demonstration n_1 and n_2 are given by (11.13) and q_1 and q_2 by (11.14). (Illustration based on [127], Copyright 1976, with permission from Elsevier.)

In the relaxation method for inequalities, see (11.9) and (11.10), if $x^{(k)}$ is in the half-space N_{i_k} then we do not change our estimate during the kth iterative step (i.e., $x^{(k+1)} = x^{(k)}$). If $x^{(k)}$ is not in the half-space N_{i_k}, then we move our estimate perpendicular to the bounding hyperplane H_{i_k} of N_{i_k} (i.e., $x^{(k+1)} - x^{(k)}$ is orthogonal to H_{i_k}). The amount of movement depends on the size of $\lambda^{(k)}$. If $\lambda^{(k)} = 1$, then by an argument identical to that given for (11.3), we can prove that $\langle n_{i_k}, x^{(k+1)} \rangle = q_{i_k}$, i.e., that $x^{(k+1)}$ is in the hyperplane H_{i_k}. The following statement can be shown in a similarly easy fashion. During the kth step of the relaxation method for inequalities with $x^{(k)}$ not in N_{i_k}, the move from $x^{(k)}$ to $x^{(k+1)}$ is perpendicular to H_{i_k} and has one of the following geometrical properties:

if $\lambda^{(k)} < 0$, the move is away from H_{i_k};
if $\lambda^{(k)} = 0$, there is no movement;
if $0 < \lambda^{(k)} < 1$, the move is toward H_{i_k}, but does not quite reach it;
if $\lambda^{(k)} = 1$, the move is to H_{i_k} exactly;
if $1 < \lambda^{(k)} < 2$, the move is past H_{i_k}, but $x^{(k+1)}$ is nearer to H_{i_k};
if $\lambda^{(k)} = 2$, $x^{(k+1)}$ is the mirror image (reflection) of $x^{(k)}$ in H_{i_k};
if $\lambda^{(k)} > 2$, $x^{(k+1)}$ is on the other side of H_{i_k} further from H_{i_k} than $x^{(k)}$.

To illustrate the relaxation method for inequalities, consider again Fig. 11.1. Two inequalities are involved (i.e., $P = 2$), and the vectors n_1, n_2 and the scalars q_1, q_2 are defined by (11.13) and (11.14), respectively. Suppose we choose $\lambda^{(k)} = 1$, for all k. We also have to choose the initial vector. If we let

$$x^{(0)} = \begin{pmatrix} 8 \\ 9 \end{pmatrix}, \tag{11.15}$$

then, as can easily be checked,

$$x^{(1)} = \begin{pmatrix} 4 \\ 8 \end{pmatrix} \quad \text{and} \quad x^{(2)} = \begin{pmatrix} 80/29 \\ 142/29 \end{pmatrix}. \tag{11.16}$$

Since $x^{(2)}$ is in both N_1 and N_2, all values of $x^{(k)}$, for $k \geq 2$, are the same as $x^{(2)}$. Hence the method converges to $x^* = x^{(2)}$, which is in N.

The convergence that occurs in this example is called *finite convergence* since the $x^{(k)}$ remain constant after a finite number of iterative steps. It is *not* the case that the relaxation method for inequalities always has finite convergence if the $\lambda^{(k)}$ are chosen according to (11.11).

Now we turn to study systems of equations. Suppose we are given J-dimensional vectors a_i and real numbers b_i for $1 \leq i \leq I$. Let,

$$L_i = \{x \mid \langle a_i, x\rangle = b_i\}, \tag{11.17}$$

and

$$L = \bigcap_{i=1}^{I} L_i. \tag{11.18}$$

We observe the following fact: L can also be expressed as the intersection of a set of half-spaces. In fact, if we let $P = 2I$ and define, for $1 \leq i \leq I$,

$$N_{2i-1} = \{x \mid \langle -a_i, x\rangle \leq -b_i\}, \tag{11.19}$$

$$N_{2i} = \{x \mid \langle a_i, x\rangle \leq b_i\}, \tag{11.20}$$

then

$$L_i = N_{2i-1} \cap N_{2i} \tag{11.21}$$

and, consequently, L defined by (11.18) is the same as N defined by (11.8), provided that the N_i are defined by (11.19) and (11.20). Hence we can apply the relaxation method for a system of inequalities to find an element of L. Here we assume that, for all $1 \leq i \leq I$, $\langle a_i, a_i \rangle > 0$.

However, note that

$$L_i = H_{2i-1} = H_{2i}, \tag{11.22}$$

where H_i denotes the bounding hyperplane of the half-space N_i, see (11.12). Hence the combined effect of the $(2k-1)$st and $(2k)$th iterative steps is to move (if at all) perpendicular to the hyperplane L_{i_k}. We can combine these two steps and obtain the following *relaxation method for systems of equalities:*

$$\begin{aligned} x^{(0)} &\text{ is arbitrary,} \\ x^{(k+1)} &= x^{(k)} + c^{(k)} a_{i_k}. \end{aligned} \tag{11.23}$$

It follows easily from the result stated for the convergence of the relaxation method for inequalities that if, for all $k \geq 0$,

$$c^{(k)} = \lambda^{(k)} \frac{b_{i_k} - \langle a_{i_k} x^{(k)} \rangle}{\langle a_{i_k}, a_{i_k} \rangle}, \tag{11.24}$$

with $\lambda^{(k)}$ satisfying (11.11), then the relaxation method for equalities produces a sequence $x^{(0)}, x^{(1)}, x^{(2)}, \ldots$ that converges to a vector in L, provided only that L is not empty.

The algorithm described by (11.1) and (11.2) is a special case of the relaxation method for equalities, with $\lambda^{(k)} = 1$, for all k. We illustrate this special case in Fig. 11.1. Defining $a_1 = n_1$, $a_2 = n_2$, $b_1 = q_1$ and $b_2 = q_2$ by (11.13) and (11.14), we see that if we start with $x^{(0)}$ defined by (11.15), then we get $x^{(1)}$ and $x^{(2)}$ as defined by (11.16). From this point on, the sequence produced by the relaxation method for equalities differs from the relaxation method for inequalities, which we discussed before. This is because $x^{(2)}$ does not lie in L_2 and so further steps are necessary to get nearer and nearer to an element of L, which, in this case, is the unique intersection x^* of the two lines L_1 and L_2. The geometrical interpretation given above shows that the sequence of vectors is produced by dropping perpendiculars alternately onto L_1 and L_2, see Fig. 11.1.

In general, L has more than one element. With a little extra care in choosing $x^{(0)}$, we can ensure that the relaxation method for equalities converges to an element of L that satisfies an optimization criterion, namely, the minimum norm criterion; see (6.37) in Section 6.4. To do this, we introduce a set S of vectors, which is the set of all linear combinations of the a_i, that is

$$S = \left\{ x \mid x = \sum_{i=1}^{I} \beta_i a_i \text{ for some real numbers } \beta_i \right\}. \tag{11.25}$$

The following result is sometimes referred to as the *minimum norm theorem*: if L is not empty, then there exists one, and only one, element x^* in $L \cap S$; furthermore, for all x in L other than x^*,

$$\|x^*\| < \|x\|, \tag{11.26}$$

where $\|x\|^2 = \langle x, x \rangle$; see (6.37). We refer to x^* as the *minimum norm element* of L. We have already discussed in Section 6.4 why choosing a minimum norm element may be considered useful in picture reconstruction.

It is clear from (11.23) that if we choose $x^{(0)}$ to be an element of S, then $x^{(k)}$ is an element of S, for all k. It follows, using basic linear algebra, that the limit x^* of the sequence $x^{(0)}, x^{(1)}, x^{(2)}, \ldots$, is also in S. Since the limit x^* is also in L (by the convergence of the relaxation method for equalities), x^* is in $L \cap S$. Hence, by the minimum norm theorem, x^* is the minimum norm element of L.

In the example for Fig. 11.1, S is the set of all two-dimensional vectors. Hence $x^{(0)}$ is in S, whichever way it is chosen. Since in that simple example there is only one solution, it is by necessity the minimum norm solution. This is, however, not typical. If there are more unknowns than equations, there will be invariably many solutions, and care has to be taken in choosing $x^{(0)}$ if the minimum norm solution is desired.

There are versions of the relaxation method that provide the minimum norm solution for a system of inequalities. These are more complex than the methods previously discussed and are beyond the scope of this book. In the next section we discuss a method whose implementation is similar to the implementation of relaxation methods for finding the minimum norm solution for a system of inequalities.

11.3 Additive ART

In this section we discuss the application of the relaxation methods of the last section to image reconstruction. Such methods are referred to as *additive* ART, since in a single iterative step the current iterate is altered by adding to it a scalar multiple of the transpose of a row of the projection matrix; see (11.1) and (11.2).

The simplest approach is to use the relaxation method for equalities, described by (11.23) and (11.24), with $a_i = r_i$ and $b_i = y_i$. By the result stated in the previous section, this generates a sequence of vectors $x^{(0)}, x^{(1)}, x^{(2)}, \ldots$ that converges to an x^* such that $Rx^* = y$, provided that there is such an x^*. The problem is that the relationship between the image vector x and the measurement vector y (6.24) is such that there may not exist such an x^* or that, even if such an x^* exists, it may not be a desirable solution to the discrete reconstruction problem. In view of this, it is pleasantly surprising that even this simple approach leads to acceptable reconstructions, especially if the relaxation parameters are chosen to be rather small (e.g., 0.05). This is illustrated in Section 11.5.

One way of making the theory of the last section applicable to the image reconstruction problem is by using the formulation that involves a system of inequalities (6.42). Much work has been done in that direction. In particular, ART-type procedures exist that find the minimum norm solution of a system of inequalities. Such procedures require a formulation more complicated than what is provided by the framework of (11.1). In addition to the sequence of J-dimensional vectors $x^{(0)}, x^{(1)}, x^{(2)}, \ldots$, they produce and use a sequence of I-dimensional vectors $u^{(0)}, u^{(1)}, u^{(2)}, \ldots$.

In this book we discuss an alternative approach, but one that has a similar implementation. We give an additive ART method for finding the Bayesian estimate (see Section 6.4) under certain restrictive assumptions.

In the terminology of Section 6.4, we make the following assumptions. Both X and E are multivariate Gaussian random variables, with μ_E the zero vector, and V_X and V_E both multiples of identity matrices of appropriate sizes. In other words, we assume that components of a sample of $X - \mu_X$ are uncorrelated, and that each component is a sample from the same Gaussian random variable; and we also assume that components of a sample of E are uncorrelated and that each component is a sample from the same zero mean Gaussian random variable.

We use t^2 to denote the diagonal entries of V_X and s^2 to denote the diagonal entries of V_E and let $r = t/s$. It follows from the discussion around (6.31) that the dimensionality of t, and hence of r, is inverse length. According to (6.33), the Bayesian estimate is the vector x that minimizes

$$r^2 \|y - Rx\|^2 + \|x - \mu_X\|^2 . \tag{11.27}$$

Note that a small value of r indicates that prior knowledge of the expected value of the image vector is important relative to the measured data, while a large value of r indicates the opposite.

What we are going to do now is essentially the following. We look at the equation $Rx + e = y$ as an equation in $I + J$ unknowns, namely all the components of x and all the components of e. This is a consistent system of equations; for any x, $e = y - Rx$ provides a solution. Methods for solving consistent systems can therefore be applied. However, in order to find the x that minimizes (11.27) a slightly more complicated approach is needed.

We denote column vectors of dimension $I + J$ by

$$\begin{pmatrix} u \\ z \end{pmatrix},$$

where u has I components and z has J components. We also use the notation

$$(U \quad rR)$$

for the $I \times (I+J)$ matrix, whose first I columns form the $I \times I$ identity matrix U and whose last J columns form the matrix R with every entry multiplied by r. The system of equations

$$(U \quad rR) \begin{pmatrix} u \\ z \end{pmatrix} = r\,(y - R\mu_X) \tag{11.28}$$

is a consistent system of equations. This is because, if we let $\hat{z}$ be an arbitrary J-dimensional vector and let

$$\hat{u} = r(y - R\mu_X - R\hat{z}), \tag{11.29}$$

then $\begin{pmatrix} \hat{u} \\ \hat{z} \end{pmatrix}$ satisfies (11.28).

The reason for introducing (11.28) is the following. If u^* and z^* are vectors such that $\begin{pmatrix} u^* \\ z^* \end{pmatrix}$ is the minimum norm solution of (11.28) and if

$$x^* = z^* + \mu_X, \tag{11.30}$$

then x^* minimizes (11.27).

In order to verify this claim consider any J-dimensional vector $\hat{x}$. Let

$$\hat{z} = \hat{x} - \mu_X \tag{11.31}$$

and define $\hat{u}$ by (11.29). Then

$$\hat{u} = r(y - R\hat{x}). \tag{11.32}$$

It follows that

$$r^2 \|y - R\hat{x}\|^2 + \|\hat{x} - \mu_X\|^2 = \|\hat{u}\|^2 + \|\hat{z}\|^2 \geq \|u^*\|^2 + \|z^*\|^2, \tag{11.33}$$

since $\begin{pmatrix} u^* \\ z^* \end{pmatrix}$ is the minimum norm solution of (11.28) and $\begin{pmatrix} \hat{u} \\ \hat{z} \end{pmatrix}$ is also a solution of (11.28).

From the fact that u^*, z^*, and x^* satisfy (11.28) and (11.30), we obtain

$$u^* = r\left(y - Rx^*\right). \tag{11.34}$$

This combined with (11.30) and (11.33) gives

$$r^2 \|y - R\hat{x}\|^2 + \|\hat{x} - \mu_X\|^2 \geq r^2 \|y - Rx^*\|^2 + \|x^* - \mu_X\|^2. \tag{11.35}$$

Since $\hat{x}$ is an arbitrary J-dimensional vector, this shows that x^* minimizes (11.27).

It follows therefore that any method that provides the minimum norm solution of (11.28) automatically gives us the vector that minimizes (11.27). One way of finding the minimum norm solution of a consistent system of equalities is the relaxation method for equalities. Note that the iterative step of (11.23) applied to (11.28) is

$$\begin{pmatrix} u^{(k+1)} \\ z^{(k+1)} \end{pmatrix} = \begin{pmatrix} u^{(k)} \\ z^{(k)} \end{pmatrix} + c^{(k)} \begin{pmatrix} e_{i_k} \\ r\, r_{i_k} \end{pmatrix}, \tag{11.36}$$

where e_i denotes the transpose of the ith row of E (which happens to be the same as the ith column of E, since E is an identity matrix), and

$$c^{(k)} = \lambda^{(k)} \frac{r\left(y_{i_k} - \langle r_{i_k}, \mu_X \rangle\right) - \left(u_{i_k}^{(k)} + r\left\langle r_{i_k}, z^{(k)}\right\rangle\right)}{1 + r^2 \left\| r_{i_k} \right\|^2}. \tag{11.37}$$

Note that, if S is defined by (11.25), then the zero vector is in S. Hence, one way of ensuring that the relaxation method for equalities, with iterative steps as in (11.36), converges to the minimum norm solution of (11.28) is to choose both $u^{(0)}$ and $z^{(0)}$ to be zero vectors of appropriate dimensions.

We define, for all k,

$$x^{(k)} = z^{(k)} + \mu_X. \tag{11.38}$$

If the sequence $z^{(0)}, z^{(1)}, z^{(2)}, \ldots$ converges to z^*, then the sequence $x^{(0)}, x^{(1)}, x^{(2)}, \ldots$ converges to x^*, defined by (11.30). This x^* minimizes (11.27).

There is in fact no need to introduce explicitly the $z^{(k)}$ into the algorithm. Combining (11.36), (11.37), and (11.38) with the fact that both $u^{(0)}$ and $z^{(0)}$ are chosen to be zero vectors, we get the following algorithm. The sequence $x^{(0)}, x^{(1)}, x^{(2)}, \ldots$ produced by it converges to the Bayesian estimate x^*, provided that the relaxation parameters $\lambda^{(k)}$ satisfy (11.11).

$$\begin{aligned}
&u^{(0)} \text{ is the } I\text{-dimensional zero vector,}\\
&x^{(0)} = \mu_X,\\
&u^{(k+1)} = u^{(k)} + c^{(k)} e_{i_k},\\
&x^{(k+1)} = x^{(k)} + r c^{(k)} r_{i_k},
\end{aligned} \tag{11.39}$$

where

$$c^{(k)} = \lambda^{(k)} \frac{r\left(y_{i_k} - \left\langle r_{i_k}, x^{(k)}\right\rangle\right) - u_{i_k}^{(k)}}{1 + r^2 \left\| r_{i_k} \right\|^2}. \tag{11.40}$$

Note that this algorithm cannot be brought into the framework of (11.1), but its implementation is hardly more complicated than the implementation of the method described by (11.2). We need an additional sequence of I-dimensional vectors $u^{(k)}$, but in the kth iterative step, only one component of $u^{(k)}$ (namely the i_kth component) is needed or altered. As pointed out in Section 11.1, in our application area the r_{i_k} are usually not stored at all, but the location and size of their nonzero elements are calculated as and when needed. Hence the algorithm described by (11.39) and (11.40) shares the storage-efficient nature of the simple ART method described in Section 11.1. It is easy to see that the computational requirements are also essentially the same.

The algorithm described by (11.39) and (11.40) is a typical additive ART algorithm. To illustrate this further, we now state, without proof, an additive ART algorithm that produces a sequence $x^{(0)}, x^{(1)}, x^{(2)}, \ldots$ that converges to the minimum norm solution of a system of two-sided inequalities

$$\gamma_i \leq \langle r_i, x \rangle \leq \delta_i, \tag{11.41}$$

$1 \leq i \leq I$; compare this with (6.40).

$$\begin{aligned} &u^{(0)} \text{ is the } I\text{-dimensional zero vector,} \\ &x^{(0)} \text{ is the } J\text{-dimensional zero vector,} \\ &u^{(k+1)} = u^{(k)} + c^{(k)} e_{i_k}, \\ &x^{(k+1)} = x^{(k)} + c^{(k)} r_{i_k}, \end{aligned} \tag{11.42}$$

where

$$c^{(k)} = \operatorname{mid}\left\{u_{i_k}^{(k)}, \left(\delta_{i_k} - \left\langle r_{i_k}, x^{(k)} \right\rangle\right) / \left\|r_{i_k}\right\|^2, \left(\gamma_{i_k} - \left\langle r_{i_k}, x^{(k)} \right\rangle\right) / \left\|r_{i_k}\right\|^2\right\}, \tag{11.43}$$

where $\operatorname{mid}\{u, v, w\}$ denotes the median of the three real numbers u, v, and w. The algorithm described by (11.42) and (11.43) has been referred to as ART4 in the literature, in order to distinguish it from other versions of ART, which have different convergence properties.

11.4 Tricks

It has been found in practice that the efficiency of iterative algorithms for image reconstruction can often be improved by applying between iterative steps certain processes to the image vectors. These processes have been referred to as *tricks* in the literature. In this section we deal with such tricks and also with other recommendations that can be made based on experience to improve the performance of ART, especially the potential usefulness of the images obtained by the early iterations of the algorithm.

Consider the iterative step in ART as described by (11.1). Let τ_k be functions mapping J-dimensional vectors into J-dimensional vectors. Then the iterative method of (11.1) combined with the sequence of tricks τ_k produces a sequence $x^{(0)}, x^{(1)}, x^{(2)}, \ldots$ defined by

$$\hat{x}^{(k+1)} = \alpha_k \left(x^{(k)}, r_{i_k}, y_{i_k}\right), \tag{11.44}$$

$$x^{(k+1)} = \tau_{k+1} \left(\hat{x}^{(k+1)}\right). \tag{11.45}$$

Tricks are useful if they incorporate prior knowledge about the desirable image vectors. Sometimes they can be used to accelerate convergence towards the image vector that satisfies the specified optimization criterion. Other times, they actually cause the process to move towards an image vector other than the one optimizing the specified criterion function, but that is nevertheless a better approximation of the picture to be reconstructed according to some evaluation criterion such as the picture distance measures of Section 5.1. The latter happens, for instance, if the desirable digitized pictures have a common property that cannot be expressed by a simple function, but that may be obtained by the application of an appropriate trick. In the discussions that follow, the intuitive justifications for all the tricks are based on the assumption that the basis functions are those associated with an $n \times n$ digitization, defined by (6.17).

One possible trick is based on the idea of *selective smoothing*, discussed in Section 5.3. It is potentially useful when the image to be reconstructed is made up from regions within which the values are largely uniform and distinguishable from those in other regions. (Figures 5.3 and 5.4 illustrate the effect of a single application of the trick of selective smoothing to the output of FBP for divergent beams. Table 5.1 shows that improvements in the picture distance measures are achieved using this trick. There was also an improvement in the HITR in our task-oriented experiment, but not in the IROI.) When this trick is used in conjunction with ART, typically we choose τ_k in (11.45) to represent selective smoothing only infrequently, e.g., only when k is a multiple of I (the number of measurements). For other values of k, we choose τ_k to be the identity function, which does not change the image vector.

In contrast, the trick of constraining is usually applied at every iterative step of ART. *Constraining* is justified in case we have prior information about the range within which the components of acceptable image vectors must lie. For example, the linear attenuation coefficient (at any energy) is always nonnegative, and in medical applications we may usually assume that it is always bounded above by the linear attenuation coefficient of compact bone. Such constraints may be introduced into series expansion methods in various ways. They may simply be made part of the set of inequalities (11.6). Or they may be introduced into the iterative algorithm as tricks. For example, if we know that, for $1 \le j \le J$,

$$\lambda \le x_j \le \mu, \tag{11.46}$$

then the following trick is appropriate.

$$\tau_k(\hat{x}) = x, \tag{11.47}$$

where, for $1 \le j \le J$,

$$x_j = \begin{cases} \lambda, & \text{if } \hat{x}_j < \lambda, \\ \hat{x}_j & \text{if } \lambda \le \hat{x}_j \le \mu, \\ \mu, & \text{if } \mu < \hat{x}_j. \end{cases} \tag{11.48}$$

Such a trick can be easily incorporated into ART. To demonstrate this, consider the relaxation method for inequalities. The following is claimed to be true. If N, as in (11.8), contains at least one vector x whose components satisfy (11.46), then the algorithm below produces a sequence $x^{(0)}, x^{(1)}, x^{(2)}, \ldots$ that converges to an element of N whose components satisfy (11.46).

$$\begin{aligned} x^{(0)} & \quad \text{is arbitrary,} \\ \hat{x}^{(k+1)} &= \alpha_k \left(x^{(k)}, n_{i_k}, q_{i_k} \right), \\ x^{(k+1)} &= \tau_{k+1} \left(\hat{x}^{(k+1)} \right), \end{aligned} \tag{11.49}$$

where α_k is defined by (11.9) with the λ_k satisfying (11.11), and τ_k is defined by (11.47) and (11.48).

The verification of this claim follows easily from the convergence of the relaxation method for inequalities. This is because the set of vectors M that satisfy (11.46) can be characterized as follows. Let, for $1 \leq j \leq J$,

$$M_{2j-1} = \{x \mid x_j \leq \mu\} \tag{11.50}$$

and

$$M_{2j} = \{x \mid -x_j \leq -\lambda\} . \tag{11.51}$$

Then

$$M = \bigcap_{j=1}^{2J} M_j . \tag{11.52}$$

Thus M, the set of vectors satisfying (11.46), can be described in a way strictly analogous to the way N is described in Section 11.2. The reader can easily check that applying the relaxation method for inequalities based on M instead of N, with relaxation parameter 1 and initial vector $\hat{x}$ produces in $2J$ iterative steps the vector $\tau_k(\hat{x})$ where τ_k is defined by (11.47) and (11.48). Thus, the trick of constraining in this case is equivalent to applying the relaxation method to a larger set of inequalities. This completes the verification of the claim on the convergence of (11.49).

There are other versions of constraining in use besides the one specified by (11.47) and (11.48). For example, there is a way of defining the constraining τ_ks so that, when used in conjunction with the algorithm described in (11.42), the method converges to the minimum norm solution of the combined system (11.41) and (11.46). Another method, which is useful when it is known a priori that there are only two different densities in the picture (as is the case in certain nondestructive testing applications), is to use τ_ks that set the values of $\hat{x}_j$ to either one or the other of the two densities.

Another trick that we have already come across is *normalization*. This is discussed in conjunction with the backprojection method in Section 7.2. Repeated normalization during the iterative procedure has sometimes been found to improve the speed of convergence of ART to a desirable result.

A trick whose use is relatively recent is referred to as *superiorization*. The idea is the following. Suppose that we have a secondary optimization criterion of the kind discussed in Section 6.4 for which we do not have an efficient algorithm that converges to the optimal solution for a given set of equality and/or inequality constraints; a possible example is total variation (6.45) minimization. Then we can select the τ_ks so that they steer the iterative process in the direction of the optimal solution. If the criterion is to find an x

satisfying the constraints for which $\phi(x)$ is small for some functional ϕ (such as provided by TV), then we can use

$$\tau_k(x) = x - \beta_k \nabla\phi(x), \tag{11.53}$$

where the vector $\nabla\phi(x)$ (called the *gradient* of ϕ at x) is the direction of greatest increase in ϕ at the vector x and the β_k are positive real numbers. For appropriate choices of the β_k it can be proved that if an ART procedure converges to a vector satisfying a set of equality/inequality constraints, then the same procedure altered by the trick of (11.53) also converges to such a vector. The expectation (validated by experience) is that for the procedure with the trick we get to an x for which $\phi(x)$ is smaller than it would be without the trick. Ideally, we would like to get to an x for which $\phi(x)$ is as small as possible, but this is not guaranteed; this is why the trick is referred to as superiorization (as opposed to optimization). In practice the trick of superiorization, just like the trick of selective smoothing, is applied only infrequently during the iterative process.

Although there are other tricks whose use has been reported in the literature, we conclude this section by a discussion of four topics related to, but somewhat different from, tricks.

An essential tool available with ART is the relaxation parameter. We have already mentioned that choosing a low value for the relaxation parameter has been found to result in good reconstructions using ART-type algorithms, even on experimentally obtained data. A low relaxation parameter, *underrelaxation*, seems to reduce the effect of inaccuracies in the equations, and prevents the noisy appearance of ART-type reconstructions when using a high relaxation parameter. This is illustrated in the next section.

In certain situations a limited use of a high relaxation parameter is advisable. When solving a system of inequalities, the process can be markedly shortened if, whenever an inequality is only slightly violated by the current iterate, a relaxation parameter with value 2 is used, resulting in a mirror *reflection* of the iterate in the bounding hyperplane associated with the inequality. Selective use of reflections can, under certain circumstances, ensure finite convergence.

The choice of *initialization* (i.e., of $x^{(0)}$) has an effect on the outcome of the iterative procedure, especially since due to time and cost constraints the number of iterative steps may be rather limited. For example, in the algorithm (11.39) $x^{(0)}$ is supposed to be μ_X. In practice, it may be very difficult to find the mean of the multivariate random variable that represents the actual situation. Instead, outputs of other methods (such as FBP) have often been used as $x^{(0)}$ for ART. Even more frequent in practice is the use of a uniformly gray picture, possibly with the estimated average density in every pixel, which is what was done in all the ART experiments reported in the next section.

Last, but not least, the order of equations (or inequalities) in the system (the data access ordering discussed in Section 11.1) can also have a significant effect on the practical performance of the algorithm, especially on the early iterates. With data collection such as our standard geometry depicted in Fig. 5.5, it is tempting to use the *sequential ordering*: access the data in the order $g(-N\lambda,0), g((-N+1)\lambda,0), \ldots, g(N\lambda,0), g(-N\lambda,\Delta), g((-N+1)\lambda,\Delta), \ldots, g(N\lambda,\Delta), \ldots, \ldots, g(-N\lambda,(M-1)\Delta), g((-N+1)\lambda,(M-1)\Delta), \ldots, g(N\lambda,(M-1)\Delta)$, where $g(\sigma,\beta)$ denotes here the measured value of what is mathematically defined in (10.2). However, this sequential ordering is inferior to what is referred to as the *efficient ordering* in which the order of projection directions $m\Delta$ and, for each view, the order of lines within the view is chosen so as to minimize the number of commonly intersected pixels by a line and the lines selected recently. This can be made mathematically precise by considering the decomposition into a product of prime numbers of M and of $2N+1$. SNARK09 calculates the efficient order, but the user needs to ensure that both M and of $2N+1$ decompose into several prime numbers, as is the case for our standard geometry for which $M = 720 = 2 \times 2 \times 2 \times 2 \times 3 \times 3 \times 5$ and $2N+1 = 345 = 3 \times 5 \times 23$. While the sequential ordering produces the sequences $m = 0,1,2,3,4,\ldots$ and $n = 0,1,2,3,4,\ldots$, the efficient ordering produces the sequences $m = 0,360,180,540,90,\ldots$ and $n = 0,115,230,23,138,\ldots$ These changes in data access ordering translate into faster initial convergence of ART, as is illustrated in Fig. 11.2 by plotting

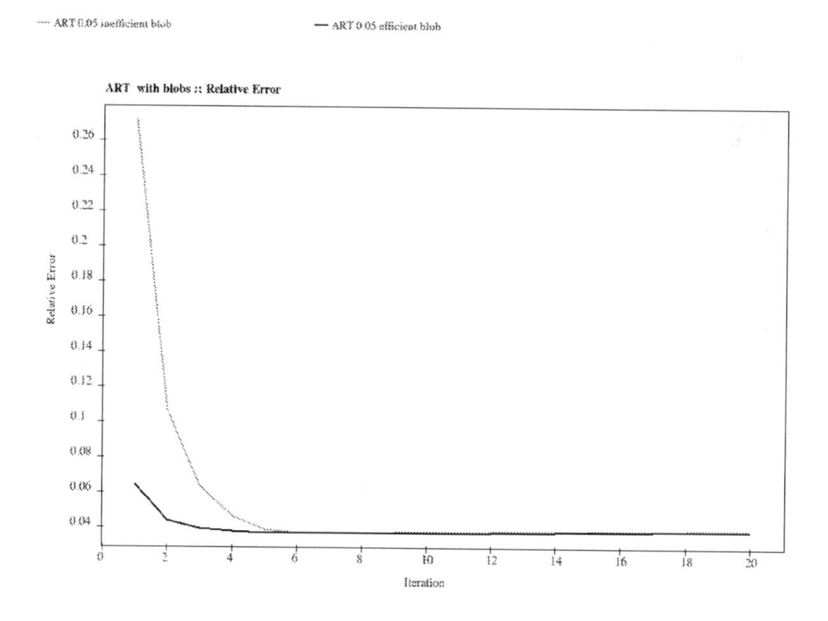

Fig. 11.2: Values of the picture distance measure r for ART reconstructions from the standard projection data with sequential ordering (light) and efficient ordering (dark), plotted at multiples of I iterations (complete cycles through the data).

the picture distance measure r against the number of times the algorithm cycled through all the data (all I equations). While it is clearly demonstrated that initially r gets reduced much faster with the efficient ordering, for this particular data set it does not seem to matter much, since both orderings need about five cycles through the data to obtain a near-minimal value of r. In other applications in which the number of projection directions is much larger (for example, in the order of 10,000 as is often the case in electron microscopy), one cycle through the data using the efficient ordering yields about as good a reconstruction as one is likely to get, but the sequential ordering needs several cycles through the data. In addition, as we demonstrate in the next section, the efficacy of the reconstruction produced by the efficient ordering may very well be superior to that produced by the sequential ordering.

11.5 Efficacy of ART

In this section we illustrate some of the algebraic reconstruction techniques. All the illustrations are done on the standard projection data. Only outputs at the end of some integer multiple of I iterations are used. This is because in I iterations the measurements for all source–detector positions have been made use of exactly once; i.e., we have cycled through the data exactly once. In all ART reconstructions reported in this section we initialized the process so that all components of x^0 are given the value of the estimated average density $\bar{x}$ based on the projection data, as specified in Section 6.4. We note that if we gave to the components of x^0 the value 0, the resulting $x^{(I)}$ would be indistinguishable from the $x^{(I)}$ we get by our selected initialization (with blobs, all $\lambda^{(k)} = 0.05$, efficient ordering, and no nonnegativity constraints).

We wish to emphasize first the importance of the basis functions. In Fig. 11.3 we plot the picture distance measure r against the number of times ART cycled through all the data, where we made the choices that the relaxation parameter is always 0.05 and the data access ordering is the efficient one. The two cases that we compare are when the basis functions are based on pixels

Table 11.1: Picture distance measures and timings (in seconds) for the reconstructions in Fig. 11.4. The last two columns report on the values of IROI and HITR for the various algorithms that were produced by a task-oriented evaluation experiment.

reconstruction in	d	r	t	IROI	HITR
Fig. 11.4(a)	0.1060	0.0423	8.7	0.1677	0.9499
Fig. 11.4(b)	0.0813	0.0327	29.4	0.1658	0.9213
Fig. 11.4(c)	0.0874	0.0470	29.2	0.1592	0.9198
Fig. 11.4(d)	0.0874	0.0373	163.7	0.1794	0.9481
Fig. 11.4(e)	0.0768	0.0488	66.2	0.1076	0.7128
Fig. 11.4(f)	0.0876	0.0391	148.9	0.1624	0.7820

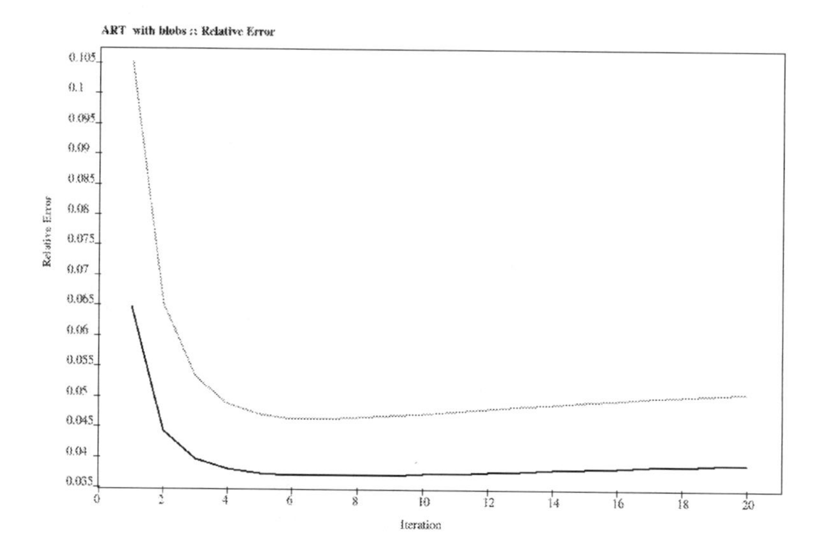

Fig. 11.3: Values of the picture distance measure r for ART reconstructions from the standard projection data with pixels (light) and blobs (dark), plotted at multiples of I iterations (complete cycles through the data).

and when they are based on blobs as specified in Section 6.5. The results are quite impressive: as measured by r, blob basis functions are much better. The result of the $5I$th iteration of the blob reconstruction is shown in Fig. 11.4(d), while that of the $5I$th iteration of the pixel reconstruction is shown in Fig. 11.4(c). The blob reconstructions appears to be clearly superior. We attempted to improve the pixel reconstruction by enforcing nonnegativity on the reconstructed values, as can be done using ART by setting $\lambda = 0$ in (11.46). This does not result in a noticeable improvement in appearance, as can be seen in Fig. 11.4(b). By looking at Table 11.1, we see great improvements in the picture distance measures r and d as a result of enforcing nonnegativity, but this is totally misleading from the point of view of our application because the improvement is due to the values being more correctly reconstructed outside the skull (where the values in the phantom are all 0). From the points of view of the task-oriented figures of merit, IROI and HITR, ART with blobs is found superior to ART with pixels, with or without nonnegativity; the relevant P-values are all less than 10^{-10}. Plots of values along the 131st column of the ART with pixels and nonnegativity reconstruction and of the ART with blobs reconstruction are compared in Fig. 11.5.

Underrelaxation is also a must when ART is applied to real, and hence imperfect, data. In the experiments reported so far $\lambda^{(k)}$ was set equal to 0.05 for all k. If we do not use underrelaxation (that is we set $\lambda^{(k)}$ to 1 for all k), we get from the standard projection data the unacceptable reconstruction shown in Fig. 11.4(e). Note that in this case we used the $2I$th iterate, further iterations give worse results. The reason for this is in the nature of ART: after one iterative step with $\lambda^{(k)} = 1$, the associated measurement is satisfied exactly as shown in (11.5) and so the process jumps around satisfying the noise in the measurements. Underrelaxation reduces the influence of the noise. The correct value of the relaxation parameter is application dependent; the noisier the data the more we should be underrelaxing. Note in Table 11.1 that the figures of merit produced by the task-oriented studies without underrelaxation are much smaller than in all the other cases with which they are compared.

We now return to the issue of data access ordering. Using $5I$ iterations with $\lambda^{(k)} = 0.05$ for all k, we get from our standard projection data using the sequential ordering the reconstruction shown in Fig. 11.4(f), which does not look very different from the reconstruction obtained using the efficient ordering that is shown in Fig. 11.4(d). However, using either IROI or HITR as the figure of merit, results in our rejecting the null hypothesis that the two data access orderings are equally good in favor of the alternative hypothesis that the the efficient ordering is better with P-value less than 10^{-9}.

For comparison, we show in Fig. 11.4(a) the reconstruction from our standard projection data obtained by FBP for divergent beams with linear interpolation and sinc window (also called the Shepp–Logan window). The visual quality is similar to the best among the ART reconstructions that are reported, which is shown in Fig. 11.4(d). According to the picture distance measures ART is superior to FBP, and the same is true according to IROI with extreme significance (the P-value is less than 10^{-13}). According to HITR, FBP appears to be superior to ART, but the result is not particularly significant (the P-value is 0.0400, which means that even if the null hypothesis that the two methods are equally good were correct, there would be a 1 in 25 chance of observing a difference greater than what we observed). This experiment confirms the reports in the literature that ART with blobs, underrelaxation and efficient ordering outperforms FBP.

Fig. 11.4: Reconstructions from the standard projection data using (a) FBP for divergent beams with linear interpolation and sinc window (also called the Shepp–Logan window), (b) ART with pixels, $\lambda^{(k)} = 0.05$, $5I$th iteration, efficient ordering and nonnegativity, (c) ART with pixels, $\lambda^{(k)} = 0.05$, $5I$th iteration, efficient ordering and no nonnegativity, (d) ART with blobs, $\lambda^{(k)} = 0.05$, $5I$th iteration, efficient ordering and no nonnegativity, (e) ART with blobs, $\lambda^{(k)} = 1.0$, $2I$th iteration, efficient ordering and no nonnegativity, (f) ART with blobs, $\lambda^{(k)} = 0.05$, $5I$th iteration, sequential ordering and no nonnegativity.

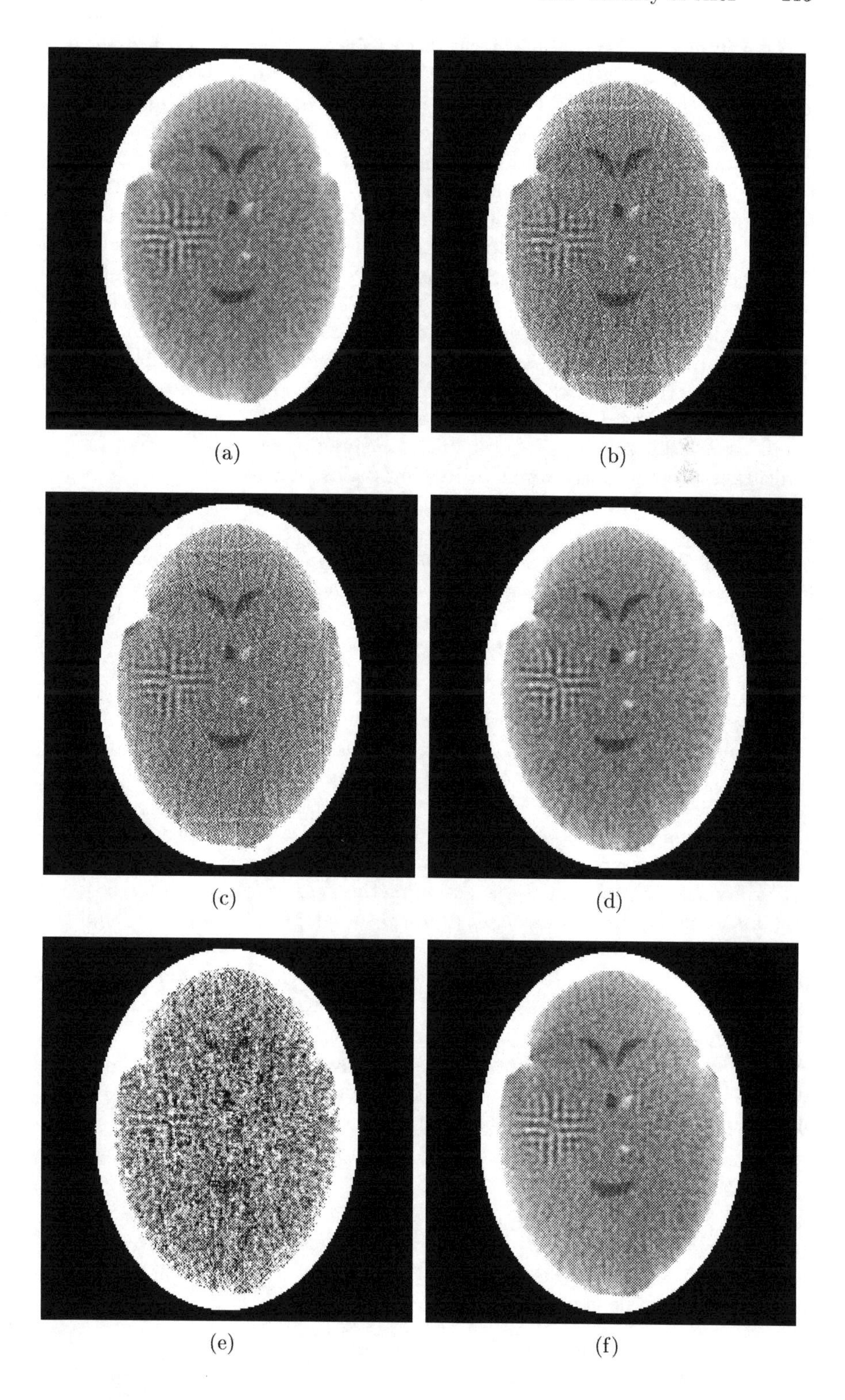
(a)
(b)
(c)
(d)
(e)
(f)

One thing is indisputable: the ART with blob reconstruction took nearly 19 times longer than FBP. However, this should not be the determining factor. The implementation of ART with blobs in SNARK09 is far from optimal and can be greatly improved. Also, computational speed keeps improving: the time reported in the first edition of this book (1980) for the ART with pixel reconstruction for a much smaller data set is 100 times longer than what we report here! A main advantage of ART over FBP is its flexibility. Even though in this section we have reported its application to data collected according to the standard geometry, the theory supports reconstruction from data collected over any set of lines. FBP-type algorithms need to be reinvented for each new mode of data collection, just as we had to do when we moved from parallel beams to divergent beams. Another aspect of the flexibility of ART is the ability to incorporate tricks and thereby steer the process towards a solution that is superior according to some criterion, such as TV.

In fact, ART can be used not only for superiorization but even for optimization of some fairly sophisticated functions. For example, the additive ART algorithm described in (11.39) and (11.40) converges to the Bayesian estimate x which minimizes (11.27). We delay the illustration of the usefulness of this until Section 13.3, where we demonstrate it on the reconstruction of a dynamic three-dimensional object, such as the heart.

Notes and References

ART for image reconstruction was first introduced into the open literature in [99]. Coincidentally, essentially the same method had been already proposed for CT in a patent specification [145], originally filed in 1968. In fact, the simple procedure expressed in (11.2) was proposed in 1937 by S. Kaczmarz [154] for solving systems of consistent linear equations. An early tutorial on ART is [98], a more recent one is [117]. The methods discussed in this chapter are examples of the so-called row-action methods for solving very large sparse systems of equations and inequalities; for a survey, see [41, 46] and Chapter 6 of [48]. Such methods can be extended from finding common points of hyperplanes and half-spaces, as we discuss in this book, to finding common points of arbitrary closed convex sets (this is often referred to as POCS, short for projections onto convex sets); see, for example, Chapter 5 of [48] and [21]. An ART algorithm of this kind with a finite convergence property is ART3, described by [110]; for a faster version with an application to intensity modulated radiation therapy see [120].

Fig. 11.5: Plots of the head phantom of Fig. 4.6(a), shown light, and its reconstructions, shown dark, from the standard projection data using ART with $\lambda^{(k)} = 0.05$, efficient ordering and (a) pixels, $5I$th iteration and nonnegativity, and (b) blobs, $5I$th iteration and no nonnegativity.

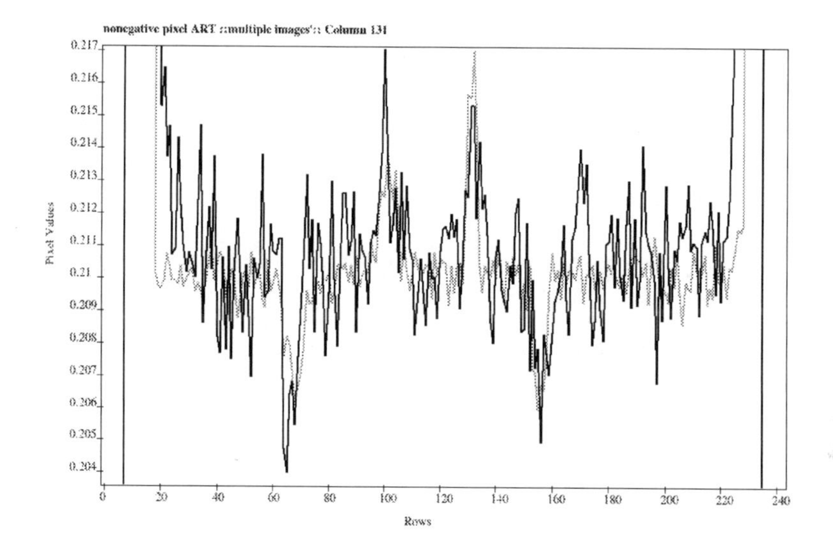
standard head phantom
standard pro_ART nonnegat_ART_0005_r_a
nonegative pixel ART ::multiple images':: Column 131
0.217
0.216
0.215
0.214
0.213
0.212
0.211
0.21
0.209
0.208
0.207
0.206
0.205
0.204
Pixel Values
0
20
40
60
80
100
120
140
160
180
200
220
240
Rows

(a)

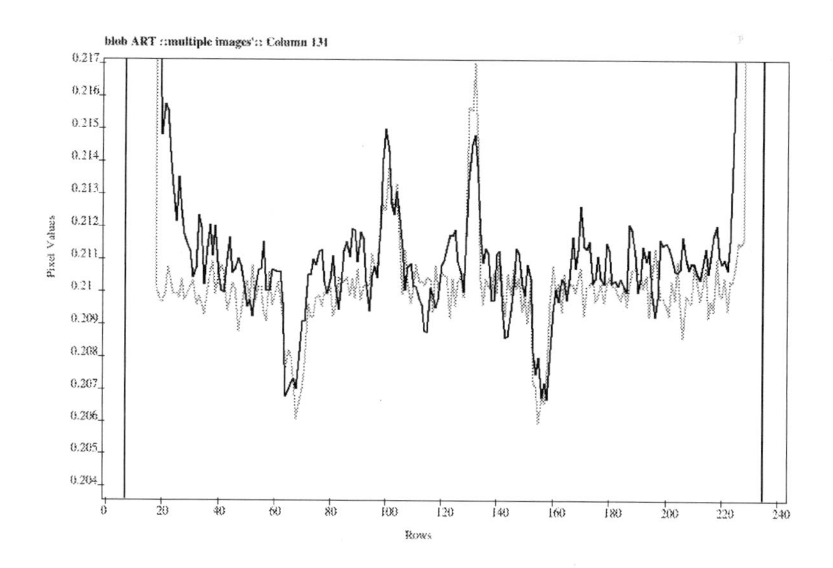
standard head phantom
standard pro_ART efficien_ART_0005_r_a
blob ART ::multiple images':: Column 131
0.217
0.216
0.215
0.214
0.213
0.212
0.211
0.21
0.209
0.208
0.207
0.206
0.205
0.204
Pixel Values
0
20
40
60
80
100
120
140
160
180
200
220
240
Rows

(b)

Our presentation of the relaxation method for solving systems of inequalities and equalities is based on [127] and [130], which reference earlier literature. The minimum norm theorem is a trivial consequence of what in optimization theory is referred to as the projection theorem (not to be confused with the theorem of the same name in image reconstruction); see, e.g., [190]. A relaxational approach to finding the minimum norm solution of systems of inequalities is presented in [177]. How such an approach translates into an algorithm for image reconstruction is discussed in [129].

Our discussion of the Bayesian approach is based on [123] and [124]; the former gives a detailed discussion of the validity of the assumptions made in the Bayesian approach. It can be generalized to minimize more complicated quadratic functions than the one in (11.27), see Appendix B of [185].

The expression "tricks" was first applied to the processes described in Section 11.4 in [127]. A treatment of the asymptotic behavior of iterative algorithms combined with the trick of selective smoothing is given in [64]. An algorithm that finds the minimum norm solution of the combined systems (11.41) and (11.46) is described in [129]; see also [220]. An algorithm for reconstructing objects with only two densities was given in [109]; the problem of reconstruction assuming only a few densities has developed into the field of discrete tomography [125]. The notion of superiorization, in particular in conjunction with total variation minimization, was introduced in [36]; see also [121]. A demonstration of the power of underrelaxation is given in [114]: it is shown that the trick of using a complimentary matrix (not discussed in this book) can be incorporated into ART as a special case of underrelaxation.

A theoretical study of the order in which views should be selected in ART was published in [106]. That paper, and its references, are also of interest, since they use a model for the image reconstruction problem different from anything discussed in this book. The outcome is an iterative procedure, which deals with pictures (as opposed to image vectors). Such procedures were referred to as continuous ART in [127]. The efficient ordering that we have proposed in Section 11.4 was first advocated in [135].

Some versions of ART that are not in this book are discussed in [98, 127]. Multiplicative ART (MART) is of particular interest, since it maximizes entropy (6.44), as proved in [176] and in [178]. MART is still the subject of active research and use [149, 162, 273, 275]. Another row-action optimization algorithm is RAMLA [34] that maximizes likelihood as defined in (6.47).

An alternative is block-ART that instead of treating single equations or inequalities one by one, tries to satisfy simultaneously a number of them (e.g., all that are associated with a single source position in the standard geometry). An early example of such an approach is [73]. The idea was rediscovered in [147], using the name ordered subsets, and became popular in emission tomography. Examples of recent papers on block-ART are [45, 47, 121].

For methods of accelerating algorithms of the type discussed above by using commonly available hardware see [23, 206, 274] and their references. For another recent implementational approach see [214].

12

Quadratic Optimization Methods

In this chapter we discuss iterative procedures for minimizing the general quadratic function that incorporates as special cases a number of different optimization criteria discussed in Section 6.4. These iterative procedures are different in nature from ART; they have been referred to in the literature as *SIRT-type methods*.

12.1 Mathematical Background to Quadratic Optimization

First we recall some terminology. A matrix M is said to be *symmetric* if it is a square matrix and $m_{i,j} = m_{j,i}$, for all entries $m_{i,j}$ of M. A matrix M is said to be *positive definite* if it is symmetric and, for every (column) vector x with at least one nonzero component, $x^T M x > 0$. Note that every positive definite matrix M has an *inverse* M^{-1}. A matrix M is said to be *nonnegative definite* if it is symmetric and, for every vector x, $x^T M x \geq 0$.

The problem we are attempting to solve has the following form. *Given* a positive definite matrix D and two nonnegative definite matrices W_1 and W_2, *find* the x in K that minimizes

$$\left\| D^{-1} x \right\|, \tag{12.1}$$

where

$$K = \{x \mid k(x) \text{ is minimum}\}, \tag{12.2}$$

$$k(x) = (y - Rx)^T W_1 (y - Rx) + (x - x_0)^T W_2 (x - x_0). \tag{12.3}$$

Note that the right-hand side of (12.3) is exactly the function (6.39), whose minimization was shown to be the general quadratic optimization criterion, provided that

$$W_1 = aA, \tag{12.4}$$

and

Table 12.1: Choices of W_1, W_2 and x_0 for obtaining various optimization criteria in Section 6.4.

equation number	W_1	W_2	x_0
(6.33)	V_E^{-1}	V_X^{-1}	μ_X
(6.34)	U_I	Θ_J	
(6.35)	Θ_I	U_J	$\bar{\mathbf{x}}$
(6.37)	Θ_I	U_J	θ
(6.38)	aU_I	$bB + U_J$	θ

$$W_2 = bB + cC^{-1}. \tag{12.5}$$

In Section 6.4, (6.39) was arrived at by generalization of (6.33), (6.34), (6.35), (6.37), and (6.38). In Table 12.1 we specify the values of W_1, W_2 and x_0 for each of these equations. In that table U_I and U_J are the identity matrices of appropriate sizes, Θ_I and Θ_J are the matrices of appropriate sizes in which all entries are zeros, θ is the vector of all zeros and $\bar{\mathbf{x}}$ is the vector of all $\bar{x}$s, where $\bar{x}$ is the estimated average density based on the measurements.

In Section 6.4 we have not discussed in detail the nature of B in (6.38). This is to be remedied below; for now we need only note that B is a nonnegative definite matrix. In view of this, W_2 is positive definite in all cases, except in (6.34), in which case $W_2 = \Theta_J$. In what follows we assume that W_2 in (12.3) is either positive definite or the matrix consisting of zeros. Note that, as discussed after (6.38), the dimensionalities of the W_1 and W_2, and hence of the $k(x)$ as defined in (12.3), are not the same for all the rows of Table 12.1. As pointed out there, this is a minor technical matter that can be resolved by division by a positive number of appropriate dimensionality.

Our basic approach is to translate the quadratic minimization problem into a problem of solving a consistent system of equations. (We have already seen an example of such an approach in Section 11.3. In fact, the function we minimize there is a special case of (12.3), with $W_1 = r^2 U_I$ and $W_2 = U_J$ and $x_0 = \mu_X$.) We treat the two cases when W_2 is positive definite and when W_2 consists only of zeros separately.

Consider first the case when W_2 is positive definite. We assume that W_2 is defined by (12.5). The reason for writing W_2 this way is that sometimes C is known, but the optimization criterion refers to C^{-1}. An example is (6.33), in which $W_2 = V_X^{-1}$ with V_X the covariance matrix of a multivariate Gaussian random variable. Since C is a large matrix ($J \times J$, where J is the number of basis functions), we do not wish to invert C if this can be avoided. Rather, we attempt to design algorithms for minimizing $k(x)$ that do not need C^{-1}.

In designing the algorithm, we assume that C is a positive definite matrix, $c > 0$, and B is a nonnegative definite matrix. (It is easy to check that all the examples in Table 12.1, except (6.34) where $W_2 = \Theta$, satisfy these assumptions.) It is a standard result of linear algebra that a nonnegative definite matrix has a *square root*; i.e., that there exists a matrix $C^{1/2}$ such that,

$$C^{1/2}C^{1/2} = C. \tag{12.6}$$

Furthermore, $C^{1/2}$ is also positive definite, and hence has an inverse $C^{-1/2}$, such that $C^{-1/2}C^{-1/2} = C^{-1}$. We do not need to calculate $C^{1/2}$ in the algorithms described in the following, but we need it to describe the rationale behind the algorithms.

We introduce a new vector variable u by

$$u = C^{-1/2}\left(x - x_0\right). \tag{12.7}$$

Then

$$x = C^{1/2}u + x_0, \tag{12.8}$$

and, from (12.3), (12.4), and (12.5),

$$\begin{aligned}
k(x) &= k\left(C^{1/2}u + x_0\right) \\
&= a\left(y - R\left(C^{1/2}u + x_0\right)\right)^T A\left(y - R\left(C^{1/2}u + x_0\right)\right) \\
&\quad + \left(C^{1/2}u\right)^T \left(bB + cC^{-1}\right)\left(C^{1/2}u\right) \\
&= u^T\left(aC^{1/2}R^TARC^{1/2} + bC^{1/2}BC^{1/2} + cU_J\right)u \\
&\quad -2au^TC^{1/2}R^TA\left(y - Rx_0\right) \\
&\quad +a\left(y - Rx_0\right)^T A\left(y - Rx_0\right).
\end{aligned} \tag{12.9}$$

Using the abbreviations

$$P = aC^{1/2}R^TARC^{1/2} + bC^{1/2}BC^{1/2} + cU_J, \tag{12.10}$$

$$z = aC^{1/2}R^TA\left(y - Rx_0\right) \tag{12.11}$$

and

$$h(u) = \frac{1}{2}u^TPu - u^Tz, \tag{12.12}$$

we see that, provided (12.8) is satisfied,

$$h(u) = \frac{1}{2}k(x) - \frac{1}{2}a\left(y - Rx_0\right)^T A\left(y - Rx_0\right). \tag{12.13}$$

It follows that x^* minimizes $k(x)$ if, and only if, $x^* = C^{1/2}u^* + x_0$, where u^* minimizes $h(u)$. Thus the problem of finding elements of the set K in (12.2) can be solved by finding vectors u that minimize h in (12.12).

Consider now the case when $W_2 = \Theta_J$. We assume that $a \neq 0$, because otherwise $W_1 = \Theta_I$, and there is nothing left to minimize. We again introduce a variable u, this time defined by

$$u = D^{-1}x. \tag{12.14}$$

Then

$$x = Du, \tag{12.15}$$

and, from (12.3) and (12.4),

$$\begin{aligned} k(x) &= k(Du) \\ &= a(y - RDu)^T A(y - RDu) \\ &= u^T \left(aDR^T ARD\right) u - 2au^T DR^T Ay + ay^T Ay. \end{aligned} \tag{12.16}$$

Using the abbreviations

$$P = DR^T ARD, \tag{12.17}$$

$$z = DR^T Ay, \tag{12.18}$$

and $h(u)$ as defined by (12.12), we see that, provided (12.15) is satisfied,

$$h(u) = \frac{1}{2a} k(x) - \frac{1}{2} y^T Ay. \tag{12.19}$$

It follows that x^* minimizes $k(x)$ if, and only if, $x^* = Du^*$, where u^* minimizes $h(u)$. So, in this case also, the problem of finding elements of K in (12.2) can be solved by finding vectors u that minimize h in (12.12).

In both cases, we get from (12.12) to a system of equations by using the following result. For any $J \times J$ nonnegative definite matrix P and any J-dimensional vector z, the vector u minimizes (12.12) if, and only if,

$$Pu = z. \tag{12.20}$$

This result is applicable to both our cases, since P (defined either by (12.10) or by (12.17)) is nonnegative definite, as is easily proved by standard techniques of linear algebra.

An interesting consequence of the result is that K is empty, unless (12.20) has a solution. However, in our two cases (12.20) is guaranteed to have a solution. If P is defined by (12.10), then P is positive definite and so it has an inverse. It is a little more complicated to show, and therefore we omit the details, that (12.20) also has a solution if P and z are defined by (12.17) and (12.18), respectively.

As just pointed out, if W_2 is positive definite, then P has an inverse. Therefore there is only one u that is a solution to (12.20), namely $u = P^{-1}z$. Therefore, in this case, there is only one u^* that minimizes $h(u)$ and, consequently, only one x^* that minimizes $k(x)$. This x^* then is the unique element of K, and the secondary optimization criterion expressed by (12.1) is irrelevant.

In case $W_2 = \Theta_J$, let u^* be the minimum norm solution of (12.20). Then among the vectors that minimize $h(u)$, u^* is the one with the smallest norm. Defining $x^* = Du^*$, we see that among the vectors x that minimize $k(x)$, x^*

is the one for which $\|D^{-1}x^*\| = \|u^*\|$ is the smallest; see comments following (12.19). Thus, x^* is the vector we set out to find.

In summary, we have shown that the quadratic optimization problem, expressed by (12.1), (12.2), and (12.3), translates into the problem of solving a system of equations (12.20). If W_2 is positive definite, then (12.20) has a unique solution. If $W_2 = \Theta_J$, then the minimum norm solution of (12.20) is needed. In the next section we discuss a class of algorithms for solving (12.20).

12.2 Richardson's Method for Solving Systems of Equations

We have already given a method for finding the minimum norm solution of a system of consistent equations in Section 11.2. This is, of course, applicable to (12.20). In this section we discuss an alternative method.

The intuitive motivation for introducing this alternative method in image reconstruction was the following. If the relaxation method is used with a relaxation parameter 1, then satisfying a single equation may result in a very noticeable stripe along the line that corresponds to the equation. Repetition of such steps results in noisy-looking pictures such as the one shown in Fig. 11.4(e). The ART approach takes care of this by the judicious use of relaxation parameters; see Fig. 11.4(d). An alternative approach is to attempt to correct for all lines simultaneously. This is why such methods are called SIRT-like, where SIRT abbreviates *simultaneous iterative reconstruction technique*. (SIRT is a name reserved for a particular one of the SIRT-type methods, whose detailed discussion we omit for reasons of space.)

One way of adjusting an iterate so that errors in all equations are corrected simultaneously is

$$u^{(k+1)} = u^{(k)} + \lambda^{(k)} \left(z - Pu^{(k)} \right). \tag{12.21}$$

Note that an iterative step of this type is applicable only if P is a square matrix, since otherwise the dimension of z and $Pu^{(k)}$ would be different from the dimension of $u^{(k)}$. An iterative method whose kth iterative step is of the type expressed in (12.21) is called in numerical analysis a *Richardson's method.* (It also goes under a number of other names, but we stick to this one, since it seems historically appropriate.) Before discussing the convergence properties of such a method, we investigate its appearance in the two cases discussed in the previous section. This provides an insight to the behavior of a Richardson's method in image reconstruction.

If W_2 is positive definite, then P and z are given by (12.10) and (12.11), respectively. We define, for $k \geq 0$,

$$x^{(k)} = C^{1/2} u^{(k)} + x_0. \tag{12.22}$$

Then, from (12.21), (12.22), (12.10) and (12.11) we get

$$\begin{aligned}
x^{(k+1)} &= C^{1/2}u^{(k+1)} + x_0 \\
&= C^{1/2}\left(u^{(k)} + \lambda^{(k)}\left(z - Pu^{(k)}\right)\right) + x_0 \\
&= C^{1/2}u^{(k)} + x_0 + \lambda^{(k)}\left(C^{1/2}z - C^{1/2}PC^{-1/2}\left(x^{(k)} - x_0\right)\right) \\
&= x^{(k)} + \lambda^{(k)}\left(aCR^T A\left(y - Rx_0\right)\right. \\
&\quad \left. - \left(aCR^T AR + bCB + cU_J\right)\left(x^{(k)} - x_0\right)\right),
\end{aligned} \tag{12.23}$$

and so

$$x^{(k+1)} = x^{(k)} + \lambda^{(k)}\left(aCR^T A\left(y - Rx^{(k)}\right) + \left(bCB + cU_J\right)\left(x_0 - x^{(k)}\right)\right). \tag{12.24}$$

It follows from the discussion of the last section, in particular from the remarks following (12.13), that if $u^{(0)}, u^{(1)}, u^{(2)}, \ldots$ converges to a solution of (12.20), then $x^{(0)}, x^{(1)}, x^{(2)}, \ldots$ converges to the unique x^* that minimizes $k(x)$. An algorithm whose iterative step is (12.24) makes no reference to $u^{(k)}$; it produces directly a sequence of image vectors $x^{(k)}$ that is supposed to converge to the sought-after image vector x^*. Note also that such an algorithm need not evaluate either C^{-1} or $C^{1/2}$, even though the definition of $k(x)$ contains C^{-1} and the mathematical justification made use of $C^{1/2}$.

As an example of an application of such a procedure in image reconstruction, consider the $k(x)$ defined by (11.27). In this case, $a = r^2$, $b = 0$, $c = 1$, $A = U_I$, $B = \Theta_J$, $C = U_J$ and $x_0 = \mu_X$, and so (12.24) yields

$$x^{(k+1)} = x^{(k)} + \lambda^{(k)}\left(r^2 R^T\left(y - Rx^{(k)}\right) + \left(\mu_X - x^{(k)}\right)\right). \tag{12.25}$$

This iterative step has a straightforward interpretation in terms of the image reconstruction problem. The present estimate of the image vector, $x^{(k)}$, is changed by the addition of another J-dimensional vector that is the sum of two terms. The first term is proportional to $R^T\left(y - Rx^{(k)}\right)$. This is nothing but the discrete backprojection (see Section 7.3) of the difference between the measurement vector and projection data associated with the present estimate. By backprojecting this difference we get a J-dimensional vector that can be used to correct the present estimate so that its projection data are nearer to the measured projection data. The second term, $\mu_X - x^{(k)}$, is nothing but the difference between the mean vector of the prior distribution and the present estimate, and so it can be used to bring the present estimate nearer to the expected value of the image vector prior to the measurements. The relative importance given to the two terms is determined by r, whose physical interpretation has been discussed in Section 11.3. Hence we see that Richardson's method leads in this case to an iterative step that operates in an intuitively reasonable fashion.

If $W_2 = \Theta_J$, then P and z are given by (12.17) and (12.18), respectively. We define, for $k \geq 0$,

$$x^{(k)} = Du^{(k)}. \tag{12.26}$$

Then, from (12.21), (12.17) and (12.18), we get

$$\begin{aligned} x^{(k+1)} &= Du^{(k+1)} \\ &= D\left(u^{(k)} + \lambda^{(k)}\left(z - Pu^{(k)}\right)\right) \\ &= Du^{(k)} + \lambda^{(k)}\left(D^2 R^T Ay - D^2 R^T ARDu^{(k)}\right), \end{aligned} \tag{12.27}$$

and so

$$x^{(k+1)} = x^{(k)} + \lambda^{(k)} D^2 R^T A\left(y - Rx^{(k)}\right). \tag{12.28}$$

It follows from the discussion of the last section that if $u^{(0)}, u^{(1)}, u^{(2)}, \ldots$ converges to the minimum norm solution of $h(u)$, then $x^{(0)}, x^{(1)}, x^{(2)}, \ldots$ converges to the x^*, which minimizes $k(x)$ and which is such that, for any other x that minimizes $k(x)$, $\left\|D^{-1}x^*\right\| \leq \left\|D^{-1}x\right\|$. Note that in this case also, an algorithm whose iterative step is (12.28) makes no reference to the $u^{(k)}$; it produces directly a sequence of image vectors $x^{(k)}$ that is supposed to converge to the sought-after image vector x^*.

Now that we have seen realizations of Richardson's method in image reconstruction, we return to the all important question: can the initial vector $u^{(0)}$ and the sequence of relaxation parameters $\lambda^{(k)}$ be chosen so that (12.21) produces a sequence of vectors that converges to the minimum norm solution of $Pu = z$?

There are a number of ways of choosing the $\lambda^{(k)}$ to ensure the convergence of (12.21) to a solution of (12.20). Here we describe a simple method, since the underlying mathematics of some of the more complicated methods is beyond the scope of this book.

A real number ρ is called an *eigenvalue* of the matrix P if there exists a nonzero vector u such that

$$Pu = \rho u. \tag{12.29}$$

It is easily seen that a nonnegative definite matrix has only nonnegative eigenvalues. We use $\rho_{\max}P$ and $\rho_{\min}P$ to denote the largest and smallest positive eigenvalues of the matrix P. There are standard methods for estimating $\rho_{\max}P$ and $\rho_{\min}P$ for any given nonnegative definite matrix P.

The following is the case. For any $u^{(0)}$, the algorithm of (12.21) produces a sequence $u^{(0)}, u^{(1)}, u^{(2)}, \ldots$ that converges to a solution of (12.20), provided that, for all $k \geq 0$,

$$\lambda^{(k)} = \lambda, \tag{12.30}$$

where

$$0 < \lambda < 2/\left(\rho_{\max}P\right). \tag{12.31}$$

Furthermore, an "optimal" choice for λ is

$$\lambda = 2/\left(\rho_{\max}P + \rho_{\min}P\right). \tag{12.32}$$

Optimality here is in a mathematical sense on the limiting behavior of the algorithm, it does not necessarily imply being the best choice for the finite number of iterations that we are willing to perform in practice.

This result, in conjunction with the minimum norm theorem in Section 11.2, shows that provided $u^{(0)}$ is chosen to be a linear combination of columns of P, Richardson's algorithm with $\lambda^{(k)}$ defined by (12.30) and (12.31) converges to the minimum norm solution of $Pu = z$.

12.3 Smoothing Matrices

We rewrite the optimization criterion (6.38) as

$$a\left\|y - Rx\right\|^2 + bx^T Bx + \left\|x\right\|^2. \tag{12.33}$$

The minimizer of this should make each of the terms small; the nonnegative weights a and b indicate the importance of keeping the first term (which measures how badly the reconstruction violates the measurements) and the second term small, relative to keeping the third term (which is the norm of the image vector) small. In this section we concentrate on the second term. Our aim is to define nonnegative definite matrices B such that

(i) $x^T Bx$ measures how unsmooth x is; in other words, minimization of $x^T Bx$ pushes us toward a smooth x (in a mathematically precise sense that is specified later in this section) and
(ii) multiplication by B (and hence the iterative step (12.24) for the special case of (12.33) in which $c = 1$, $C = U_J$ and $x_0 = \theta$) can be carried out very efficiently.

We refer to such matrices B as *smoothing matrices.*

Since B is a $J \times J$ matrix, it maps image vectors into image vectors. Let us assume that the image vectors represent $n \times n$ digitized pictures; i.e., that the components represent densities in pixels. A smoothing matrix is determined by three *smoothing weights* that are denoted by w_1, w_2, and w_3. This has a superficial similarity to the idea of smoothing weights used in selective smoothing as defined in Section 5.3, but as we now make precise, the use of the weights in this section is quite different. In particular, in contrast to what was done in Section 5.3, here we do not require the smoothing weights to be nonnegative; in fact, to achieve our aim it is desirable that w_2 and w_3 be negative.

Let, for $1 \le j \le J$, E_j denote the set of indices of the pixels that have exactly one edge in common with the jth pixel and let V_j denote the set of indices of pixels that have exactly one vertex in common with the jth pixel in the $n \times n$ digitization. We now define a matrix S, called the *basic smoothing matrix* associated with the triple (w_1, w_2, w_3) of smoothing weights, as follows: S is the $J \times J$ matrix whose (j,k)th entry $s_{j,k}$ is defined by

$$s_{j,k} = \begin{cases} w_1, & \text{if } k = j, \\ w_2, & \text{if } k \in E_j, \\ w_3, & \text{if } k \in V_j, \\ 0, & \text{otherwise.} \end{cases} \tag{12.34}$$

Note that a basic smoothing matrix is symmetric.

We get from S to a smoothing matrix B via an intermediate step. Let K denote the set of indices of pixels that are not on the border of the $n \times n$ digitization. Let Z be the $J \times J$ diagonal matrix, whose (j,j)th element is

$$z_{j,j} = \begin{cases} 1, & \text{if } j \in K, \\ 0, & \text{otherwise.} \end{cases} \tag{12.35}$$

Clearly, if x is an image vector, then Zx is an image vector representing the same digitized picture as x, except that the densities in the border pixels have been set to zero. The *smoothing matrix* associated with the triple (w_1, w_2, w_3) of smoothing weights is defined by

$$SZS, \tag{12.36}$$

where S is the basic smoothing matrix associated with (w_1, w_2, w_3).

Returning now to the original motivation for smoothing matrices, suppose that we desire a solution of the discrete image reconstruction problem in which the values x_j assigned to neighboring pixels are close to one another on the average. Such a condition can be expressed mathematically by requiring that

$$\sum_{j \in K} \left(x_j - \frac{1}{8} \sum_{k \in N_j} x_k \right)^2 \tag{12.37}$$

should be as small as possible, where

$$N_j = E_j \cup V_j, \tag{12.38}$$

for $1 \le j \le J$, i.e., N_j is the set of indices of pixels neighboring the jth pixel.

Let S be the basic smoothing matrix associated with $\left(1, -\frac{1}{8}, -\frac{1}{8}\right)$, and let s_j denote the transpose of the jth row of S. It is easy to check that, for $j \in K$,

$$\left(x_j - \frac{1}{8} \sum_{k \in N_j} x_k \right)^2 = \left(s_j^T x \right)^2 = x^T s_j s_j^T x. \tag{12.39}$$

Therefore,

$$\sum_{j \in K} \left(x_j - \frac{1}{8} \sum_{k \in N_j} x_k \right)^2 = x^T B x, \tag{12.40}$$

where

$$B = \sum_{j \in K} s_j s_j^T . \tag{12.41}$$

So far we have succeeded in showing that minimizing (12.37) is in fact minimizing the quadratic form $x^T Bx$. Clearly, B is symmetric, and in view of (12.40), it is nonnegative definite. We now show that B is the smoothing matrix associated with $\left(1, -\frac{1}{8}, -\frac{1}{8}\right)$.

Define T by

$$T = SZ, \tag{12.42}$$

where S is the basic smoothing matrix associated with $\left(1, -\frac{1}{8}, -\frac{1}{8}\right)$ and Z is the diagonal matrix defined by (12.35). Then the (j, k)th entry of T is

$$t_{j,k} = \begin{cases} s_{j,k}, & \text{if } k \in K, \\ 0, & \text{otherwise.} \end{cases} \tag{12.43}$$

Hence, the (i, j)th element of SZS is

$$(SZS)_{i,j} = (SZS)_{j,i} = \sum_{k=1}^{J} t_{j,k} s_{k,i} = \sum_{k \in K} s_{j,k} s_{k,i} = \sum_{k \in K} \left(s_k s_k^T\right)_{i,j} = B_{i,j}, \tag{12.44}$$

where $B_{i,j}$ denotes the (i, j)th element of B. This proves that

$$B = SZS \tag{12.45}$$

is the smoothing matrix associated with $\left(1, -\frac{1}{8}, -\frac{1}{8}\right)$.

In general, multiplication of a J-dimensional vector x by a $J \times J$ matrix S requires J^2 scalar multiplications. However, if the vector is an image vector representing an $n \times n$ digitization ($J = n^2$), then the number of scalar multiplications required to evaluate Bx is approximately $6J$. This is easily seen by looking at the mechanism described by (5.6). In our application, with J typically well over 50,000, there is a very significant difference between the computational requirements for the evaluation of Bx when B is a general matrix and when B is a smoothing matrix.

12.4 Implementation of Richardson's Methods for Image Reconstruction

The iterative step of Richardson's algorithm as applied to the image reconstruction problem is described by (12.24) and (12.28). In both cases, the iterative step requires the evaluation of

$$R^T A \left(y - Rx^{(k)}\right). \tag{12.46}$$

This appears at first sight to be quite a difficult computational task. We now show that under an acceptable assumption, the evaluation of (12.46) is not nearly as expensive as the size of the matrices imply.

The assumption we make is that A is a diagonal matrix. The reasonableness of this assumption in our application area follows from the fact that in Table 12.1 the only case in which A is not diagonal is provided by the Bayesian estimation, for which $A = V_E^{-1}$. But V_E is the covariance matrix of the random variable whose samples are the error vectors in the measurements. The assumption that A (and hence V_E) is diagonal is equivalent to assuming that the errors in the physical estimation of $\langle r_i, x \rangle$ (r_i^T is the ith row of the projection matrix R) are not correlated with each other. Physical and simulation experiments confirm that this is not an unreasonable assumption.

If A is a diagonal matrix with entries $a_{i,i}$, then

$$R^T A \left(y - Rx^{(k)} \right) = \sum_{i=1}^{I} a_{i,i} \left(y_i - \left\langle r_i, x^{(k)} \right\rangle \right) r_i. \tag{12.47}$$

The right-hand side of (12.47) can be evaluated in I stages, adding at each stage an extra term to the accumulating sum. The computational process at each stage is very similar to a single iterative step of ART (see Section 11.1). At any stage only one row of the matrix R is needed, and only the nonzero entries of this row need to be used explicitly. These can be obtained efficiently using the DDA of Section 4.6. The only essential difference between the process of evaluating (12.47) in this way and I steps of ART is that while in ART the image vector is updated at each step (and hence only one J-dimensional vector needs to be stored), in evaluating (12.47) we need to keep two J-dimensional vectors: $x^{(k)}$ and the sum we are evaluating.

If we assume that D is a smoothing matrix (in practice D is usually a diagonal matrix, see Section 6.4), then all other operations in (12.24) and (12.28) are either a multiplication of a J-dimensional vector by a smoothing matrix, or a multiplication of a J-dimensional vector by a scalar, or an addition of two J-dimensional vectors. All these are likely to be computationally even less expensive than the evaluation of (12.47). Thus, the computation of one iterative step of Richardson's method takes about as long as I steps of ART. Since a SIRT-type method takes all the I measurements into consideration during one iterative step (while ART only uses one) this is to be expected. A slight disadvantage of Richardson's method is the additional storage requirement.

Since Richardson's method is an iterative process, many of the tricks in Section 11.4 can be applied to it with only minor alterations.

12.5 A Demonstration of Quadratic Optimization

We illustrate quadratic optimization for the special case when the function to be minimized is the one given in (11.27), so that we can compare the performance of SIRT-type methods with that of additive ART for minimizing the same function as specified in (11.39) and (11.40). As discussed in Section 12.2, the iterative formula for Richardson's method in this case is (12.25). We applied all methods discussed in this section to the standard projection data. We chose $a = r^2 = 100$, the blob basis functions, and $x^{(0)} = \mu_X = \bar{\mathbf{x}}$.

We decided to keep the $\lambda^{(k)}$ constant over all iterations. In ART the constant value was 0.05, as found appropriate in the previous chapter. For Richardson's method we considered the "optimal" value provided by (12.32) to be too large; in early iterations it seems to "over-correct," which results, for example, in a nonmonotonic decrease in the picture distance measures as the iterations progress. This can be overcome by choosing smaller constant values for the $\lambda^{(k)}$, such as 0.00001 or 0.000015, as illustrated in Fig. 12.1.

The plots in Fig. 12.1 show that Richardson's method is very slow: it requires many iterations to reach a near minimal value of the picture distance measure r. Since, as discussed in the last section, one iterative step of Richardson's method takes about as long as I iterative steps of ART, this is a serious consideration even for those of us who generally do not pay much attention to computer time. That we cannot possibly get away with using an early iterate of the Richardson's method is illustrated in Fig. 12.2(a). That image

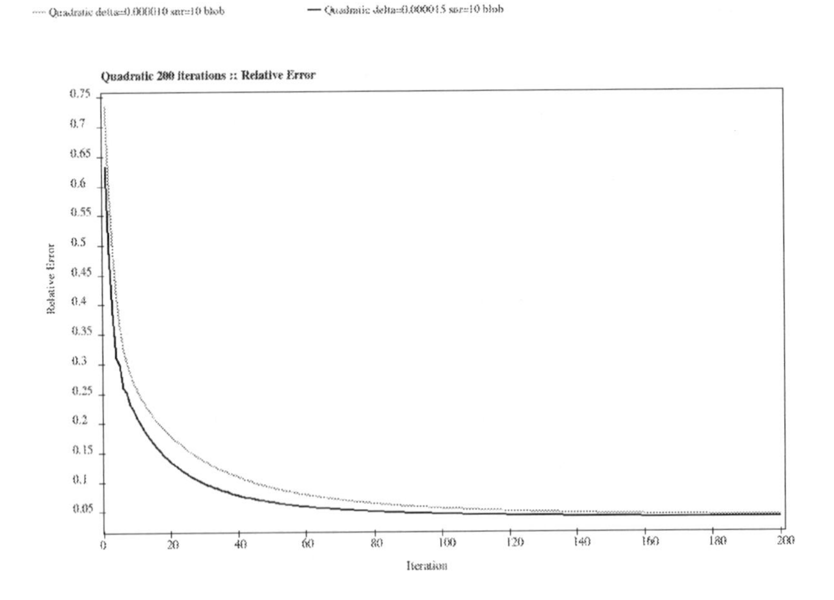

Fig. 12.1: Values of the picture distance measure r for Richardson's method reconstructions from the standard projection data with $\lambda^{(k)} = 0.00001$ (light) and $\lambda^{(k)} = 0.000015$ (dark).

is of the 10th iterate, which is essentially useless, but by the time we get to the 100th iterate we get the reasonably high-quality reconstruction shown in Fig. 12.2(b). It can be compared with Fig. 12.2(c), which is the additive ART reconstruction after $5I$ iterations.

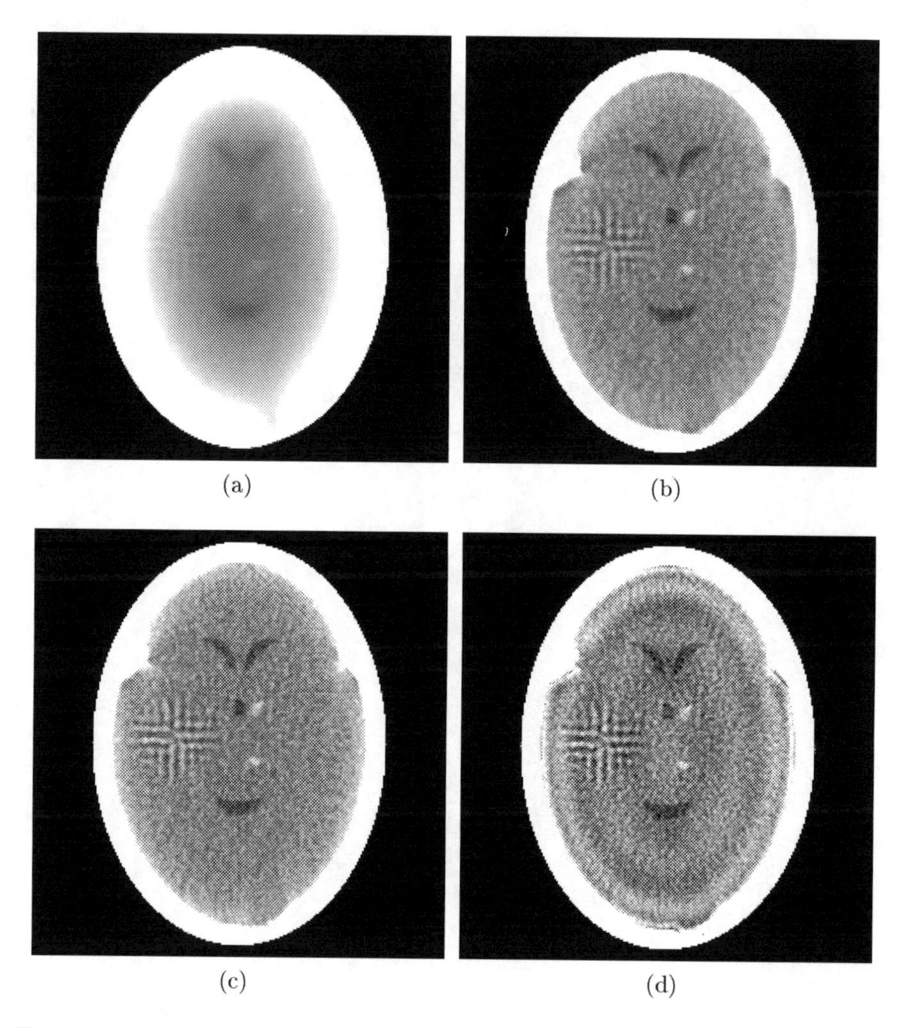

Fig. 12.2: Reconstructions from the standard projection data using iterative methods that minimize (11.27). (a) Richardson's method with $\lambda^{(k)} = 0.000015$, 10th iterate. (b) Richardson's method with $\lambda^{(k)} = 0.000015$, 100th iterate. (c) Additive ART with $\lambda^{(k)} = 0.05$, $5I$th iterate. (d) Conjugate gradient method, 20th iterate.

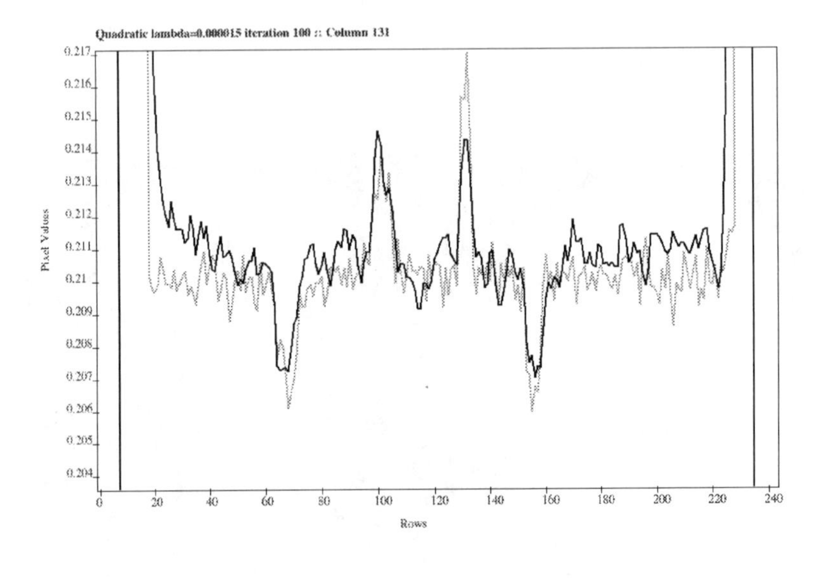

standard head phantom
standard pro_Quadratic de_QUAD_0100_r_a
Quadratic lambda=0.000015 iteration 100 :: Column 131
Pixel Values
0.217
0.216
0.215
0.214
0.213
0.212
0.211
0.21
0.209
0.208
0.207
0.206
0.205
0.204
0 20 40 60 80 100 120 140 160 180 200 220 240
Rows

(a)

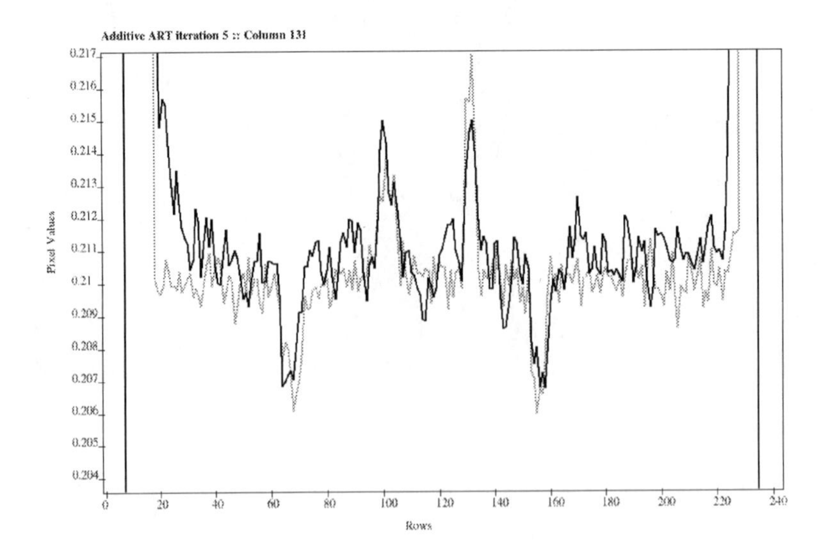

standard head phantom
standard pro_Bayesian ART_ART_0005_r_a
Additive ART iteration 5 :: Column 131
Pixel Values
0.217
0.216
0.215
0.214
0.213
0.212
0.211
0.21
0.209
0.208
0.207
0.206
0.205
0.204
0 20 40 60 80 100 120 140 160 180 200 220 240
Rows

(b)

Table 12.2: Picture distance measures and timings (in seconds) for the reconstructions that minimize (11.27).

algorithm	d	r	t
Richardson's method, $\lambda^{(k)} = 0.000015$, 100th iterate	0.1186	0.0449	2407.9
additive ART, $\lambda^{(k)} = 0.05$, $5I$th iterate	0.0878	0.0374	166.5
conjugate gradient method, 20th iterate	0.0799	0.0387	489.1

The quality of these two reconstructions is also compared in Fig. 12.3. Such visual inspections do not indicate a definite superiority by either of these methods, and neither do the picture distance measures that are reported in Table 12.2. The more noticeable difference between the methods is the timing: Richardson's method requires more than an order of magnitude more computer time than additive ART. This would not be important if for this extra cost we gained something, but that does not seem to be the case here.

Richardson's method is only one of the SIRT-type methods that can be used for quadratic optimization; there are others that are computationally more efficient. We give one example, which is a version of the *conjugate gradient method.* In this method (12.21) is replaced by the following more complicated looking, but nevertheless easily implementable, iterative process. This process involves, in addition to the $u^{(k)}$, two sequences $v^{(k)}$ and $w^{(k)}$ of vectors of the same size as the $u^{(k)}$ and two sequences $\lambda^{(k)}$ and $\kappa^{(k)}$ of scalars.

$$\begin{aligned} w^{(0)} &= v^{(0)} = z - Pu^{(0)}, \\ u^{(k+1)} &= u^{(k)} + \lambda^{(k)} w^{(k)}, \\ v^{(k+1)} &= v^{(k)} - \lambda^{(k)} P w^{(k)}, \\ w^{(k+1)} &= v^{(k+1)} + \kappa^{(k)} w^{(k)}, \end{aligned} \tag{12.48}$$

with

$$\lambda^{(k)} = \frac{\langle v^{(k)}, v^{(k)} \rangle}{\langle w^{(k)}, P w^{(k)} \rangle} \quad \text{and} \quad \kappa^{(k)} = \frac{\langle v^{(k+1)}, v^{(k+1)} \rangle}{\langle v^{(k)}, v^{(k)} \rangle}. \tag{12.49}$$

Note that as opposed to the $\lambda^{(k)}$ in (12.21), whose choice may be restricted as in (12.30) and (12.31) but is not fixed, the $\lambda^{(k)}$ and $\kappa^{(k)}$ of the conjugate gradient algorithm are totally determined by (12.49).

The faster initial convergence of the conjugate gradient method as opposed to Richardson's method can be seen by comparing the plot for the conjugate

Fig. 12.3: Plots of the head phantom of Fig. 4.6(a), shown light, and its reconstructions, shown dark, from the standard projection data using iterative methods that minimize (11.27). (a) Richardson's method with $\lambda^{(k)} = 0.000015$, 100th iterate. (b) Additive ART with $\lambda^{(k)} = 0.05$, $5I$th iterate.

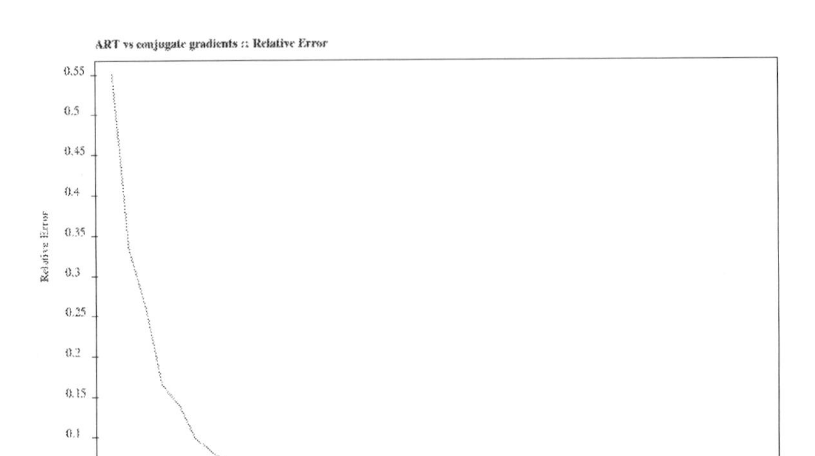

Fig. 12.4: Values of the picture distance measure r for reconstructions from the standard projection data using the conjugate gradient method (light) and additive ART (dark).

gradient method in Fig. 12.4 with the plots for the Richardson method in Fig. 12.1. Figure 12.4 and the picture distance measures in Table 12.2 imply that the quality of the reconstruction obtained by the 20th iterate of the conjugate gradient method should be as good as that obtained by the $5I$th iterate of additive ART. However this is not really so, as can be seen by looking at the reconstructed image in Fig. 12.2(d). Indeed it needs another 20 iterations of the conjugate gradient method before the visual quality of the reconstruction matches that of additive ART after $5I$ iterations. So, at least for the standard projection data, the conjugate gradient method has a faster initial convergence than Richardson's method, but it is still not as fast as additive ART. While there are further variations that may speed up the initial convergence of the SIRT-type approach to quadratic optimization, we do not discuss them here.

The comments near the end of Section 11.5 regarding the efficacy of ART as opposed to the FBP method apply nearly verbatim to the efficacy of quadratic optimization as opposed to FBP. As far as comparing ART-type methods with SIRT-type methods is concerned, we find that ART-type methods require less storage and get much further in a single cycle through the data. On the other hand, a larger selection of quadratic functions can be optimized within the framework of SIRT-type methods than with ART-type methods, and (although this is unlikely to be of great significance) an iterative step of Richardson's or of the conjugate gradient method takes somewhat less computer time than I iterations of additive ART.

Notes and References

The reason for calling the methods described in this chapter SIRT-type is that the first method of this type proposed for image reconstruction is the simultaneous iterative reconstruction technique (SIRT) of [93]. A paper that discusses SIRT in the more general context of least squares methods is [166]. In fact, just as ART has a mathematical precursor from the 1930s in the work of S. Kaczmarz [154] (and for this reason some people refer to ART as Kaczmarz's method), SIRT also has a mathematical precursor from the 1930s in the work of G. Cimmino [55] (and for this reason SIRT is often referred to as the Cimmino algorithm, see for example [6, 36, 43, 45]).

Definitions and results of linear algebra that we have used can be found in such standard texts as [105]. Our derivation of the appropriate forms for P and z follows [128]. That paper can be used to fill in the few gaps in our discussion. A follow-up to that work is [11], which discusses smoothing matrices, as well as two non-Richardson type methods for solving the system $Pu = z$, namely the conjugate gradient method and Chebyshev semi-iteration. We use the term "Richardson's method" in the general sense, as has been done, for example, in [276], which gives background references. The most commonly used alternate name for this method is "Landweber algorithm," see [167].

Quadratic optimization is widely used in many applications of image reconstruction; recent examples from electron paramagnetic resonance imaging and from electron tomography of silicon crystals are [259] and [256], respectively.

13

Truly Three-Dimensional Reconstruction

If we wish to reconstruct a three-dimensional body by the methods discussed in the previous chapters, the only option available to us is to reconstruct the body cross section by cross section and then stack the cross sections to form the three-dimensional density distribution. This may cause a number of problems, the most important of which are associated with time requirements. During the time needed to collect all the data, the patient may move, causing a misalignment between the cross sections. More basically, in moving organs such as the lungs (and even more so, the heart), changes in the organ over time are unavoidable, and it is desirable (but often not possible) to collect data for all cross sections simultaneously.

Sometimes, it is actually the change in the object over time that is the desired information. If we wish to see cardiac wall motion or the spread of radiopaque dye in a part of the circulatory system, then it is essential that we reconstruct the whole three-dimensional object at short time intervals. One may consider this as a four-dimensional (spatio-temporal) reconstruction. Of all the scanning modes discussed in Section 3.4, only the one depicted in Fig. 3.3(e) is capable of producing exactly the data that we would like. However, that scanning mode has not turned into a clinically-used reality and so we look instead at data that can be collected by helical CT, see Fig. 3.4. In this chapter we discuss reconstruction algorithms for data collected by such a device. One approach to obtaining reconstructions of dynamically moving objects, such as the heart, is to assume that the movement is cyclic. Assuming also that there exists a way of recording where we are in the cyclic movement as we take the 2D *views* of the moving 3D object, it is possible to bin the views into subsets such that all views that are binned into any one of the subsets have been taken at approximately the same phase of the cyclic movement, and so they are views of approximately the same (time frozen) 3D object. In the case of the heart this can be done by recording the electrocardiogram and noting on it the times when views have been taken. These views can then be binned, after the fact, according to the phases of the cardiac cycle.

13.1 Three-Dimensional Series Expansion

We use *rectangular coordinates* to describe three-dimensional space. That is, a point is represented by a triple of numbers (v_1, v_2, v_3). Each cross section is a plane for a fixed value of v_3, and the value of the three-dimensional function restricted to this plane is a function of the two rectangular variables (v_1, v_2). We assume that all the objects we wish to reconstruct are of a limited physical size; stated more precisely, we assume that there exists a constant E such that

$$f(v_1, v_2, v_3) = 0, \quad \text{if} \quad \max\{|v_1|, |v_2|, |v_3|\} > E, \tag{13.1}$$

where $f(v_1, v_2, v_3)$ is the value at the point (v_1, v_2, v_3) of the object that we wish to reconstruct. This equation is the three-dimensional analog of (6.1); it says that the object f (which can be thought of as a "3D picture") is zero-valued outside the *object region* that is a cube of size $2E \times 2E \times 2E$ whose center is at the origin of the coordinate system.

In this book we concentrate on series expansion methods for truly three-dimensional reconstructions. Just as in the case of two-dimensional reconstruction, we assume a fixed set of J *basis functions* $\{b_1, \ldots, b_J\}$, whose linear combinations give us an adequate approximation to any object f we may wish to reconstruct.

An example of such an approach that corresponds to $n \times n$ digitization as introduced in Section 4.1 is the following. For any positive real number d, we define the *cubic grid* C_d by

$$C_d = \{(dc_1, dc_2, dc_3) |\, c_1,\ c_2 \text{ and } c_3 \text{ are integers}\}, \tag{13.2}$$

compare this with (6.51). Note that a point (dc_1, dc_2, dc_3) of C_d is in the object region if, and only if, $|dc_i| \leq E$, for $1 \leq i \leq 3$. Each of these finitely many grid points gives rise to a *cubic voxel*, which is defined as the set

$$\left\{(v_1, v_2, v_3) |\, \max\{|v_1 - dc_1|, |v_2 - dc_2|, |v_3 - dc_3|\} \leq \frac{d}{2}\right\} \tag{13.3}$$

of points in the three-dimensional space. We number the voxels from 1 to J, and define

$$b_j(v_1, v_2, v_3) = \begin{cases} 1, & \text{if } (v_1, v_2, v_3) \text{ is in the } j\text{th voxel}, \\ 0, & \text{otherwise}. \end{cases} \tag{13.4}$$

Such a tessellation into cubic voxels is often referred to as a *cubrille*.

Irrespective of how we have selected the J basis functions, they can be used to associate with any J-dimensional vector x of real numbers an object $\hat{f}$ that is defined by

$$\hat{f}(v_1, v_2, v_3) = \sum_{j=1}^{J} x_j b_j(v_1, v_2, v_3), \tag{13.5}$$

where x_j is the jth component of x. Following the development in Section 6.3, we assume that we have a set of I linear continuous functionals $\mathscr{R}_i$ that map objects into real numbers. Denoting by R the $I \times J$ matrix whose (i, j)th element is $\mathscr{R}_i b_j$, we end up with

$$y = Rx + e, \tag{13.6}$$

which is the same as (6.24), where y is an I-dimensional *measurement vector* whose ith component is the measured value of $\mathscr{R}_i f$, x is the J-dimensional *image vector* that we wish to find so that we can use it in (13.5) for estimating the object f, and e is an I-dimensional *error vector*. The problem is again of the form:

given the data y, **estimate** the image vector x.

In CT, the $\mathscr{R}_i$ are usually defined as follows. We assume that there are I straight lines connecting source and detector positions in three-dimensional space. We refer to these lines as rays, and number them from 1 to I. For any object f, $\mathscr{R}_i f$ is the line integral of f along the ith ray. (The comment in Section 6.3 about the continuity assumption not always being satisfied by such $\mathscr{R}_i$ is valid here as well. The same goes for the advice that when using other than voxel-based basis functions, it is important not to include in (13.6) any equation that is associated with a line that misses the object region.) All methods previously discussed for solving (13.6) are in principle applicable to the three-dimensional case as well. However, the sizes of the problems to be solved are even greater now than before, since the values of I and J are likely to be 10 to 100 times larger in the three-dimensional case than in the two-dimensional case. The extra complication that we are interested in reconstructing time-varying objects results in the problem becoming even larger by at least another order of magnitude.

13.2 Dynamically Changing 3D Phantoms and Their Projections

To test algorithms for "four-dimensional" (spatio-temporal) reconstructions, we need the capability of generating appropriate phantoms and projection data. Similar methodology has been discussed for the two-dimensional case; in this section we discuss and illustrate a four-dimensional extension. While there are a number of applications, we restrict our discussion to helical CT, see Fig. 3.4 and the discussion that follows it.

In order to test an algorithm for a helical CT scanner, we need the capability of generating the type of data expected from it on known objects. Computer software has been developed for mathematically describing a dynamically changing three-dimensional object and then simulating the process of helical x-ray CT projection taking.

In this software, phantoms are described by a collection of time-varying elemental objects, which are essentially four-dimensional generalizations of the two-dimensional elemental objects introduced in Section 4.2. For our illustration, we designed a phantom of the human thorax based on the description of the FORBILD thorax phantom. We added to that stationary phantom two dynamically changing spheres representing the myocardium and a single contrast material filled cavity. We assumed that we are interested in this phantom at 24 equally-spaced (in time) phases of the cardiac cycle, whose total length was assumed to be 0.9375 second. Figure 13.1 shows a central cross section of this dynamic phantom at the two extremes of the 24 phases. In calculating the density in the phantom within a voxel, we subsampled the voxel at $5 \times 5 \times 5$ uniformly-spaced points, in a manner analogous to (4.1). The number of voxels in the three-dimensional phantom was $128 \times 128 \times 128$, but only the central 17 of the 128 cross-sectional slices intersected the "heart" in any one of its 24 phases. The E defining the size of the object region as in (13.1) was 25 cm.

Projection taking was done by integrating the density of the phantom along lines between the x-ray source position and detectors in a two-dimensional array. For every source position, data were collected for 384 equally-spaced detectors in each of 16 rows in the array. The size of each detector was assumed to be 0.425 cm $\times$ 0.425 cm. Data were collected (i.e., the pulsing of the x-ray source was simulated) at every 0.0015 second, using a total of 8,400 pulses. The number of turns of the helix in which the x-ray source moved during the data collection was 30. The radius of the helix was 57 cm, and the total movement parallel to the axis of the helix was 17.28 cm. The distance from the source to the detector array was 104 cm. Integrals of the density were collected for $I = 51,609,600$ rays (8,400 pulses times 16 rows of 384 detectors). Detector area was simulated similarly to what is described in Section 5.7, by placing a uniform square array of 2×2 points on each detector and calculating the number of photons reaching the detector as the sum of the number of photons reaching each of the four sub-detectors. The effect of photon statistics was simulated as in Section 5.5, assuming (in the notation of that section) that $\lambda = 1,000,000$ and $\lambda_c = 300,000,000$. The numbers used in this paragraph are not inappropriate for helical CT, but a state-of-the-art helical CT scanner would have more and smaller detectors and would be pulsed more frequently.

Fig. 13.1: The central cross section of the thorax phantom at the two extreme phases of the cardiac cycle. First row: the phantom. Second row: reconstruction from data collected at the time when the heart was in the appropriate phase after five cycles of ART. Third row: reconstructions from all the data after $2I$ (on the left) and $5I$ (on the right) iterations of ART. Fourth row: reconstruction from data collected at the time when the heart was in the appropriate phase after three cycles of Bayesian ART initialized with the reconstruction in the third row left.

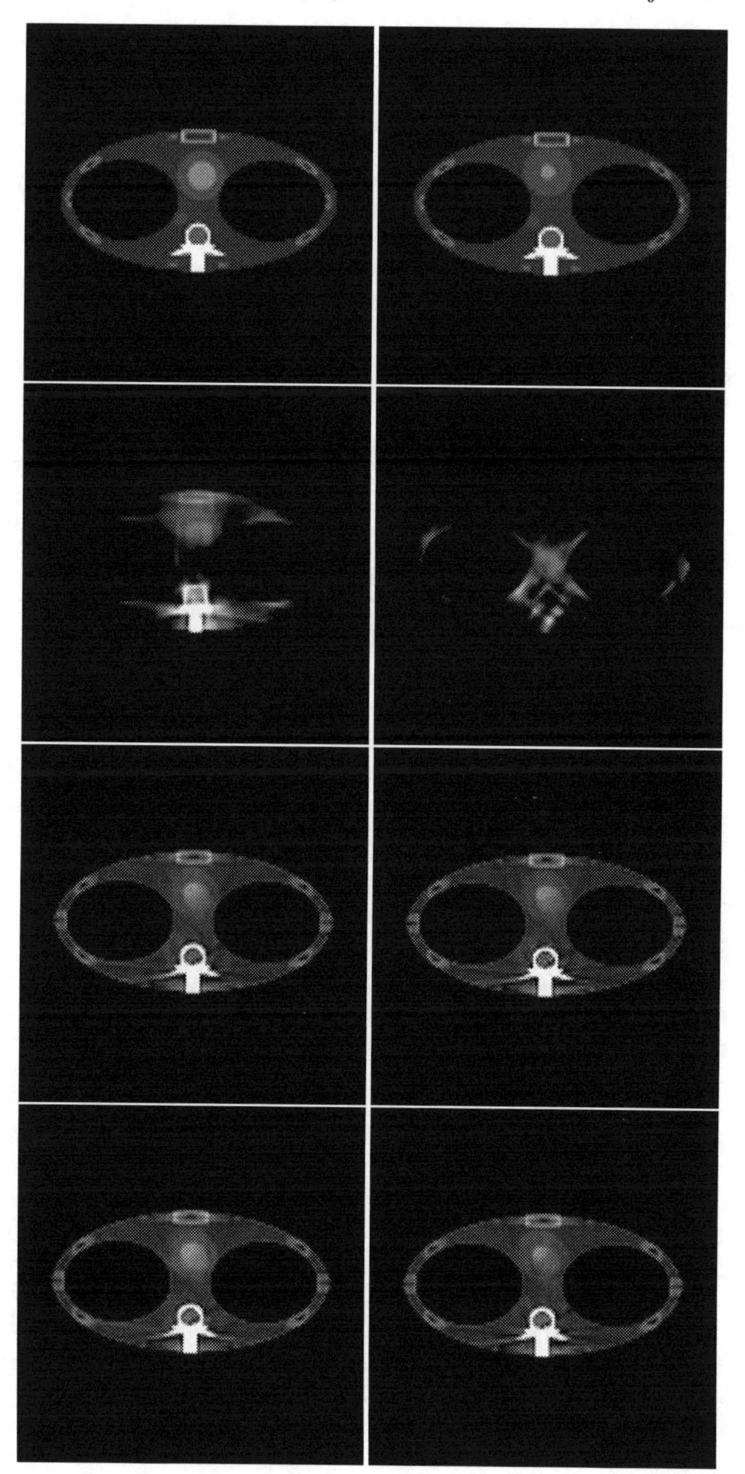

13.3 Three-Dimensional Reconstructions of the Dynamic Phantom

We report on three reconstructions from the data collected as described in the previous section. All three reconstructions used ART with three-dimensional blob basis functions. The computational costs of the three reconstructions were approximately the same, since for each a total of $5I$ iterative steps of ART were performed. Nevertheless, as shown below, the quality of the reconstructions are quite different.

Before getting into the details of the three algorithms, we say a bit more about three-dimensional blobs. The definition (6.50) given for the two-dimensional case carries over without change to define a function $b_{a,\alpha,\delta}$ of three variables. (The original variable r has to be reinterpreted as the distance $\sqrt{v_1^2 + v_2^2 + v_3^2}$ from the origin and the constant $C_{\alpha,a,\delta}$ needs to be defined slightly differently.) The recommended grids in this case are the so-called *body-centered cubic grids*

$$B_\delta = \{ (\ell\delta, m\delta, n\delta) | \, \ell, \, m \text{ and } n \text{ are either all even or all odd integers} \}, \tag{13.7}$$

where δ is a positive number. Just as in the two-dimensional case, the selection of the blob parameters is important for achieving high-quality reconstructions; for example, it is recommended that they should be chosen so that

$$\alpha = \sqrt{2\,(a/\delta)^2\,\pi^2 - 6.987932^2}. \tag{13.8}$$

The set $G = \{g_1, \ldots, g_J\}$ of *grid points* is chosen as the subset of those points in B_δ that fall within the object region defined by (13.1). Then, for $1 \le j \le J$, b_j is obtained from $b_{a,\alpha,\delta}$ by shifting its center from the origin to g_j. In all our experiments we had $J = 2,153,935$.

In the first experiment we reconstructed the 24 phases of the cardiac cycle independently of each other. This was done by subdividing all the projection data into 24 subsets, each corresponding to one of the phases. A ray sum was put into a particular subset if it was collected due to a pulsing of the x-ray source at a time nearer to the central time for that phase than to the central time of any other phase. This results in a number of consecutive pulses producing data for the same phase and then there is a relatively large gap before the collected data are again used for that phase. This very nonuniform mode of data collection results in unacceptably bad reconstructions, two of which are demonstrated in the second row of Fig. 13.1. These reconstructions were produced using ART with the three-dimensional blob basis functions, with all components of x^0 given the value $\bar{x}$, which is the estimated average density based on the projection data, all $\lambda^{(k)} = 0.05$, efficient ordering, and no nonnegativity constraints. The results are shown at the end of the fifth cycle through the data associated with the particular phase of the cardiac cycle.

In the second reconstruction we illustrate the other extreme: all the data were combined into a single projection data set, without any attention paid to the phases of the cardiac cycle. Because of the stationarity of most of the phantom and the overabundance of the projection data, we get (using the same choices for ART as in the previous paragraph) reconstructions that are good overall. They are illustrated in the third row of Fig. 13.1. The problem is that the movement of the heart is blurred out due to the various views used in the reconstruction having been taken all through the cardiac cycle. We note that in this case there is no need to cycle through the data five times: the reconstruction at the end of the second cycle through the data (on the left) is just about indistinguishable from the reconstruction at the end of the fifth cycle through the data (on the right). With a state-of-the-art helical CT scanner (that would have more and smaller detectors and would be pulsed more often) we would get even better reconstructions of the human thorax.

However, our main aim here is to see the changes in the heart over its cycle. This can be achieved by using the Bayesian approach of Section 11.3. We selected in (11.27) μ_X as the reconstruction obtained at the end of the second ART cycle through all the data as described in the previous paragraph and $r = 0.8$. For each separate phase of the cardiac cycle, we used the algorithm specified by (11.39) and (11.40) for a further three cycles through the data that are associated with that particular phase. The relaxation parameter was again the constant 0.05. The results, for the two extreme phases of the cardiac cycle, are shown in the last row of Fig. 13.1. Here the overall reconstruction of the thorax is every bit as good as in the third row, but at the same time one can observe that the heart is dynamically changing.

Notes and References

There have been a number of methods proposed for truly three-dimensional reconstruction. For an overview of early work, see [5], which also surveys approaches to reconstruction from both limited range of view data and from limited field of view data. Truly 3D reconstruction is a very much pursued topic, due to the prevalence of imaging devices that collect their data in a truly 3D fashion; such as the helical CT scanner of Fig. 3.4. As a few examples from the very large relevant literature, both on transform methods and on series expansion methods, we list [16, 39, 79, 156, 157, 212, 266, 279] for cone-beam CT, [24, 198] for positron emission tomography, and [194, 195, 196, 224, 236, 237, 249] for electron microscopy. As an interesting sample application see [193], in which radionuclide transmission cone-beam CT from data collected by a rotating gamma camera is used to improve single-photon emission computerized tomography imaging by providing attenuation maps for attenuation compensation and for anatomical correlation.

For a detailed description of the DSR, as well as a discussion of its applications in physiology and medicine, see [231, 272]. For a detailed discussion of a rapid hardware implementation for the DSR of an "unaltered divergent beam convolution algorithm" see [92].

For the work reported in this chapter, the generation of the dynamically-varying phantom, its projection data, the reconstructions from the data and the display of the results were all done using the software package jSNARK that is currently being developed by S.W. Rowland. Many of the specific parameters, both for helical CT and for heart motion, were based on choices reported in [148]. Description of the FORBILD thorax phantom was taken from http://www.imp.uni-erlangen.de/phantoms/thorax/thorax.htm.

For the technical details on how the parameters of three-dimensional blobs should be selected to achieve efficacious reconstructions see [199, 200].

The algorithm to reconstruct the beating heart based on Bayesian optimization in which the mean of the prior distribution is the reconstruction produced from all the data taken over several heart cycles was proposed and demonstrated in [4]. The same basic idea has been rediscovered and applied; see, for example, the recent publications [174, 175]. An alternative, in which an iterative method uses "adapted blobs" as basis functions, is demonstrated in [148] to produce accurate reconstructions from cone-beam x-ray projections of the beating heart.

An approach that is similar in spirit, but different in details, to what is discussed in this chapter is described in [277]. There the aim is to achieve CT perfusion studies at a low dose. The suggestion is to take a complete projection data set at a normal dose at the beginning and low-dose data sets at later times and track perfusion over time by altering the reconstruction from the normal-dose data according to the information collected at low dose. Such approaches seem to be also applicable to other problems, such as the imaging of the growth of crystals [251].

A recent paper that describes the use in electron microscopy of a complete truly three-dimensional reconstruction software package is [239]. That package incorporates a truly three-dimensional ART using blobs as the basis function [194]. This algorithm has been shown to be efficacious in numerous applications in electron microscopy (for example, in [196, 236, 237]) and recently for the reconstruction of whole cells from projections taken using soft (517 Ev) x-rays [216]. A comparison of it with SIRT and weighted backprojection in the case of overabundant projections directions is reported in [249].

The use of truly 3D ART in x-ray diffraction contrast tomography is suggested in [189].

14

Three-Dimensional Display of Organs

In the previous chapter we have discussed methods that can be used to produce a three-dimensional array of numbers, each number representing the average density (relative linear attenuation) in a voxel at an appropriate location. Even if two-dimensional reconstruction techniques are used, from a sequence of computed tomograms of transverse slices one can build up a three-dimensional array of numbers containing spatial rather than cross-sectional information.

Given such an array, it is easy to display coronal and sagittal sections of the body; see Figs. 1.9 and 1.11. Using linear interpolation one can calculate densities at arbitrary points inside the body, and thus produce displays of a slice at any desired orientation through the object. Such techniques are simple in conception (although they may require clever implementation when dealing with large arrays), and we do not discuss them in detail in this book.

We concentrate instead on methods that, based on the reconstructed three-dimensional array of densities, display what organs would look like if they were removed from the body. There are many ways of achieving this; broadly speaking, the approaches fall into two categories: *volume rendering* and *surface rendering*. We present here an example of the latter, but it is by no means the only one. In volume rendering a display is produced based on the densities assigned by the reconstruction to all voxels (similarly to what is produced in a projection image as in Fig. 1.5(a), but using the computer to emphasize the organs of interest while calculating the projections), whereas in surface rendering one first detects the surfaces of the organs of interest and then displays these surfaces (as, for example, in Fig. 2.1). The combination of computerized tomography with 3D display techniques has been aptly named as "noninvasive vivisection."

14.1 The Basic Approach

We assume that the region of interest is subdivided into voxels, as described in Section 13.1; in other words, we assume that we are working with a cubrille.

Each voxel has a density associated with it; these are the x_js of (13.5). We also assume that in the resulting three-dimensional array of numbers the objects of interest can be identified; such an assignment of voxels to specific objects of interest is usually referred to as a *segmentation*. There exist a large variety of segmentation methods, we now give a simple example.

Our example is illustrated by Fig. 14.1, which shows one of a stack of two-dimensional CT images in which bone appears light, softer tissues appear gray, and air appears dark. In this figure a cursor is placed at the right edge of a large piece of bone in the upper part of the image. Since this CT scan was taken of a trauma victim, an important question to ask is: are all other bones that are normally "connected" to this main piece of bone still connected for this patient? For example, the biggish piece of bone just to the right and below the cursor (it is the mandible) is not connected to any other bone in this cross section, but it should be connected to the rest of the skull (at our resolution) somewhere in the whole three-dimensional array.

The overall aim of the type of work on which we are reporting in this chapter is the display of selected objects based on the estimated densities in voxels. Examples for bones in the head are shown in Fig. 14.2. On the top we show a computer graphic display of the boundary of the connected piece of bone that is indicated by the cursor in Fig. 14.1. (The cursor location in

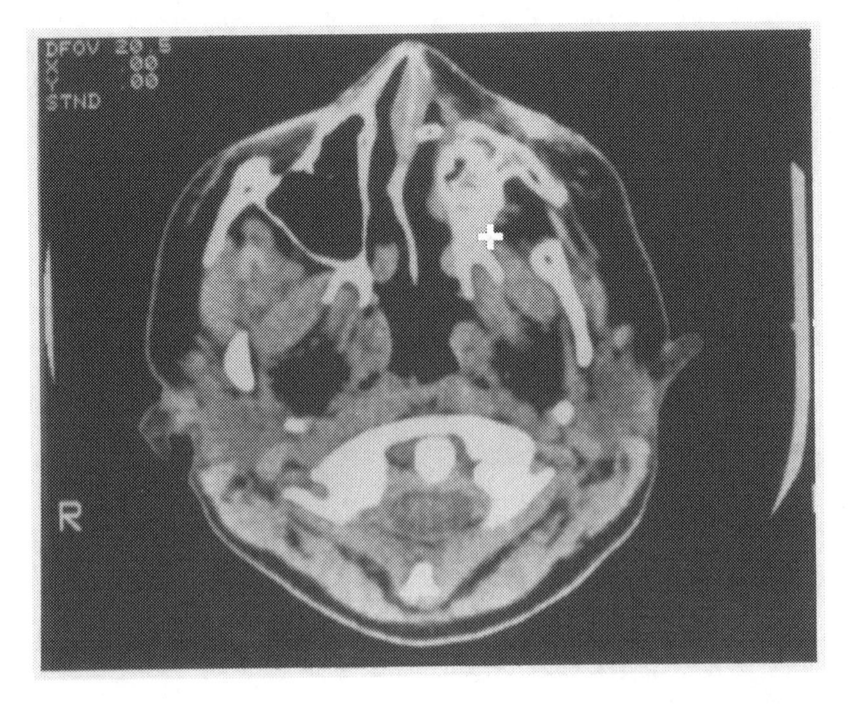

Fig. 14.1: A cross section from a CT scan of the head of a trauma victim.

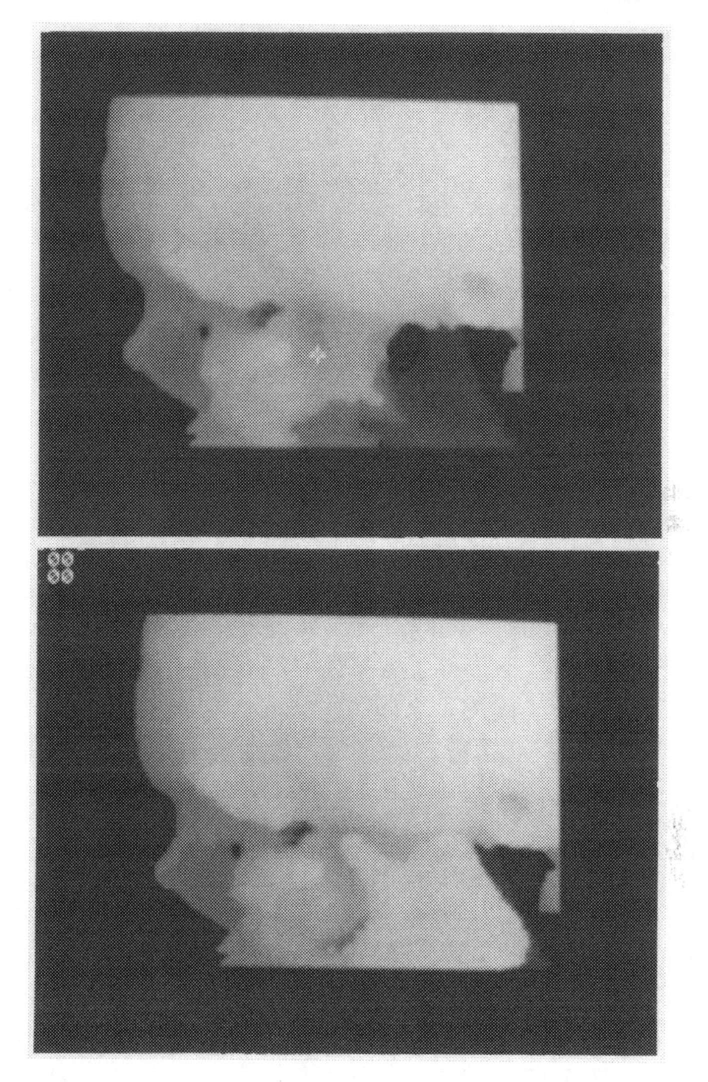

Fig. 14.2: Computer graphic displays of detected boundaries of bones in the head, based on the CT reconstruction that contains the cross section shown in Figure 14.1.

the top image in Fig. 14.2 corresponds to the cursor location in Fig. 14.1.) We now see that the mandible is disconnected from this bone in the whole three-dimensional data set. The boundary of the mandible can be extracted separately, and then the two boundaries can be displayed together in their correct relative locations, as shown in the bottom image of Fig. 14.2.

As mentioned above, the first step in the process that is reported here (which is the one that we used to get from Fig. 14.1 to Fig. 14.2) is segmentation, which in this case is the identification of the voxels that are occupied by bone. In this particular example segmentation is an easy task: since bone attenuates x-rays more than any other type of tissue in the human body, we may say that if the reconstructed value assigned to a voxel is above a certain level (referred to as the *threshold*), then that voxel is bone containing. So, as an approximation, the part of space that is occupied by bone may be considered to be the union of the voxels associated with those pixels for which the estimated x-ray attenuation coefficient is above the threshold for bone.

In many applications of image reconstruction from projections efficacious segmentation cannot be achieved by simple thresholding. We do not give details in this book of the more sophisticated segmentation methods that may be applicable under such circumstances.

14.2 Boundary Detection

As mentioned above, we are discussing in detail a surface-rendering approach; that is, one in which we first detect the surfaces of the organs of interest and then display these surfaces. In this section we concentrate on a particular way of detecting the surface of an object of interest, motivating our precise mathematical approach by giving first a much less precise discussion based on the example given in the last section and illustrated in Figs. 14.1 and 14.2. Our initial aim is to work towards making precise, in our environment, the notion of "a surface of an object."

The union of voxels that are identified by the segmentation process does not necessarily form a connected subset of the three-dimensional space; as seen in Fig. 14.2, some pieces of bone may be disconnected from the rest. Let us assume, for now, that the object surfaces that we wish to display are unions of voxel faces separating a component (i.e., a maximal connected subset) of "bone" voxels from adjacent "not bone" voxels.

Even this specification is not precise enough to describe the intuitive notion of "a boundary" of an object. This is because an object of the kind we have described in the previous paragraph may have cavities inside it (just look at Fig. 14.1; the inside of bones contains lots of less x-ray attenuating tissue and may well be identified as a result of thresholding as "not bone") and so an object may have multiple boundaries (an exterior one and possibly many interior ones). Let us say that our task is to identify exactly one of these boundaries.

How do we specify which one? One way is to point at a boundary face, that is at a face that separates a bone voxel from a not-bone voxel, and say that we wish to display that boundary of the object that contains that boundary face. (At this point, it is not even clear that this specification is legitimate. Is the "boundary containing a boundary face" a well-defined concept? In fact, it is; we will define things so that, for any boundary face, there will be one and only one boundary containing it.)

An intuitively useful picture is the following. We consider the tessellation of the three-dimensional space into cubic voxels. A finite number of these voxels are occupied by sugar cubes of just the right size; these indicate the voxels that have been identified by the segmentation process. We point at an uncovered face of one of these sugar cubes (that is, a face such that the voxel on the other side of it is not occupied by a sugar cube) and ask that there be delivered to us the boundary surface that contains that face. The problems are to make this intuitive aim mathematically precise and then to design an algorithm that is guaranteed to deliver the desired boundary surface for all possible arrangements of the sugar cubes.

To solve these problems we work with the infinite set V of voxels, its elements are defined by (13.3), one voxel for each of the infinitely many elements of C_d as defined in (13.2). A set ρ of ordered pairs of elements of V with the property that $(c, d) \in \rho$ if, and only if, $(d, c) \in \rho$ is referred to as an *adjacency* on V. If ρ is an adjacency on V and $(c, d) \in \rho$. then we say that c and d are *ρ-adjacent*. We will be dealing with two specific adjacencies: ω and δ. For any two voxels c and d, $(c, d) \in \omega$ if, and only if, c and d have a face in common, while $(c, d) \in \delta$ if, and only if, c and d have either a face or an edge in common. These are illustrated in Fig. 14.3. For obvious reasons, ω is often referred to as *face-adjacency* and δ is often referred to as *face-or-edge-adjacency.*

For any c and d in V, we call a sequence $\langle c^{(0)}, \ldots, c^{(K)} \rangle$ of voxels a *ρ-path connecting c to d*, if $c^{(0)} = c$, $c^{(K)} = d$ and, for $1 \leq k \leq K$, $c^{(k-1)}$ is ρ-adjacent to $c^{(k)}$. For a nonempty subset A of V and c, $d \in A$, we say that *c is ρ-connected in A to d* if there is ρ-path $\langle c^{(0)}, \ldots, c^{(K)} \rangle$ connecting c to d such that $c^{(k)} \in A$, for $0 \leq k \leq K$. We say that A is *ρ-connected* if, for any c and d in A, c is ρ-connected in A to d. A *ρ-component* of A is a ρ-connected subset of A that is not a proper subset of any other ρ-connected subset of A. For any subset A of V, we denote the set of voxels not in A by $\bar{A}$, and call it the *complement* of A.

For any two subsets O and Q of V we define the *boundary* between them by:

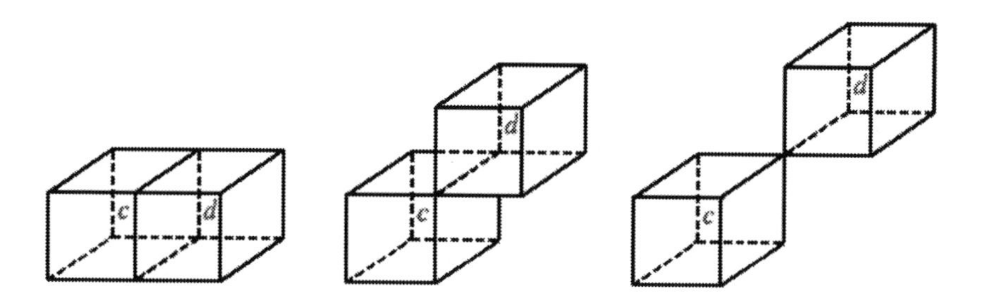

Fig. 14.3: The voxels c and d on the left are both δ- and ω-adjacent; those in the middle are δ-adjacent but not ω-adjacent; those on the right are neither δ-adjacent nor ω-adjacent.

$$\vartheta(O,Q) = \{(c,d) \mid c \in O,\ d \in Q,\ (c,d) \in \omega\}. \tag{14.1}$$

Note that a boundary is defined as a subset of ω. This is reasonable, since each element of ω is a pair (c,d) of face-adjacent voxels and so it can be geometrically interpreted as the oriented face that is crossed when we move from c to d. Let $\langle c^{(0)}, \ldots, c^{(K)} \rangle$ be an ω-path and S be any subset of ω. We say that $\langle c^{(0)}, \ldots, c^{(K)} \rangle$ *crosses* S, if there is a k, $1 \le k \le K$, such that either $(c^{(k-1)}, c^{(k)}) \in S$ or $(c^{(k)}, c^{(k-1)}) \in S$.

With this terminology we are now in position to state a rather remarkable fact. For any nonempty finite subset A of V, let O be any δ-component of A and Q be any ω-component of $\bar{A}$ such that $\vartheta(O,Q)$ is not empty. Then there exist two uniquely defined subsets I and E of V with the following properties.

(i) $O \subseteq I$ and $Q \subseteq E$.
(ii) $\vartheta(O,Q) = \vartheta(I,E)$.
(iii) $I \cup E = V$ and $I \cap E = \emptyset$.
(iv) I is δ-connected and E is ω-connected.
(v) Every ω-path connecting an element of I to an element of E crosses $\vartheta(O,Q)$.

We do not prove this result in this book, but we give an interpretation of it in the terminology of our earlier discussion.

The subset A is the output of the segmentation procedure: it would be the set of all bone voxels identified by thresholding in the example illustrated by Figs. 14.1 and 14.2, or the set of all voxels occupied by sugar cubes in the intuitive picture given earlier. Consider now an uncovered face of one of these sugar cubes, let us say that it is the one associated with voxel g. Let us denote by h the voxel on the other side of the face; it is not occupied by a sugar cube. Mathematically, $g \in A$ and $h \in \bar{A}$. If we now let O be the δ-component of A that contains g and Q be the ω-component of $\bar{A}$ that contains h, then we see that the boundary $\vartheta(O,Q)$ is not empty since it contains (g,h). This is the boundary that we wish to display.

The rest of the result stated above implies that we have now achieved not only a precise mathematical definition of the boundary to be displayed, but also that this boundary has some very attractive properties. In words, the boundary $\vartheta(O,Q)$ has an *interior* I and an *exterior* E such that (i) O is a subset of the interior and Q is a subset of the exterior, (ii) the boundary between the interior and the exterior is exactly $\vartheta(O,Q)$, (iii) the interior and exterior partition the whole space V, (iv) both the interior and the exterior are connected in some sense, but (v) one cannot get from the interior to the exterior without crossing the boundary. These properties are reminiscent of the famous *Jordan curve theorem*. According to that theorem, the set of all points in the plane that are not on a simple closed curve can be partitioned into two subsets, one may be called the interior and the other the exterior. Both of these are connected sets in the sense that we can get from any point of the interior, respectively the exterior, to any other point by drawing continuously a curve between them that never leaves the interior, respectively the exterior, but one cannot draw continuously a curve from a point in the interior to a point in the exterior that does not contain at least one point of the simple closed curve, which is in fact the boundary between the interior and the exterior. For this reason we refer to a boundary that satisfies (i)–(v) above as a *Jordan surface.*

Now we come to the solution of the second of the two problems stated above, which is to design an algorithm that is guaranteed to deliver $\vartheta(O,Q)$ given any nonempty finite subset A of V and any $g \in A$ and $h \in \bar{A}$ such that $(g,h) \in \omega$. We need to introduce a bit more terminology. For the purpose of the following discussion the set A is considered fixed (as it is indeed fixed by the segmentation process).

For any two ω-adjacent voxels c and d, we say that (c,d) is a *bel* (short for *boundary element*), if $c \in A$ and $d \in \bar{A}$. Note that the (g,h) of the previous paragraph is a bel. Our boundary tracking algorithm will start with (g,h) and will keep finding extra bels until all bels that are in $\vartheta(O,Q)$ are found. This is done by making use of the notion of *bel-adjacency*, which is defined so that for every bel there are exactly two bels bel-adjacent from it. We do not give the precise definition of bel-adjacency in this book, but illustrate the definition by Figs. 14.4 and 14.5. The important computational observation here is that, for any bel (c,d), the two bels bel-adjacent from it can be determined by simple checking on whether or not some voxels that are ω-adjacent to c or d are in A.

We are now ready to state our boundary tracking algorithm. Its input is the set A and a bel (g,h). It works with three sets of bels: S, L, and T. The set S contains all the detected bels in the boundary; when the algorithm terminates the set S is exactly $\vartheta(O,Q)$. The set L contains all the loose ends; since the computer can do only one thing at a time and to every bel there are two bels bel-adjacent from it, we need to keep a record of all the bels that have been

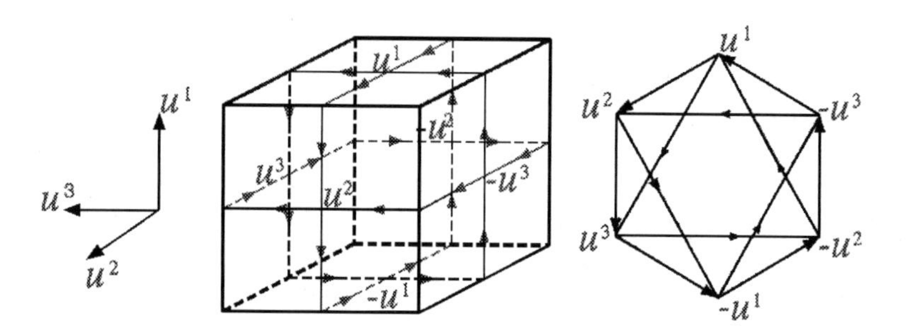

Fig. 14.4: Illustration of a directed graph (on the right) and its interpretation as a set of directions taken while tracking the boundary between a single voxel and the set of all other voxels in V (in the middle).

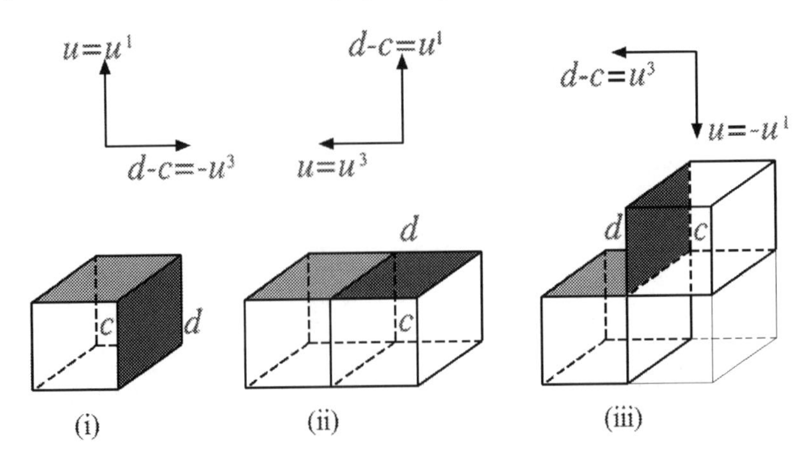

Fig. 14.5: Illustration of the definition of bel-adjacency using the directed graph of Fig. 14.4. In each case, the lightly-shaded bel is bel-adjacent from the darkly-shaded one. (Note that there is also a second bel, not indicated in this figure, that is bel-adjacent from the darkly-shaded one.)

identified as being in the boundary but for which we have not yet investigated which other bels bel-adjacent from it are also in the boundary. The set T provides a clever mechanism, at a relatively small cost, of avoiding infinite loops (in which the same bels in the boundary would be detected again and again); we return to discussing the nature of T below. The boundary tracking algorithm that we used to find the surfaces displayed in Figs. 2.1 and 14.2 is as follows:

1. Put (g, h) into L and S and put two copies of (g, h) into T.
2. Remove a bel a from L. For both bels b that are bel-adjacent from a, try to find one copy of b in T.
   a) If successful, then remove this copy of b from T.
   b) If not, then put b into L, S and T.
3. Check if L is empty.
   a) If it is, STOP.
   b) If it is not, go back to Step 2.

In this book we do not give the proof of correctness for this algorithm (it is correct in the sense that, for any finite nonempty subset A of V and for any bel (g, h), the algorithm will STOP and, at that time, S will contain exactly all the elements of $\vartheta(O, Q)$), but restrict ourselves to discussing the role of T in achieving performance efficiency. A correct algorithm could have been given without using T and using S instead of T to avoid getting into infinite loops. The practical problem with that is that S eventually contains the whole boundary, which may be very large, millions of bels are quite typical in the medical application. By proving mathematically that in such an algorithm each bel is visited exactly twice, we can replace checking membership in S by checking membership in the much smaller set T. This is the set of once-visited bels: the first time we visit a bel we put it into T in Step 2(b), and the next time we visit it we remove it from T in Step 2(a) (since we know that it will never be visited again). This way the largest size of T during the execution of the algorithm tends to be orders of magnitude smaller than the eventual size of S, resulting in an efficient algorithm.

14.3 Hidden Surface Removal

As discussed in the previous section, the boundary detection algorithm produces a set $S = \vartheta(O, Q)$ of faces. A face is represented as an ordered pair of voxels, but it is best thought of from now on as a square-shaped *surface element* that lies in one of six possible orientations (the directed normal to a bel from the interior to the exterior must be in one of three mutually perpendicular pairs of opposing directions, see Fig. 14.4).

The mathematics of the last section is equally applicable to finding internal and external boundaries. For example, if the segmentation identifies all voxels that are in the heart muscle and we start the boundary tracking process with a bel that separates a voxel in the muscle from one in a cavity, then the boundary produced should be that of the cavity. However, our mathematical definitions lead to a counter-intuitive terminology: what we have defined as the exterior of the boundary consists in this case of the voxels in the cavity and the interior is the set of all other voxels. To simplify our discussion, we assume that we are not dealing with such a case and that the exterior of the surface surrounds its interior. (This can always be achieved by switching the roles of A and $\bar{A}$ in the mathematical definitions.) We further assume that there is a display screen that is placed in a fixed position in space, so that the plane of the screen is entirely in the exterior of the surface. Our display of the surface is a projection of the appearance of the surface onto the screen.

In displaying surfaces we use here *orthogonal projections*. That is, we assume that a point P on the screen displays the point Q on the surface such that

(i) the line segment QP is perpendicular to the screen;
(ii) the interior of the line segment QP does not contain any point of the surface;

see Fig. 14.6. A little reflection is sufficient here to realize that in order for a point Q to be displayed on the screen at all it is necessary that the orientation of the face a on which Q lies is such that the directed normal to the face a from the interior to the exterior meets the plane of the screen (this is partly due to the fact that our detected boundaries are Jordan surfaces). We call faces that satisfy this condition *potentially visible*.

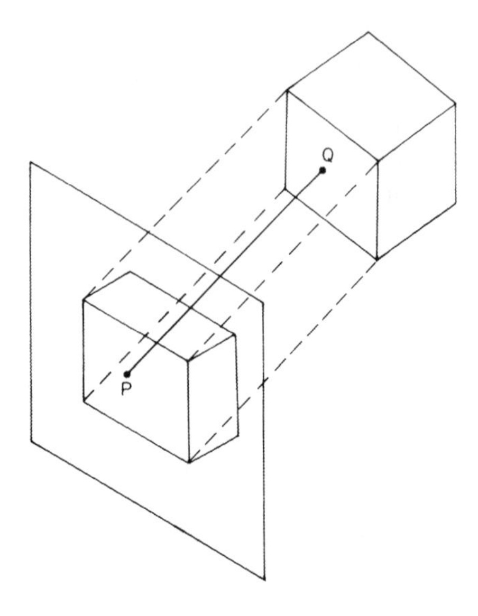

Fig. 14.6: Orthogonal projection.

Note that an orthogonal projection does not make any use of perspective. Organs being fairly small objects, an orthogonal projection gives a realistic appearance, which is not improved noticeably by the introduction of perspective.

There are two separate questions involved in the display method just described. The first is: by what intensity should the point Q on the surface be displayed at the point P on the screen? The second is: if there are several points on the surface that lie on the line perpendicular to the screen at the point P, how should the correct point Q be selected? In this section we deal with the latter question, which is the problem of *hidden surface removal* or, equivalently, *visible surface display*. We leave the discussion of the first question until the next section.

There are many techniques for hidden surface removal. Here we discuss one that appears to be particularly appropriate for the environment in which we are working. This method is generally referred to as the *z-buffer algorithm* and it works as follows.

With each point (raster element) P on the display screen we associate two numbers: *brightness* $b(P)$ and *distance from the screen* $z(P)$. Initially, for each point we assign zero (dark) to the brightness and a very large number (essentially infinity) to the distance from the screen. If a face a is not potentially visible, then it is not displayed. All other faces making up our surface are displayed one by one, according to the following procedure.

For each potentially visible face a, we locate all the points P on the screen that would be used if that face alone were to be displayed. These points then are treated one by one as follows.

For each point P, we find the point Q on the face a such that PQ is perpendicular to the screen. Let $\bar{z}(Q)$ be the distance of Q from the screen (that is, the distance from P to Q) and let $\bar{b}(Q)$ be the brightness that would be assigned to P if the face a alone were to be displayed. If $\bar{z}(Q)$ is less than $z(P)$, then we change the value of $b(P)$ to that of $\bar{b}(Q)$ and the value of $z(P)$ to that of $\bar{z}(Q)$. However, if $\bar{z}(Q)$ is not less than $z(P)$, we do not change the values of $b(P)$ and $z(P)$.

In this fashion, by the time we have dealt with all the faces, brightnesses are displayed for the visible faces, and the hidden faces (or parts of faces) do not influence the display. There are two ways that the general z-buffer algorithm, as just described, can be made to work faster in our special environment.

(i) We can make use of the following result, whose somewhat messy proof we omit. For any two potentially visible faces a and b, if A is a point inside a (i.e., on a but not on an edge of a) and B is a point inside b such that the line AB is perpendicular to the screen, then $\bar{z}(A) < \bar{z}(B)$ if, only if, $\bar{z}(C(a)) < \bar{z}(C(b))$, where $C(a)$ and $C(b)$ denote the center points on the faces a and b, respectively. This result tells us that we can approximate, for any point Q on a, $\bar{z}(Q)$ by $\bar{z}(C(a))$ in the z-buffer algorithm, and yet end up with the same display.

(ii) Since each of the faces is small, we may also assume that all points on the face would be displayed by the same brightness, and so approximate for any point Q on a, $\bar{b}(Q)$ by $\bar{b}(C(a))$.

14.4 Shading

We desire to display the visible part of a detected surface on the screen of our computer in such a way that its appearance resembles the appearance of the surface of the original object in the same orientation. This three-dimensional appearance on a raster graphics device is attempted by *shading*; that is, by assigning different gray levels to the display points on the screen. A number of depth and shape cues exists. Here we discuss only two of them: z-distance and orientation.

The underlying assumption in this simple case is that light travels in parallel rays perpendicular to the screen from a plane source that is parallel to the screen. The intensity assigned to a point P on the screen, which is displaying a point Q on a surface element in three-dimensional space, depends on the distance of Q from the light source and on the angle between the normal to the surface element at Q and the direction of the light.

Computationally, cube-shaped voxels are very appropriate for such calculations. Each surface element is a square in one of three pairs of orientations, and so only three normals need to be calculated. Since the surface elements are small, one may assume, without appreciably affecting the output, that all points on a surface element a are at the same z-distance, namely the $\bar{z}(C(a))$ of its center, which has already been established during the hidden surface removal process.

In practice, something further has to be done, because of the limited number of orientations of the faces of the detected surface. The original surface is likely to have been quite smooth, but the displayed surface often looks jagged.

We list three techniques that have been proposed and used to overcome this, either individually or in combination with each other.

(i) Put the final image through a low-pass filter in order to smooth its appearance (i.e., convolve it with a function that has no high-frequency components).
(ii) Assume a virtual display screen of higher resolution than the actual screen and display on the actual screen by averaging the values on the virtual screen.
(iii) Make the influence of the angle between the light and surface normal unimportant as compared with the z-distance.

None of these solutions is entirely satisfactory. The third one essentially removes the important depth cue provided by the angle between the direction of light and the surface normal. The other two do nothing to resolve the type of difficulty that we now describe.

Consider a part of the surface of the original object that is flat and is perpendicular to the light. If the orientation of two voxel faces is also perpendicular to the light, then the above-mentioned flat surface is approximated by faces of voxels all parallel to each other (and perpendicular to the light direction). In this case, at every point, the normal to the detected surface makes an angle zero with the direction of light. and the surface will appear uniformly very bright. If the orientation of the voxels happens to be chosen at 45° to the flat part of the surface of the original object, then the flat surface is approximated by faces of voxels that make an angle 45° with it (and hence an angle 45° with the light direction). In this case, at every point, the normal to the detected surface makes an angle 45° with the direction of light, and the surface will appear uniformly lit, but not as bright as in the previous case.

This is a serious drawback. It can, in principle, be overcome either by determining shading based on the orientation of a face and its neighbors and/or by using surface elements more complex than squares. The first of these alternatives has been demonstrated to be quite successful; in fact, the images in Figs. 2.1 and 14.2 were all produced by calculating for display purposes a normal to a surface element using a weighted average of the normals to that face and the normals to the other faces that share an edge with it. The use of more complicate surface elements than square appears intuitively attractive, but tends not to deliver the hoped-for improvement. For example, by using instead of the cubic grid of (13.2) a *face-centered cubic grid,* we get "voxels" in

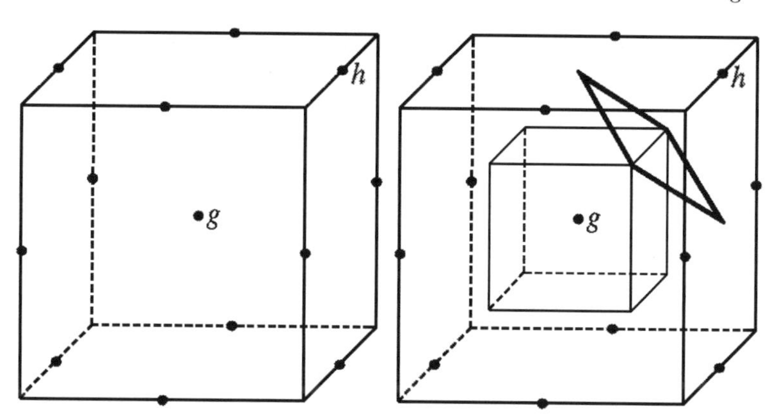

Fig. 14.7: The face-centered cubic grid (on the left) and a typical face of the associated rhombic dodecahedral voxels (drawn heavily on the right).

the shape of rhombic dodecahedra (see Fig. 14.7) and our boundary detection algorithm can be adapted with very minor alterations to detect surfaces consisting of faces of such "voxels." This seems promising, since the angle between the normals of the faces that share an edge in a face-centered cubic grid is always 60°, while it is often 90° in the case of the cubic grid (see Figs. 14.5(i) and (iii)). However, when one compares the quality of displays produced based on these two grids, there is not really an appreciable difference between them,

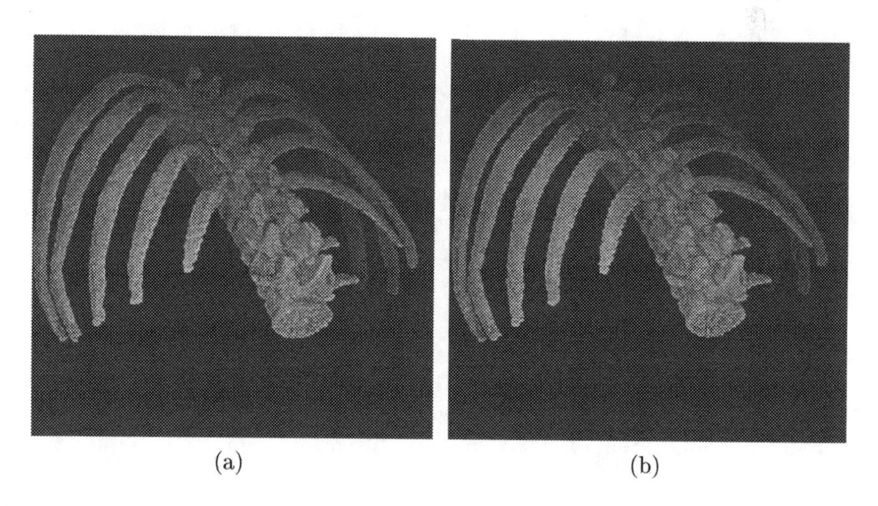

Fig. 14.8: Three-dimensional displays of the spine and ribs of a patient (seen from behind and downward from the vertical vertebrae) approximated as a collection of (a) 1,661,728 faces of cubic voxels and (b) 1,258,482 faces of rhombic dodecahedral voxels. (The areas of the individual faces are the same in the two cases.)

as is demonstrated in Fig. 14.8. (Note, however, that fewer faces are needed to approximate the object in the case of the rhombic dodecahedral voxels.)

Notes and References

The phrase "noninvasive vivisection" was used in [271] to describe the potential for the study of structural and functional dynamics of the heart, lungs and circulation of techniques that display reconstructed dynamic structures.

A particular method for displaying arbitrary sections through the body based on a sequence of computed tomograms of transverse sections is described by [132]. That paper also gives references to earlier literature both on sectional display and three-dimensional boundary detection and display, using methods that are in some cases quite different from what has been described in this chapter. Some other early references are [86, 94, 102, 186, 261]. A quite comprehensive and up-to-date coverage of the field of 3D imaging in medicine, including both volume rendering and surface rendering, is given in [260].

Of the many sophisticated methods for segmentation we mention the approach of fuzzy segmentation that is based on the concept of fuzzy connectedness of voxels, originally proposed in [262] for segmenting an object in an array of densities. For extension of this approach to simultaneous segmentation of multiple objects and for implementation on parallel computers see [40, 90]. This approach has been found very efficacious in practice. For an example of a recent paper validating its use in a medical application see [76].

The material in the present chapter is based on the early ideas in [12, 133]. The section on boundary tracking follows in many of its particulars the much further developed approach presented in [118, 119]. (These works discuss, in particular, the adaptation of our presented boundary tracking algorithm to tracking boundaries when the voxels are rhombic dodecahedra.) As we have seen, our boundary detection approach produces a single boundary of a single component, specified by a user-supplied initial face in the boundary. As opposed to this, the very popular marching cubes algorithm [187] automatically detects all surfaces of all components. It is not clear that this is really an advantage: after all, in practical visualization only a few of these surfaces should be displayed (as in Fig. 14.2). Besides, the mathematical property of the boundary detected by our algorithm that it has a well-defined interior and exterior allows us to detect automatically all boundaries by repeated applications of the algorithm for the tracking of a single boundary. In fact, as discussed in [165], the set of all surfaces produced by the marching cubes algorithm can also be produced by creating "continuous analogs" of the boundaries produced by the algorithm of Section 14.2, and the total process of tracking all the boundaries (in our sense) and creating their continuous analogs requires less computer time than what is needed by the marching cubes algorithm when the number of voxels occupied by the objects of interest is as large as what is typical in an application of image reconstruction from projections.

For a very recent paper on the marching cubes algorithm see [67] and for a recently-developed surface-based system for topological analysis, quantization and visualization of voxel data see [56].

One of the many ways of producing esthetically pleasing smooth-looking displays is provided by an idea of R.M. Lewitt, who suggested that the blobs of [183] advocated by him for image reconstruction can also be used to produce smooth thresholded surfaces, the normals to which can be easily identified. An implementation of this idea is reported in [89]. However, as mentioned in the last paragraph of Section 14.4, smooth-looking displays can be produced also for boundaries consisting of faces of cubic voxels by estimating normals by considering each surface element in combination with others near it in the surface. This idea originates from [51]; the current state of the art can be seen from [81].

15

Mathematical Background

Throughout the previous chapters we repeatedly omitted proofs of mathematical claims, since we did not want such proofs to interfere with the flow of the main argument. In this chapter we fill in some of these gaps, in the order in which they appear in the previous text. In order to do this in not too excessive space we occasionally have to assume greater mathematical knowledge than what was assumed until now.

15.1 The Dimensionality of the Linear Attenuation Coefficient

In Section 2.4 the claim is made that the linear attenuation coefficient has to be measured in units of inverse length; that is, its dimensionality is inverse length (see also Sections 6.3, 6.4 and 7.1). We now justify this claim.

Let $\mu_e(z)$ denote the linear attenuation coefficient at energy e at the point z between the source ($z = z_s \leq 0$) and the detector ($z = z_d \geq D$), see Fig. 2.4. Let $p_e(z)$ denote the probability that a photon of energy e that leaves the source in the direction of the detector gets as far as the point z without being removed from the beam. Let $q_e(z, \Delta z)$ denote the probability that a photon of energy e that made it as far as a distance z from the source is removed before it gets to a distance $z + \Delta z$ from the source. As can be easily worked out, the relationship between $\mu_e(z)$ and $q_e(z, \Delta z)$ is given by

$$p_e(z + \Delta z) = p_e(z) - p_e(z)q_e(z, \Delta z). \tag{15.1}$$

More importantly, we now show that

$$\mu_e(z) = \lim_{\Delta z \to 0} \left(q_e(z, \Delta z)/\Delta z\right). \tag{15.2}$$

In order to prove (15.2) let us use $v_e(z)$ to denote the right-hand side of the equation. Observe that $v_e(z)$ is a property of the tissue t occupying the point z, and so may be written as v_e^t. Thus our aim is to prove that, for any tissue t, $\mu_e^t = v_e^t$.

From (15.1) it follows that

$$\frac{p_e(z+\Delta z) - p_e(z)}{\Delta z} \frac{1}{p_e(z)} = -\frac{q_e(z,\Delta z)}{\Delta z}. \tag{15.3}$$

Taking the limit as $\Delta z \to 0$, we get

$$p_e'(z)/p_e(z) = -v_e(z). \tag{15.4}$$

Integration of both sides from z_s to z_d (source to detector) leads to

$$\ln p_e(z_d) - \ln p_e(z_s) = -\int_{z_s}^{z_d} v_e(z)\,dz. \tag{15.5}$$

Recalling the definition of $p_e(z)$, we see that $p_e(z_s) = 1$ (and, hence, $\ln p_e(z_s) = 0$), and so

$$-\ln p_e(z_d) = \int_{z_s}^{z_d} v_e(z)\,dz. \tag{15.6}$$

Now we show that $v_e(z) = \mu_e(z)$ for whatever tissue t occupies the position z along the line L.

Suppose that the object between the source and detector is a uniform slab of unit thickness of the tissue t and that the line L is perpendicular to the face of the slab (see Fig. 1.20). In this case $\int_{z_s}^{z_d} v_e(z)\,dz = v_e^t$, since $v_e(z) = 0$ at points not occupied by the slab. Using (15.6) we see that $v_e^t = -\ln p_e(z_d)$, where $p_e(z_d)$ is the probability that a photon at energy e that approaches the slab along the line L will not get removed from the line before exiting through the other side of the slab. Hence, by the definition of the linear attenuation coefficient (2.1), $v_e^t = \mu_e^t$.

Since the probability $q_e(z,\Delta z)$ is dimensionless and Δz is a length, the validity of (15.2) justifies our claim that the linear attenuation coefficient is measured in units of inverse length.

15.2 The Line Integral of the Relative Linear Attenuation

In this section we prove that

$$-\ln\frac{\rho_a}{\rho_c} = \int_0^D \mu_{\bar{e}}(x,y)\,dz, \tag{15.7}$$

where, based on Fig. 2.4, ρ_a is the transmittance along the line L during the monochromatic actual measurement, ρ_c is the transmittance along L during the monochromatic calibration measurement, and the right-hand side of (15.7) is the line integral along L of the relative linear attenuation. Equation (15.7) is exactly (3.5). Using (3.4), (15.7) also gives rise to (2.4).

To prove (15.7), let $\mu_{\bar{e}}^{a}(z)$ and $\mu_{\bar{e}}^{c}(z)$ be the linear attenuation coefficients along the line L (see Fig. 2.4).

$$\mu_{\bar{e}}^{a}(z) = \mu_{\bar{e}}^{c}(z), \quad \text{if} \quad z < 0 \quad \text{or} \quad z > D \tag{15.8}$$

and

$$\mu_{\bar{e}}(x,y) = \mu_{\bar{e}}^{a}(z) - \mu_{\bar{e}}^{c}(z), \ \text{if } 0 \le z \le D, \tag{15.9}$$

where (x,y) are the coordinates of the point z along the line L. Hence, we get (15.7) from

$$\begin{aligned}\int_0^D \mu_{\bar{e}}(x,y)\,dz &= \int_{z_s}^{z_d} \left(\mu_{\bar{e}}^{a}(z) - \mu_{\bar{e}}^{c}(z)\right) dz \\ &= -\ln \rho_a + \ln \rho_c,\end{aligned} \tag{15.10}$$

where the last step follows from (15.6).

15.3 The Radon Inversion Formula

The most important single fact for image reconstruction by transform methods is that there exists a closed-form formula that expresses a function in terms of its Radon transform. In this section we derive such a formula.

In fact, there are two different formulations of the Radon inversion formula that appear in the earlier text. One is (2.5) and the other is (6.10). We prove the validity of both of them.

We follow closely Radon's original proof. We do this both because of its historical interest and because it uses only basic calculus. The only objection that can be reasonably raised against it is that the same result can be proved using less restrictive assumptions, but such considerations are beyond the scope of this book.

In this section we assume that the picture function f is continuous and bounded. Recall also that $f(r,\phi) = 0$, if $r > E$.

For any point (r,ϕ) in the picture region (in particular, $|r| \le E$), we define a function $\bar{F}_{(r,\phi)}$ of one variable by

$$\bar{F}_{(r,\phi)}(q) = \frac{1}{2\pi} \int_0^{2\pi} [\mathscr{R}f]\left(r\cos(\theta-\phi) + q, \theta\right) d\theta. \tag{15.11}$$

Since $[\mathscr{R}f](\ell,\theta) = 0$, if $|\ell| \ge E$, we have that, for $|r| \le E$,

$$\bar{F}_{(r,\phi)}(q) = 0, \quad \text{if } q \ge 2E. \tag{15.12}$$

Radon proved that

$$f(r,\phi) = \frac{1}{\pi} \lim_{\varepsilon \to 0} \left(\frac{1}{\varepsilon} \bar{F}_{(r,\phi)}(\varepsilon) - \int_{\varepsilon}^{\infty} \frac{1}{q^2} \bar{F}_{(r,\phi)}(q)\, dq \right). \tag{15.13}$$

We are interested in the validity of this result for all (r, ϕ)s in the picture region. Prior to giving the proof, we show how the formulas used in the previous chapters can be derived from (15.13). For this we have to make an additional assumption, namely that $\mathscr{R}f$ has a continuous first derivative; i.e., that $\mathscr{D}_Y \mathscr{R} f$ exists and is continuous in its first variable (see (6.11) for the definition of $\mathscr{D}_Y$). In what follows we make repeated use of (15.12).

$$\begin{aligned} \int_{\varepsilon}^{\infty} & \frac{1}{q^2} \bar{F}_{(r,\phi)}(q)\, dq \\ &= \int_{\varepsilon}^{2E} \frac{1}{q^2} \left(\frac{1}{2\pi} \int_0^{2\pi} [\mathscr{R}f]\,(r\cos(\theta - \phi) + q, \theta)\, d\theta \right) dq \\ &= \frac{1}{2\pi} \int_0^{2\pi} \left(\int_{\varepsilon}^{2E} \frac{1}{q^2} [\mathscr{R}f]\,(r\cos(\theta - \phi) + q, \theta)\, dq \right) d\theta. \end{aligned} \tag{15.14}$$

Using integration by parts, we get

$$\begin{aligned} \int_{\varepsilon}^{2E} & \frac{1}{q^2} [\mathscr{R}f]\,(r\cos(\theta - \phi) + q, \theta)\, dq \\ &= \left[-\frac{1}{q} [\mathscr{R}f]\,(r\cos(\theta - \phi) + q, \theta) \right]_{q=\varepsilon}^{q=2E} \\ &\quad - \int_{\varepsilon}^{2E} -\frac{1}{q} [\mathscr{D}_Y \mathscr{R} f]\,(r\cos(\theta - \phi) + q, \theta)\, dq. \end{aligned} \tag{15.15}$$

Substituting this into (15.14), we obtain

$$\begin{aligned} \int_{\varepsilon}^{\infty} & \frac{1}{q^2} \bar{F}_{(r,\phi)}(q)\, dq \\ &= \frac{1}{\varepsilon} \bar{F}_{(r,\phi)}(\varepsilon) + \frac{1}{2\pi} \int_0^{2\pi} \int_{\varepsilon}^{2E} \frac{1}{q} [\mathscr{D}_Y \mathscr{R} f]\,(r\cos(\theta - \phi) + q, \theta)\, dq\, d\theta. \end{aligned} \tag{15.16}$$

Changing the order of integration in the second term and substituting into (15.13), we get

$$f(r,\phi) = -\frac{1}{2\pi^2} \lim_{\varepsilon \to 0} \int_{\varepsilon}^{\infty} \frac{1}{q} \int_0^{2\pi} [\mathscr{D}_Y \mathscr{R} f]\,(r\cos(\theta - \phi) + q, \theta)\, d\theta\, dq, \tag{15.17}$$

which is (2.5), but with polar coordinates instead of rectangular coordinates.

Next we derive (6.10) from (15.17). First note that, for all ℓ and θ,

$$[\mathscr{D}_Y \mathscr{R} f]\,(\ell, \theta) = [\mathscr{D}_Y \mathscr{R} f]\,(-\ell, \theta - \pi). \tag{15.18}$$

Using this fact and the change of variables $\theta' = \theta - \pi$ and $q' = -q$, we get

$$\begin{aligned} &\int_{\varepsilon}^{\infty} \frac{1}{q} \int_{\pi}^{2\pi} [\mathscr{D}_Y \mathscr{R} f]\,(r\cos(\theta-\phi)+q,\theta)\,d\theta\,dq \\ &\quad = \int_{-\varepsilon}^{-\infty} -\frac{1}{q'} \int_{0}^{\pi} [\mathscr{D}_Y \mathscr{R} f]\,(-r\cos(\theta'-\phi)-q',\theta'+\pi)\,d\theta'(-dq') \\ &\quad = \int_{-\infty}^{-\varepsilon} \frac{1}{q} \int_{0}^{\pi} [\mathscr{D}_Y \mathscr{R} f]\,(r\cos(\theta-\phi)+q,\theta)\,d\theta\,dq. \end{aligned} \tag{15.19}$$

Substituting into (15.17) provides

$$\begin{aligned} f(r,\phi) &= -\frac{1}{2\pi^2} \lim_{\varepsilon\to 0} \left[\int_{-\infty}^{-\varepsilon} \frac{1}{q} \int_{0}^{\pi} [\mathscr{D}_Y \mathscr{R} f]\,(r\cos(\theta-\phi)+q,\theta)\,d\theta\,dq \right. \\ &\quad \left. + \int_{\varepsilon}^{\infty} \frac{1}{q} \int_{0}^{\pi} [\mathscr{D}_Y \mathscr{R} f]\,(r\cos(\theta-\phi)+q,\theta)\,d\theta\,dq \right] \\ &= -\frac{1}{2\pi^2} \int_{0}^{\pi} \lim_{\varepsilon\to 0} \left[\int_{-\infty}^{-\varepsilon} \frac{1}{q} [\mathscr{D}_Y \mathscr{R} f]\,(r\cos(\theta-\phi)+q,\theta)\,dq \right. \\ &\quad \left. + \int_{\varepsilon}^{\infty} \frac{1}{q} [\mathscr{D}_Y \mathscr{R} f]\,(r\cos(\theta-\phi)+q,\theta)\,dq \right] d\theta, \end{aligned} \tag{15.20}$$

where the last step is justified by the assumed continuity of $\mathscr{D}_Y \mathscr{R} f$ in its first variable. The integrand of the outer integral can also be written as an improper integral from $-\infty$ to ∞ (equivalently, from $-2E$ to $2E$), which is to be evaluated in its Cauchy principle value sense. By changing the variable, $q = \ell - r\cos(\theta-\phi)$, we get

$$f(r,\phi) = \frac{1}{2\pi^2} \int_{0}^{\pi} \int_{-E}^{E} \frac{1}{r\cos(\theta-\phi)-\ell} [\mathscr{D}_Y \mathscr{R} f]\,(\ell,\theta)\,d\ell\,d\theta, \tag{15.21}$$

which is (6.10), bearing in mind (6.9) and (6.11).

All that is left is to prove (15.13). First note that it is sufficient to prove (15.13) for the case $r = 0$ and $\phi = 0$, since its validity in the general case then follows by shifting the origin of the coordinate system. We denote $\bar{F}_{(0,0)}$ by $\bar{F}$, i.e.,

$$\bar{F}(q) = \frac{1}{2\pi} \int_{0}^{2\pi} [\mathscr{R} f]\,(q,\theta)\,d\theta. \tag{15.22}$$

We also define $\bar{f}$ by

$$\bar{f}(r) = \frac{1}{2\pi} \int_{0}^{2\pi} f(r,\phi)\,d\phi. \tag{15.23}$$

The following basic relationship between $\bar{F}$ and $\bar{f}$ is essential to our proof. For any $q > 0$,

$$\bar{F}(q) = 2 \int_{q}^{\infty} \frac{r\bar{f}(r)}{\sqrt{r^2-q^2}}\,dr. \tag{15.24}$$

The proof of (15.24) is by the following sequence of steps that makes use of (6.4) and the change of variables $s = \sqrt{r^2 - q^2}$.

$$
\begin{aligned}
\bar{F}(q) &= \frac{1}{2\pi} \int_0^{2\pi} \int_{-\infty}^{\infty} f\left(\sqrt{q^2 + s^2}, \theta + \tan^{-1}(s/q)\right) ds\, d\theta \\
&= \frac{1}{2\pi} \int_{-\infty}^{\infty} \int_0^{2\pi} f\left(\sqrt{q^2 + s^2}, \theta\right) d\theta\, ds \\
&= 2 \int_0^{\infty} \bar{f}\left(\sqrt{q^2 + s^2}\right) ds \\
&= 2 \int_q^{\infty} \frac{r}{\sqrt{r^2 - q^2}} \bar{f}(r)\, dr. \qquad (15.25)
\end{aligned}
$$

Substituting (15.24) into the right-hand side of (15.13) we get

$$
\frac{2}{\pi} \lim_{\varepsilon \to 0} \left(\frac{1}{\varepsilon} \int_{\varepsilon}^{\infty} \frac{r\bar{f}(r)}{\sqrt{r^2 - \varepsilon^2}}\, dr - \int_{\varepsilon}^{\infty} \frac{1}{q^2} \int_q^{\infty} \frac{r\bar{f}(r)}{\sqrt{r^2 - q^2}}\, dr\, dq \right). \qquad (15.26)
$$

The last double integral simplifies as follows.

$$
\begin{aligned}
\int_{\varepsilon}^{\infty} \frac{1}{q^2} \int_q^{\infty} \frac{r\bar{f}(r)}{\sqrt{r^2 - q^2}}\, dr\, dq &= \int_{\varepsilon}^{\infty} \int_{\varepsilon}^{r} \frac{r\bar{f}(r)}{q^2\sqrt{r^2 - q^2}}\, dq\, dr \\
&= \int_{\varepsilon}^{\infty} r\bar{f}(r) \left[-\frac{\sqrt{r^2 - q^2}}{r^2 q} \right]_{q=\varepsilon}^{q=r} dr \\
&= \frac{1}{\varepsilon} \int_{\varepsilon}^{\infty} \frac{\sqrt{r^2 - \varepsilon^2}}{r} \bar{f}(r)\, dr. \qquad (15.27)
\end{aligned}
$$

Substituting this into (15.26) we get that

$$
\frac{2}{\pi} \lim_{\varepsilon \to 0} \left(\varepsilon \int_{\varepsilon}^{\infty} \frac{1}{r\sqrt{r^2 - \varepsilon^2}} \bar{f}(r)\, dr \right) \qquad (15.28)
$$

is equal to the right-hand side of (15.13). To complete our proof we need to show that (15.28) is equal to $f(0,0)$.

First note that $\bar{f}(r)$ is continuous and $\bar{f}(0) = f(0,0)$. Hence, for any $\eta > 0$, there exists a $\delta > 0$ such that

$$
\left| \bar{f}(r) - f(0,0) \right| < \eta, \quad \text{if } |r| \le \delta. \qquad (15.29)
$$

Also,

$$
\frac{2}{\pi} \lim_{\varepsilon \to 0} \varepsilon \int_{\varepsilon}^{\delta} \frac{1}{r\sqrt{r^2 - \varepsilon^2}}\, dr = \frac{2}{\pi} \lim_{\varepsilon \to 0} \cos^{-1} \frac{\varepsilon}{\delta} = 1. \qquad (15.30)
$$

Combining (15.29) and (15.30) we get that, for an arbitrary $\eta > 0$,

$$\begin{aligned}
&\left| \frac{2}{\pi} \lim_{\varepsilon \to 0} \left(\varepsilon \int_{\varepsilon}^{\infty} \frac{1}{r\sqrt{r^2 - \varepsilon^2}} \bar{f}(r)\, dr \right) - f(0,0) \right| \\
&\quad \le \left| f(0,0) \left(\frac{2}{\pi} \lim_{\varepsilon \to 0} \left(\varepsilon \int_{\varepsilon}^{\delta} \frac{1}{r\sqrt{r^2 - \varepsilon^2}}\, dr \right) - 1 \right) \right| \\
&\quad + \left| \eta \frac{2}{\pi} \lim_{\varepsilon \to 0} \left(\varepsilon \int_{\varepsilon}^{\delta} \frac{1}{r\sqrt{r^2 - \varepsilon^2}}\, dr \right) \right| \\
&\quad + \left| \frac{2}{\pi} \lim_{\varepsilon \to 0} \left(\varepsilon \int_{\delta}^{\infty} \frac{\bar{f}(r)}{r\sqrt{r^2 - \varepsilon^2}}\, dr \right) \right| \\
&\quad \le \eta.
\end{aligned} \tag{15.31}$$

This completes the proof of the Radon inversion formula.

15.4 A Picture Is Not Uniquely Determined by a Finite Number of Its Views

In the previous section it is shown that if the picture function f has certain mathematical properties (for example, it is continuous), then it is uniquely determined by its Radon transform $\mathscr{R}f$. In practice we have available estimates of $[\mathscr{R}f](\ell, \theta)$ for a finite number of values of ℓ and θ. In this section we show that the finiteness of the data alone is a source of a fundamental nondeterminacy. We prove the following result.

Let M and K be any positive integers. For $1 \le k \le K$, let (r_k, ϕ_k) be arbitrary distinct points in the interior of the picture region and let L_k be arbitrary real numbers. Then there exists a continuous picture function e such that, for $1 \le k \le K$,

$$e(r_k, \phi_k) = L_k \tag{15.32}$$

and, for $1 \le m \le M - 1$ and for all ℓ,

$$[\mathscr{R}e](\ell, m\pi/M) = 0. \tag{15.33}$$

In other words, e is a *ghost* for the views at angles $0, \pi/M, \ldots, (M-1)\pi/M$.

The significance of this result is the following. For any continuous picture function f, there exists another continuous picture function, $f + e$, such that f and $f + e$ have the same line integrals for all lines that lie in one of the given M equally-spaced directions, and yet f and $f + e$ may differ from each other in an arbitrary fashion at each of an arbitrary large finite set of given points. We first prove this result and then further discuss its practical significance.

As a preliminary result we show the following. Let M be any positive integer and δ be any real number such that $0 < \delta < E/\sqrt{2}$, where $E/\sqrt{2}$ is the side of the square that is the picture region as in Section 6.1. Let d be the function defined by

$$d(r, \phi) = \begin{cases} \sin(\pi |r| / \delta) \sin(M\phi), & \text{if } 0 \leq r \leq \delta, \\ 0, & \text{if } r > \delta, \\ d(-r, \phi - \pi), & \text{if } r < 0. \end{cases} \tag{15.34}$$

Then, for $1 \leq m < M$ and for all ℓ,

$$[\mathscr{R}d](\ell, m\pi/M) = 0. \tag{15.35}$$

In order to see the validity of this result, recall the definition of the Radon transform, as given by (6.4).

First consider the case when $\ell \neq 0$.

$$[\mathscr{R}d](\ell, m\pi/M) = \int_{-\infty}^{\infty} d\left(\sqrt{\ell^2 + z^2}, (m\pi/M) + \tan^{-1}(z/\ell)\right) dz \tag{15.36}$$

$$= \begin{cases} 0, & \text{if } \ell \geq \delta, \\ \int_{-\sqrt{\delta^2-\ell^2}}^{\sqrt{\delta^2-\ell^2}} \sin\left(\frac{\pi\sqrt{\ell^2+z^2}}{\delta}\right) \sin\left(m\pi + M \tan^{-1} \frac{z}{\ell}\right) dz, & \text{if } 0 < \ell < \delta. \end{cases}$$

It is easy to see that in the second case in (15.36), the integrand is an odd function of z (i.e., its value for $-z$ is minus its value for z), and so this integral is equal to zero.

Second, if $\ell = 0$, then using (15.34) we get

$$[\mathscr{R}d](\ell, m\pi/M) = \int_{-\infty}^{\infty} d\left(z, (m\pi/M) + \frac{1}{2}\pi\right) dz$$

$$\begin{aligned} &= \int_{-\delta}^{0} d\left(-z, (m\pi/M) - \frac{1}{2}\pi\right) dz \\ &\quad + \int_{0}^{\delta} d\left(z, (m\pi/M) + \frac{1}{2}\pi\right) dz \\ &= \int_{-\delta}^{0} \sin(\pi |z| / \delta) \sin\left(m\pi - \frac{1}{2}M\pi\right) dz \\ &\quad + \int_{0}^{\delta} \sin(\pi |z| / \delta) \sin\left(m\pi + \frac{1}{2}M\pi\right) dz \\ &= 0. \end{aligned} \tag{15.37}$$

Thus we have proved the validity of (15.35) for $1 \leq m \leq M$ and for all ℓ.

Now note that d is a continuous picture function and

$$d(\delta/2, \pi/2M) = 1. \tag{15.38}$$

Furthermore, multiplication by a constant (scaling) and/or translation in the plane does not change the property of d expressed by (15.35). Hence, by choosing δ sufficiently small, we can define a continuous picture function e

satisfying (15.32) and (15.33) as a sum of K scaled and translated versions of d.

At first sight, the result we have just proved seems to imply that reconstruction from a finite number of views is a hopeless task. This contradicts the already well-illustrated practical experience of successful reconstructions from a finite number of views.

The resolution of this apparent contradiction between theory and practice comes by investigating the nature of the function d defined by (15.34). We see that, for a large M, it is a highly oscillatory function: on a circle of radius $\delta/2$ it defines a harmonic function of ϕ of frequency $M/2\pi$ (or, equivalently, period $2\pi/M$). If we choose M so large that the objects we are interested in are unlikely to have regions with such oscillatory properties (and even if they do, we do not care to reproduce such fine oscillations), then there is a hope that algorithms may produce from the potential infinity of solutions one that is similar to the sought-after picture. In particular, if we demand that our reconstruction be similar to the original only after both the original and reconstruction have been blurred (say, by repeated applications of selective smoothing, see Section 5.3, or preferably by a corresponding continuous operation), addition of a function such as d to f would not make any difference, since the blurred versions of f and $f + d$ are likely to be indistinguishable. Similar arguments apply to other mathematical results showing the impossibility of reconstructing from a finite number of views; see the Notes and References at the end of this chapter.

15.5 Analysis of the Photon Statistics

In this section we derive the mathematical claims made in Section 3.1 regarding the nature of photon statistics.

First we show that the number of photons, which (a) are at a fixed energy $\bar{e}$, (b) reach the detector without having been absorbed or scattered, and (c) are counted by the detector, is a sample of a Poisson random variable with parameter $\lambda\rho\sigma$. (For definitions and notation see Section 3.1.)

As stated in (3.1), the probability that exactly y photons at energy $\bar{e}$ are emitted by the source in one unit of time is

$$p_{Y_\lambda}(y) = \frac{\lambda^y \exp(-\lambda)}{y!}. \tag{15.39}$$

The probability that one of these photons is counted by the detector without having been absorbed or scattered is $\rho\sigma$. Hence, the probability that x of the y photons are counted by the detector without having been absorbed or scattered is given by, see (1.3),

$$p_{y,\rho\sigma}(x) = \begin{cases} 0, & \text{if } x < 0 \text{ or } x > y, \\ \frac{y!}{x!(y-x)!}(\rho\sigma)^x(1-\rho\sigma)^{y-x}, & \text{if } 0 \le x \le y. \end{cases} \tag{15.40}$$

Hence the combined probability $p_X(x)$ that in one unit of time exactly x photons of energy $\bar{e}$ are counted by the detector without having been absorbed or scattered is

$$\begin{aligned}
p_X(x) &= \sum_{y=0}^{\infty} p_Y(y) p_{y,\rho\sigma}(x) \\
&= \sum_{y=x}^{\infty} \exp(-\lambda) \frac{\lambda^y}{y!} \frac{y!}{x!(y-x)!} (\rho\sigma)^x (1-\rho\sigma)^{y-x} \\
&= \exp(-\lambda) \frac{(\rho\sigma)^x}{x!} \sum_{y=x}^{\infty} \frac{1}{(y-x)!} \lambda^y (1-\rho\sigma)^{y-x} \\
&= \exp(-\lambda) \frac{(\lambda\rho\sigma)^x}{x!} \sum_{t=0}^{\infty} \frac{\lambda^t (1-\rho\sigma)^t}{t!} \\
&= \exp(-\lambda) \frac{(\lambda\rho\sigma)^x}{x!} \exp(\lambda - \lambda\rho\sigma) \\
&= \exp(-\lambda\rho\sigma) \frac{(\lambda\rho\sigma)^x}{x!},
\end{aligned} \tag{15.41}$$

where we have made use of the infinite expansion of $\exp(z)$ in powers of z. This shows, as required, that x is a sample of the Poisson random variable with parameter $\lambda\rho\sigma$.

Next we derive (3.6) and (3.7). In order to do this we need to discuss the random variable that is the natural logarithm of the Poisson random variable (see Section 1.2). However, there is a basic difficulty here. The number zero is a possible sample of the Poisson variable, and the natural logarithm function ln is undefined for zero. For practical purposes, we usually deal with a Poisson random variable whose parameter λ is very large and, hence, the probability of zero as a sample (namely, $\exp(-\lambda)$) is very small. We may therefore introduce an altered Poisson random variable Z whose outcomes are all positive integers and such that $p_X(x)$ and $p_Z(x)$ are very similar for all positive integers x. A simple way of doing this is to define $p_Z(1) = p_X(0) + p_X(1)$. We refer to such a random variable Z as the *truncated Poisson random variable* with parameter λ. The following holds.

If Z_λ is a truncated Poisson random variable with a large parameter λ, and if $T_\lambda = \ln Z_\lambda$, then

$$\mu_{T_\lambda} \simeq \ln \lambda - 1/(2\lambda) \tag{15.42}$$

and

$$V_{T_\lambda} \simeq 1/\lambda. \tag{15.43}$$

The precise interpretation of this result is that there are constants c and Λ, such that for all $\lambda > \Lambda$, the absolute values of the differences between the two sides (15.42) and (15.43) are less than c/λ^2. The proof of this result is beyond the scope of this book.

Combining (2.2) with the discussion in Section 3.1 and the result proved at the beginning of the current section, we see that the monochromatic ray sum m can be written as

$$m = -\ln \frac{(z_1/z_2)}{(z_3/z_4)} = -\ln z_1 + \ln z_2 + \ln z_3 - \ln z_4, \tag{15.44}$$

where z_1, z_2, z_3, and z_4 are samples of the truncated Poisson random variables Z_{λ_1}, Z_{λ_2}, Z_{λ_3}, and Z_{λ_4} with parameters $\lambda_1 = \phi_d \lambda_a \rho_a \sigma_d$, $\lambda_2 = \phi_r \lambda_a \rho_r \sigma_r$, $\lambda_3 = \phi_d \lambda_c \rho_c \sigma_d$ and $\lambda_4 = \phi_r \lambda_c \rho_r \sigma_r$, respectively. We see that m is a sample of a random variable M, where

$$M = -\ln Z_1 + \ln Z_2 + \ln Z_3 - \ln Z_4. \tag{15.45}$$

From (15.42) and (1.13) we get

$$\mu_M \simeq -\ln \frac{(\lambda_1/\lambda_2)}{(\lambda_3/\lambda_4)} - \frac{1}{2}\left(-\frac{1}{\lambda_1} + \frac{1}{\lambda_2} + \frac{1}{\lambda_3} - \frac{1}{\lambda_4}\right). \tag{15.46}$$

Rewriting (3.8) as

$$S = \frac{1}{\lambda_1} + \frac{1}{\lambda_2} + \frac{1}{\lambda_3} + \frac{1}{\lambda_4} \tag{15.47}$$

yields (3.6).

Getting (3.7) is trickier, due to the fact that Z_1 and Z_2 are not independent and also Z_3 and Z_4 are not independent, see the discussion in Section 3.1. If it were not for this, it would immediately follow from (1.14) and the fact that the variance of the negative of a random variable is clearly the same as the variance of the random variable ($V_X = V_{-X}$), that

$$V_M \simeq \frac{1}{\lambda_1} + \frac{1}{\lambda_2} + \frac{1}{\lambda_3} + \frac{1}{\lambda_4}, \tag{15.48}$$

which is the same as (3.7). That this result still holds in spite of the lack of independence has been validated by experimental sampling of the random variables in question. It turns out that with the large number of photons involved in x-ray CT, it makes practically no difference to V_M whether in sampling the random variable M of (15.45) one samples Z_1, Z_2, Z_3 and Z_4 independently or in the more accurate fashion described in Section 3.1.

15.6 The Integral Expression for Polychromatic Ray Sums

In this section we prove (3.10). Assume that in the polychromatic x-ray beam, the number of photons of energy e that leave the source towards the detector during both the calibration measurement and the actual measurement is approximately S_e. (This assumption says, in particular, that the normalization by the readings of the reference detector works perfectly and totally eliminates any differences between the strengths of the x-ray pulses at the times of the actual and of the calibration measurements.) By (15.6) the number of photons at energy e counted by the detector during the calibration measurement is

$$T_e \simeq S_e \sigma_e \kappa_e \exp\left(-\int_0^D \mu_e^a \, dz\right), \tag{15.49}$$

where σ_e is the detector efficiency at energy e and κ_e is used as the abbreviation

$$\kappa_e = \exp\left(-\int_{Z_s}^0 \mu_e(z)\, dz\right) \exp\left(-\int_D^{Z_d} \mu_e(z)\, dz\right); \tag{15.50}$$

for the definitions of Z_s and Z_d see Fig. 2.4 and for those of μ_e^a and $\mu_e(z)$ see Section 3.2.

Since C_p is the total number of photons (at any energy) detected during the calibration measurement, the detected spectrum during the calibration is

$$\tau_e = T_e / C_p. \tag{15.51}$$

Hence

$$\begin{aligned} p = -\ln\left(A_p/C_p\right) &\simeq -\ln\left(\int_0^E S_e \sigma_e \kappa_e \exp\left(-\int_0^D \mu_e(z) dz\right) de/C_p\right) \quad (15.52) \\ &\simeq -\ln\left(\int_0^E T_e \exp\left(-\int_0^D \left(\mu_e(z) - \mu_e^a\right) dz\right) de/C_p\right), \end{aligned}$$

which, in view of (15.51), provides us with (3.10).

15.7 Proof of the Regularization Theorem

In this section we prove the regularization theorem stated in Section 8.1. We first need to define what it means for a function ϕ to be reasonable at a point v.

A function ϕ is said to be *reasonable at a point* v if the following conditions are satisfied:

$$\phi(u) = 0, \quad \text{if } |u| \geq E, \tag{15.53}$$

$$\int_{-E}^{E} \phi(u)\, du \text{ exists}, \tag{15.54}$$

$$\lim_{\varepsilon \to 0} \int_\varepsilon^\infty \frac{|\phi(v-t) - \phi(v+t)|}{t}\, dt \text{ exists}. \tag{15.55}$$

(Here, and in the rest of this section, all integrals can be interpreted as Riemann integrals.)

We first show that if ϕ is reasonable at the point v, then $[\mathscr{H}\phi](v)$, as defined by (8.7), exists.

$$\begin{aligned}[\mathscr{H}\phi](v) &= -\frac{1}{\pi}\lim_{\varepsilon\to 0}\left(\int_{-\infty}^{v-\varepsilon}\frac{\phi(u)}{v-u}\,du + \int_{v+\varepsilon}^{\infty}\frac{\phi(u)}{v-u}\,du\right) \\ &= -\frac{1}{\pi}\lim_{\varepsilon\to 0}\int_{\varepsilon}^{\infty}\frac{\phi(v-t)-\phi(v+t)}{t}\,dt,\end{aligned} \tag{15.56}$$

which exists in view of (15.55). The last line in (15.56) is obtained by changes of variable $u = v - t$ and $u = v + t$, respectively, in the two integrals in the previous line.

It is an easily derivable consequence of what is known in analysis as the *Riemann–Lebesgue lemma for absolutely integrable functions* that

$$\lim_{B\to\infty}\int_{-\infty}^{\infty}\phi(v-t)\frac{1-\cos 2\pi Bt}{t}\,dt = \int_{0}^{\infty}\frac{\phi(v-t)-\phi(v+t)}{t}\,dt, \tag{15.57}$$

which, combined with (15.56), gives us an alternative expression for $[\mathscr{H}\phi](v)$. We work on this further, to obtain an expression for $[\mathscr{H}\phi](v)$ that is particularly useful for proving the regularization theorem.

Let G_v be the function defined by

$$G_v(U) = -2\int_{-\infty}^{\infty}\phi(u)\sin\left(2\pi(v-u)U\right)du. \tag{15.58}$$

Using (15.53) and (15.54) we get that, for any $B > 0$,

$$\begin{aligned}\int_0^B G_v(U)\,dU &= -2\int_0^B\left(\int_{-E}^{E}\phi(u)\sin\left(2\pi(v-u)U\right)du\right)dU \\ &= -2\int_{-E}^{E}\phi(u)\left(\int_0^B \sin\left(2\pi(v-u)U\right)dU\right)du \\ &= -\frac{1}{\pi}\int_{-\infty}^{\infty}\phi(u)\frac{1-\cos 2\pi B(v-u)}{(v-u)}\,du \\ &= -\frac{1}{\pi}\int_{-\infty}^{\infty}\phi(v-t)\frac{1-\cos 2\pi Bt}{t}\,dt,\end{aligned} \tag{15.59}$$

where the last equality is obtained by the change of variable $u = v - t$.

So, by (15.57) the limit as $B \to \infty$ of the left-hand side of (15.59) exists, and using (15.56) we get

$$\int_0^{\infty} G_v(U)\,dU = [\mathscr{H}\phi](v). \tag{15.60}$$

The right-hand side of (15.60) is the same as the right-hand side of (8.9). What we now have to prove is that the left-hand sides are also equal. A step, using (8.10), in this direction is the following.

$$
\begin{aligned}
[\phi * \rho_A](v) &= \int_{-\infty}^{\infty} \rho_A(v-u)\phi(u)\,du \\
&= \int_{-E}^{E} \left[-2 \int_0^{A/2} F_A(U) \sin\left(2\pi U(v-u)\right) dU \right] \phi(u)\,du \\
&= \int_0^{A/2} F_A(U) \left[-2 \int_{-\infty}^{\infty} \phi(u) \sin\left(2\pi U(v-u)U\right) du \right] dU \\
&= \int_0^{A/2} F_A(U) G_v(U) dU. \qquad (15.61)
\end{aligned}
$$

We have to show that the right-hand side of (15.61) tends to the left-hand side of (15.60) as $A \to \infty$, i.e., that

$$\lim_{A\to\infty} \psi_A(v) = 0, \qquad (15.62)$$

where

$$
\begin{aligned}
\psi_A(v) &= \int_0^{\infty} G_v(U)\,dU - \int_0^{A/2} F_A(U) G_v(U)\,dU \\
&= \int_0^{A/2} \left(1 - F_A(U)\right) G_v(U)\,dU + \int_{A/2}^{\infty} G_v(U)\,dU. \qquad (15.63)
\end{aligned}
$$

Let ε be an arbitrary but fixed positive real number. There exists a real number $N(\varepsilon)$ such that, for any $C \geq N(\varepsilon)$,

$$\int_C^{\infty} G_v(U)\,dU \leq \varepsilon. \qquad (15.64)$$

Letting $A > 2N(\varepsilon)$, we have

$$
\begin{aligned}
\psi_A(v) = &\int_0^{N(\varepsilon)} \left(1 - F_A(U)\right) G_v(U)\,dU + \int_{N(\varepsilon)}^{A/2} \left(1 - F_A(U)\right) G_v(U)\,dU \\
&+ \int_{A/2}^{\infty} G_v(U)\,dU. \qquad (15.65)
\end{aligned}
$$

By the statement of the regularization theorem, $0 \leq F_A(U) \leq 1$ and $F_A(U)$ is monotonically nonincreasing. It follows that $0 \leq (1 - F_A(U)) \leq 1$ and $1 - F_A(U)$ is monotonically nondecreasing. Furthermore $G_v(U)$ is continuous. Hence we can apply the second mean value theorem for Riemann integrals and obtain

$$\int_0^{N(\varepsilon)} (1 - F_A(U))\, G_v(U)\, dU = (1 - F_A(N(\varepsilon))) \int_a^{N(\varepsilon)} G_v(U)\, dU, \quad (15.66)$$

for some a, $0 \le a \le N(\varepsilon)$, and

$$\int_{N(\varepsilon)}^{A/2} (1 - F_A(U))\, G_v(U)\, dU = (1 - F_A(A/2)) \int_b^{A/2} G_v(U)\, dU, \quad (15.67)$$

for some b, $N(\varepsilon) \le b \le A/2$.

From (15.65), (15.66), and (15.67) we get

$$\begin{aligned}|\psi_A(v)| \le{}& (1 - F_A(N(\varepsilon))) \left| \int_a^{N(\varepsilon)} G_v(U)\, dU \right| \\ &+ (1 - F_A(A/2)) \left| \int_b^{A/2} G_v(U)\, dU \right| \\ &+ \left| \int_{A/2}^{\infty} G_v(U)\, dU \right| \\ \le{}& (1 - F_A(N(\varepsilon))) \left| \int_a^{N(\varepsilon)} G_v(U)\, dU \right| + 3\varepsilon; \end{aligned} \quad (15.68)$$

recall (15.64).

Note that $N(\varepsilon)$ does *not* depend on A. Hence $\int_a^{N(\varepsilon)} G_v(U)\, dU$ does not depend on A. According to the conditions of the regularization theorem $\lim_{A\to\infty} F_A(N(\varepsilon)) = 1$, and so the first term on the right-hand side of (15.68) converges to zero as A tends to infinity. Since ε was arbitrary, (15.62) holds and the proof of the regularization theorem is complete.

15.8 Convergence of the Relaxation Method for Inequalities

In this section we prove that the algorithm described by (11.9), (11.10), and (11.11) converges to an element of N, defined by (11.7) and (11.8).

Following Chapter 11, we assume that, for $1 \le i \le P$, $\|n_i\| \ne 0$. The notation of Section 11.2 is adopted without further notice.

Let k be a nonnegative integer such that $x^{(k)} \notin N_{i_k}$. Then

$$\begin{aligned}\left\| x^{(k+1)} - x^{(k)} \right\|^2 &= \left\| \lambda^{(k)} \frac{q_{i_k} - \langle n_{i_k}, x^{(k)} \rangle}{\|n_{i_k}\|^2} n_{i_k} \right\|^2 \\ &= \left(\lambda^{(k)}\right)^2 \frac{\left(q_{i_k} - \langle n_{i_k}, x^{(k)} \rangle\right)^2}{\|n_{i_k}\|^2}. \end{aligned} \quad (15.69)$$

Let z be any vector in N. Using the positivity of $\lambda^{(k)}$ and the facts that $\langle n_{i_k}, z\rangle \leq q_{i_k}$ and $\left\langle n_{i_k}, x^{(k)}\right\rangle > q_{i_k}$, we get that

$$-\lambda^{(k)} \frac{q_{i_k} - \left\langle n_{i_k}, x^{(k)}\right\rangle}{\left\|n_{i_k}\right\|^2} \langle n_{i_k}, z\rangle \leq -\lambda^{(k)} \frac{q_{i_k} - \left\langle n_{i_k}, x^{(k)}\right\rangle}{\left\|n_{i_k}\right\|^2} q_{i_k}. \tag{15.70}$$

Combining the last two equations provides

$$\begin{aligned}\left\langle x^{(k+1)} - x^{(k)}, x^{(k)} - z\right\rangle &= \lambda^{(k)} \frac{q_{i_k} - \left\langle n_{i_k}, x^{(k)}\right\rangle}{\left\|n_{i_k}\right\|^2} \left\langle n_{i_k}, x^{(k)} - z\right\rangle \\ &\leq \lambda^{(k)} \frac{q_{i_k} - \left\langle n_{i_k}, x^{(k)}\right\rangle}{\left\|n_{i_k}\right\|^2} \left(\left\langle n_{i_k}, x^{(k)}\right\rangle - q_{i_k}\right) \\ &= -\lambda^{(k)} \frac{\left(q_{i_k} - \left\langle n_{i_k}, x^{(k)}\right\rangle\right)^2}{\left\|n_{i_k}\right\|^2} \\ &= -\frac{1}{\lambda^{(k)}} \left\|x^{(k+1)} - x^{(k)}\right\|^2.\end{aligned} \tag{15.71}$$

From this we obtain that

$$\begin{aligned}\left\|x^{(k+1)} - z\right\|^2 &= \left\|x^{(k+1)} - x^{(k)} + x^{(k)} - z\right\|^2 \\ &= \left\|x^{(k+1)} - x^{(k)}\right\|^2 + 2\left\langle x^{(k+1)} - x^{(k)}, x^{(k)} - z\right\rangle + \left\|x^{(k)} - z\right\|^2 \\ &\leq \left(1 - \left(2/\lambda^{(k)}\right)\right) \left\|x^{(k+1)} - x^{(k)}\right\|^2 + \left\|x^{(k)} - z\right\|^2.\end{aligned} \tag{15.72}$$

Hence,

$$\left\|x^{(k+1)} - z\right\|^2 + \left(\left(2/\lambda^{(k)}\right) - 1\right) \left\|x^{(k+1)} - x^{(k)}\right\|^2 \leq \left\|x^{(k)} - z\right\|^2. \tag{15.73}$$

We proved (15.73) under the assumption $x^{(k)} \notin N_{i_k}$. However, if $x^{(k)} \in N_{i_k}$, then $x^{(k+1)} = x^{(k)}$ and (15.73) is trivially satisfied.

From (11.11) we obtain

$$\left(\frac{2}{\lambda^{(k)}} - 1\right) \geq \left(\frac{2}{\varepsilon_2} - 1\right) = \frac{2 - \varepsilon_2}{\varepsilon_2} > 0, \tag{15.74}$$

and so the sequence $\left\|x^{(k)} - z\right\|^2$, for $k = 0, 1, 2, \ldots$, is never increasing. Since it is bounded below, $\lim_{k\to\infty} \left\|x^{(k)} - z\right\|^2$ exists. Hence (15.73) and (15.74) imply that

$$\lim_{k\to\infty} \left\|x^{(k+1)} - x^{(k)}\right\|^2 = 0. \tag{15.75}$$

We also obtain that the sequence $x^{(0)}, x^{(1)}, x^{(2)}, \ldots$ is bounded.

Since the sequence $x^{(0)}, x^{(1)}, x^{(2)}, \ldots$ is bounded, there is at least one infinite subsequence that converges to some vector, y, say. We show that y is in N

and that y is independent of the subsequence that is used in its construction. This will complete the proof.

Consider an infinite subsequence of $x^{(0)}, x^{(1)}, x^{(2)}, \ldots$ that converges to a vector y. Let i be any integer, $1 \leq i \leq P$. We now show that $y \in N_i$, by proving that, for any $\varepsilon > 0$,

$$\langle n_i, y \rangle - q_i < \varepsilon. \tag{15.76}$$

Let

$$f = \min \{1, \varepsilon_1\} / \|n_i\|. \tag{15.77}$$

For any $\varepsilon > 0$, there is an element $x^{(t)}$, say, in the infinite subsequence of $x^{(0)}, x^{(1)}, x^{(2)}, \ldots$ that converges to y, such that

$$\left\| y - x^{(t)} \right\| < (f/2P)\varepsilon. \tag{15.78}$$

Because of (15.75), this element $x^{(t)}$ can be chosen so that

$$\left\| x^{(s+1)} - x^{(s)} \right\| < (f/2P)\varepsilon, \tag{15.79}$$

for all $s \geq t$. There exists an s such that $t \leq s < t + P$ and $i = i_s$. For this s,

$$\left\| y - x^{(s)} \right\| < P \frac{f}{2P} \varepsilon \leq \frac{1}{2\|n_i\|} \varepsilon. \tag{15.80}$$

If $x^{(s)} \notin N_i$, then by (15.69)

$$\begin{aligned} \left\langle n_i, x^{(s)} \right\rangle - q_i &= \frac{\|n_i\|}{\lambda^{(s)}} \left\| x^{(s+1)} - x^{(s)} \right\| < \frac{\|n_i\|}{\lambda^{(s)}} \frac{f}{2P} \varepsilon \\ &\leq \frac{\|n_i\|}{\lambda^{(s)}} \frac{\varepsilon_1}{\|n_i\|} \frac{\varepsilon}{2P} \leq \frac{1}{2} \varepsilon. \end{aligned} \tag{15.81}$$

If $x^{(s)} \in N$, then (15.81) is trivially true. Using (15.80) and (15.81), we get

$$\begin{aligned} \langle n_i, y \rangle - q_i &= \left\langle n_i, y - x^{(s)} + x^{(s)} \right\rangle - q_i \\ &= \left\langle n_i, x^{(s)} \right\rangle - q_i + \left\langle n_i, y - x^{(s)} \right\rangle \\ &\leq \frac{1}{2} \varepsilon + \|n_i\| \left\| y - x^{(s)} \right\| < \varepsilon, \end{aligned} \tag{15.82}$$

proving (15.76). Since $y \in N_i$ for an arbitrary i, $1 \leq i \leq P$, we get that $y \in N$.

Suppose that there exists another subsequence of $x^{(0)}, x^{(1)}, x^{(2)}, \ldots$ that converges to y'. As above, we can show that $y' \in N$. Recalling that, for any $z \in N$, $\lim_{k\to\infty}(\left\| x^{(k)} - z \right\|^2)$ exists, let

$$\alpha = \lim_{k\to\infty} \left(\left\| x^{(k)} - y \right\|^2 - \left\| x^{(k)} - y' \right\|^2 \right). \tag{15.83}$$

Using the subsequence that converges to y we get

$$\alpha = -\left\|y - y'\right\|^2, \tag{15.84}$$

and using the other subsequence we get

$$\alpha = \left\|y' - y\right\|^2. \tag{15.85}$$

Hence $\alpha = 0$ and $y = y'$, completing our proof.

Notes and References

Sections 15.1 and 15.2 are based on [111].

Section 15.3 follows [225] very closely. The continuity of f is not necessary for the existence of the inverse Radon transform. Inversion formulas and proofs exist for many large classes of functions; see, for example, [142, 188, 211, 244]. Also, inversion of the Radon transform is possible (at least in principle) if the Radon transform is known only in parts of its domain, see, for example, [179, 182, 208], and the references in those papers.

A much stronger version of the result in Section 15.4 exists. See, e.g., Theorem 4.3 of [244]. The authors summarize this result by saying "a finite set of radiographs tells us nothing at all." However, this is a somewhat extreme rephrasing of the precise mathematical statement. In particular, just assuming that all picture functions are bounded by the same value (a blatantly reasonable assumption in CT), allows one to give error estimates of the convolution method that are picture independent and converge to zero as the finite number of views increases; see, e.g., [63]. Resolution of such apparent contradictions can be given along the lines suggested at the end of Section 15.4. See also [158]. An alternative method for producing ghosts is described in [121]; it is the method that was used to produce the "large tumor" in Fig. 4.5(b) that happens to be a ghost for 22 views.

The estimates for the mean and the variance of the natural logarithm of a truncated Poisson random variable with a large parameter λ that are provided by (15.42) and (15.43), respectively, can be derived by standard techniques of probability theory, as described, e.g., in [217]. A discussion in the framework of CT is given in Appendix B of [19], wich provides some earlier references.

Section 15.6 is based on [111].

The results of mathematical analysis used in Section 15.7 can be found, for example, in [10]. The proof of the regularization theorem follows that given in [49].

The convergence of the relaxation methods for inequalities (under the general conditions stated in Section 11.2) follows from the results of [103]. Our proof in Section 15.8 is in line with [130], which gives some additional relevant references.

For up-to-date information (at the time of writing) on mathematical matters related to CT, the reader may consult the books [48, 75, 143, 211].

References

1. A.O. Allen. *Probability, Statistics, and Queueing Theory with Computer Science Applications.* Academic Press, 2nd edition, 1990.
2. A. Alpers, L. Rodek, H.F. Poulsen, E. Knudsen, and G.T. Herman. Discrete tomography for generating grain maps of polycrystals. In G.T. Herman and A. Kuba, editors, *Advances in Discrete Tomography and Its Applications*, pages 303–331. Birkhäuser, 2007.
3. M.D. Altschuler. Reconstruction of the global-scale three-dimensional solar corona. In G.T. Herman, editor, *Image Reconstruction Implementation and Applications*, pages 105–145. Springer-Verlag, 1979.
4. M.D. Altschuler, Y. Censor, P.P.B. Eggermont, G.T. Herman, Y.H. Kuo, R.M. Lewitt, M. McKay, H.K. Tuy, J.K. Udupa, and M.M. Yau. Demonstration of a software package for the reconstruction of the dynamically changing structure of the human heart from cone-beam x-ray projections. *J. Med. Syst.*, 4:289–304, 1980.
5. M.D. Altschuler, Y. Censor, G.T. Herman, A. Lent, R.M. Lewitt, S.N. Srihari, H.K. Tuy, and J.K. Udupa. Mathematical aspects of image reconstruction from projections. In L.N. Kanal and A. Rosenfeld, editors, *Progress in Pattern Recognition*, pages 323–375. North-Holland, 1981.
6. M.D. Altschuler, T.C. Zhu, J. Li, and A.S.M. Hahn. Optimized interstitial PDT prostrate treatment planning with the Cimmino feasibility algorithm. *Med. Phys.*, 32:3524–3536, 2005.
7. R.E. Alvarez and A. Macovski. Energy-selective reconstructions in x-ray computerized tomography. *Phys. Med. Biol.*, 21:733–744, 1976.
8. H.C. Andrews and B.R. Hunt. *Digital Image Restoration.* Prentice-Hall, 1977.
9. D. Andronico, R.A. Corsaro, A. Cristaldi, and M. Polacci. Characterizing high energy explosive eruptions at Stromboli volcano using multidisciplinary data: An example from the 9 January 2005 explosion. *J. Volcanol. Geotherm. Res.*, 176:541–550, 2008.
10. T.M. Apostol. *Mathematical Analysis.* Addison-Wesley, 2nd edition, 1974.
11. E. Artzy, T. Elfving, and G.T. Herman. Quadratic optimization for image reconstruction II. *Comput. Vision Graph.*, 11:242–261, 1979.
12. E. Artzy, G. Frieder, and G.T. Herman. The theory, design, implementation and evaluation of a three-dimensional surface detection algorithm. *Comput. Graph. Image Proc.*, 15:1–24, 1981.

13. S.W. Atlas. *Magnetic Resonance Imaging of the Brain and Spine.* Lippincott Williams & Wilkins, 3rd edition, 2001.
14. T. Austin, A.P. Gibson, G. Branco, R.M. Yusof, S.R. Arridge, J.H. Meek, J.S. Wyatt, D.T. Delpy, and J.C. Hebden. Three dimensional optical imaging of blood volume and oxygenation in the neonatal brain. *NeuroImage*, 31:1426–1433, 2006.
15. L. Axel, G.T. Herman, D.A. Roberts, and L. Dougherty. Linogram reconstruction for magnetic resonance imging (MRI). *IEEE T. Med. Imag.*, 9:447–449, 1990.
16. C. Axelsson and P. Danielsson. Three-dimensional reconstruction from cone-beam data in O(N^3logN) time. *Phys. Med. Biol.*, 39:477–491, 1994.
17. D.L. Bailey, D.W. Townsend, P.E. Valk, and M.N. Maisey. *Positron Emission Tomography: Basic Sciences.* Springer-Verlag, 2005.
18. J. Banhart. *Advanced Tomographic Methods in Materials Research and Engineering.* Oxford University Press, 2008.
19. H.H. Barrett, S.K. Gordon, and R.S. Hershel. Statistical limitations in transaxial tomography. *Comput. Biol. Med.*, 6:307–323, 1976.
20. J. Baumann, Z. Kiss, S. Krimmel, A. Kuba, A. Nagy, L. Rodek, B. Schillinger, and J. Stephan. Discrete tomography methods for nondestructive testing. In G.T. Herman and A. Kuba, editors, *Advances in Discrete Tomography and Its Applications*, pages 303–331. Birkhäuser, 2007.
21. H.H. Bauschke and J.M. Borwein. On projections algorithms for solving convex feasibility problems. *SIAM Rev.*, 38:367–426, 1996.
22. W.T. Baxter, R.A. Grassucci, H. Gao, and J. Frank. Determination of signal-to-noise ratios and spectral SNRs in cryo-EM low-dose imaging of molecules. *J. Struct. Biol.*, 166:126–132, 2009.
23. J.R. Bilbao-Castro, R. Marabini, C.O.S. Sorzano, I. García, J.M. Carazo, and J.J. Fernández. Exploiting desktop supercomputing for three-dimensional electron microscopy reconstructions using ART with blobs. *J. Struct. Biol.*, 165:19–26, 2009.
24. F.B. Bouallegue, J.F. Crouzet, and D. Mariano-Goulart. Evaluation of a new gridding method for fully 3D direct Fourier PET reconstruction based on a two-plane geometry. *Comput. Med. Imag. Graph.*, 32:580–589, 2008.
25. R.N. Bracewell. Strip integration in radio astronomy. *Aust. J. Phys.*, 9:198–217, 1956.
26. R.N. Bracewell. Correction for collimator width (restoration) in reconstructive x-ray tomography. *J. Comput. Assist. Tomo.*, 1:6–15, 1977.
27. R.N. Bracewell. Image reconstruction in radio astronomy. In G.T. Herman, editor, *Image Reconstruction from Projections: Implementation and Applications*, pages 81–104. Springer-Verlag, 1979.
28. R.N. Bracewell. *The Fourier Transform and Its Applications.* McGraw-Hill, 3rd edition, 1999.
29. R.N. Bracewell and A.C. Riddle. Inversion of fanbeam scans in radio astronomy. *Astrophys. J.*, 150:427–434, 1967.
30. J.E. Bresenham. Algorithm for computer control of a digital plotter. *IBM Systems J.*, 4:25–30, 1965.
31. E.O. Brigham. *The Fast Fourier Transform and Its Applications.* Prentice-Hall, 1988.

32. R.A. Brooks and G. DiChiro. Principles of computer assisted tomography (CAT) in radiographic and radioisotopic imaging. *Phys. Med. Biol.*, 21:689–732, 1976.
33. R.A. Brooks and G.H. Weiss. Interpolation problems in image reconstruction. *Proc. SPIE*, 96:313–319, 1976.
34. J.A. Browne and A.R. De Pierro. A row-action alternative to the EM algorithm for maximizing likelihood in emission tomography. *IEEE T. Med. Imag.*, 15:687–699, 1996.
35. T.F. Budinger, G.T. Gullberg, and R.H. Huesman. Emission computed tomography. In G.T. Herman, editor, *Image Reconstruction from Projections: Implementation and Applications*, pages 147–246. Springer-Verlag, 1979.
36. D. Butnariu, R. Davidi, G.T. Herman, and I.G. Kazansev. Stable convergence behavior under summable perturbations of a class of projection methods for convex feasibility and optimization problems. *IEEE J. Select. Topics Signal Proc.*, 1:540–547, 2007.
37. P.L. Butzer and R.J. Nessel. *Fourier Analysis and Approximation*, volume 1. Academic Press, 1971.
38. J.-M. Carazo, G.T. Herman, C.O.S. Sorzano, and R. Marabini. Algorithms for thee-dimensional reconstruction from the imperfect projection data provided by electron microscopy. In J. Frank, editor, *Electron Tomography: Methods for Three-Dimensional Visualization of Structures in the Cell*, pages 217–244. Springer, 2nd edition, 2006.
39. B.M. Carvalho and G.T. Herman. Low-dose, large-angled cone-beam helical CT data reconstruction using algebraic reconstruction techniques. *Imag. Vision Comput.*, 25:78–94, 2007.
40. B.M. Carvalho, G.T. Herman, and T.Y. Kong. Simultaneous fuzzy segmentation of multiple objects. *Discrete Appl. Math.*, 151:55–77, 2005.
41. Y. Censor. Row-action methods for huge and sparse systems and their applications. *SIAM Rev.*, 23:444–466, 1981.
42. Y. Censor. Mathematical optimization for the inverse problem of intensity-modulated radiation therapy. In J.R. Palta and T.R. Mackie, editors, *Intensity-Modulated Radiation Therapy: The State of the Art*, pages 25–49. Medical Physics Publishing, 2003.
43. Y. Censor, M.D. Altschuler, and W.D. Powlis. On the use of Cimmino's simultaneous projections method for computing a solution of the inverse problem in radiation therapy treatment planning. *Inverse Problems*, 4:607–623, 1988.
44. Y. Censor, T. Elfving, and G.T. Herman. A method of iterative data refinement and it applications. *Math. Methods Appl. Sci*, 7:108–123, 1985.
45. Y. Censor, T. Elfving, G.T. Herman, and T. Nikazad. On diagonally-relaxed orthogonal projection methods. *SIAM J. Sci. Comput.*, 30:473–504, 2008.
46. Y. Censor and G.T. Herman. Row-generation methods for feasibility and optimization problems involving sparse matrices and their applications. In I.S. Duff and G.W. Stewart, editors, *Sparse Matrix Proceedings 1978*, pages 197–219. SIAM, 1979.
47. Y. Censor and G.T. Herman. Block-iterative algorithms with underrelaxed Bregman projections. *SIAM J. Opt.*, 13:283–297, 2002.
48. Y. Censor and S.A. Zenios. *Parallel Optimization: Theory, Algorithms and Applications*. Oxford University Press, 1998.
49. T. Chang and G.T. Herman. A scientific study of filter selection for a fan-beam convolution algorithm. *SIAM J. Appl. Math.*, 39:83–105, 1980.

50. A.C.M. Chen, W.H. Berninger, R.W. Redington, R. Godbarsen, and P. Barrett. Five-second fan beam CT scanner. *Proc. SPIE*, 96:294–298, 1976.
51. L.S. Chen, G.T. Herman, R.A. Reynolds, and J.K. Udupa. Surface shading in the cuberille environment (erratum appeared in 6(2):67-69, 1986). *IEEE Comput. Graph. Appl.*, 5(12):33–43, 1985.
52. D.A. Chesler and S.J. Riederer. Ripple suppression during reconstruction in transverse tomography. *Phys. Med. Biol.*, 20:632–636, 1975.
53. S. Chiang, C. Cardi, S. Matej, H. Zhuang, A. Newberg, A. Alavi, and J.S. Karp. Clinical validation of fully 3-D versus 2.5-D RAMLA reconstruction on the Phillips-ADAC CPET PET scanner. *Nucl. Med. Comm.*, 25:1103–1107, 2004.
54. E.E. Christensen, T.S. Curry III, and J. Nunnally. *An Introduction to the Physics of Diagnostic Radiology.* Lea and Febiger, 1973.
55. G. Cimmino. Calcolo approssimato per le soluzioni dei sistemi di equazioni lineari. *La Ricerca Scientifica, XVI, Series II, Anno IX*, 1:326–333, 1938.
56. I. Cohen and D. Gordon. VS: A surface-based system for topological analysis, quantization and visualization of voxel data. *Med. Image Anal.*, 13:245–256, 2009.
57. A.M. Cormack. Representation of a function by its line integrals, with some radiological applications. *J. Appl. Phys.*, 34:2722–2727, 1963.
58. C.R. Crawford and K.F. King. Computed-tomography scanning with simultaneous patient motion. *Med. Phys.*, 17:967–982, 1990.
59. F. Crepaldi and A.R. De Pierro. Activity and attenuation reconstruction for positron emission tomography using emission data only via maximum likelihood and iterative data refinement. *IEEE T. Nucl. Sci.*, 54:100–106, 2007.
60. R.A. Crowther, D.J. DeRosier, and A. Klug. The reconstruction of a three-dimensional structure from projections and its application to electron microscopy. *Proc. R. Soc. Lon. Ser.-A*, A317:319–340, 1970.
61. R. Davidi, G.T. Herman, and J. Klukowska. SNARK09: A Programming System for the Reconstruction of 2D Images from 1D Projections. Technical report, The CUNY Institute for Software Design and Development, http://www.snark09.com/SNARK09.pdf, 2009.
62. P.J. Davis and P. Rabinowitz. *Methods of Numerical Integration.* Academic Press, 2nd edition, 1967.
63. E. Davison and F.A. Grunbaum. Convolution algorithms for arbitrary projection angles. *IEEE T. Nucl. Sci.*, 26:2670–2673, 1979.
64. A.R. De Pierro and A.N. Iusem. On the asymptotic behavior of some alternate smoothing series expansion iterative methods. *Lin. Alg. Appl.*, 130:3–24, 1990.
65. D.J. DeRosier and A. Klug. Reconstruction of three-dimensional structures from electron micrographs. *Nature*, 217:130–134, 1968.
66. N.A. Diakopoulos and P.D. Stephenson. Anti-aliased lines using run-masks. *Comput. Graph. Forum*, 24:165–172, 2005.
67. C.A. Dietrich, C.E. Scheidegger, J. Schreiner, J.L.D. Comba, L.P. Nedel, and C.T. Silva. Edge transformations for improving mesh quality of marching cubes. *IEEE T. Visual. Comput. Graph.*, 15:150–159, 2009.
68. J.T. Dobbins III and D.J. Godfrey. Digital x-ray tomosynthesis: Current state of the art and clinical potential. *Phys. Med. Biol.*, 48:R65–R106, 2003.
69. P. Dreike and D.P. Boyd. Convolution reconstruction of fan beam projections. *Comput. Graph. Image Proc.*, 5:459–469, 1976.

70. L.S. Edelheit, G.T. Herman, and A.V. Lakshminarayanan. Reconstruction of objects from diverging x-rays. *Med. Phys.*, 4:226–231, 1977.
71. P. Edholm, G.T. Herman, and D.A. Roberts. Image reconstruction from linograms: Implementation and evaluation. *IEEE T. Med. Imag.*, 7:239–246, 1988.
72. P.R. Edholm and G.T. Herman. Linograms in image reconstruction from projections. *IEEE T. Med. Imag.*, 6:301–307, 1987.
73. P.P.B. Eggermont, G.T. Herman, and A. Lent. Iterative algorithms for large partitioned linear systems, with applications to image reconstruction. *Lin. Alg. Appl.*, 40:37–67, 1981.
74. T. Elfving. On some methods for entropy maximization and matrix scaling. *Lin. Alg. Appl.*, 34:321–339, 1980.
75. C.S. Epstein. *Introduction to the Mathematics of Medical Imaging.* SIAM, 2nd edition, 2007.
76. B.B. Ertl-Wagner, J.D. Blume, D. Peck, J.K. Udupa, B. Herman, A. Levering, and I.M. Schmalfuss. Reliability of tumor volume estimation from MR images in patients with malignant glioma. Results from the American College of Radiology Imaging Network (ACRIN) 6662 Trial. *Euro. Radiol.*, 19:599–609, 2009.
77. R.D. Evans. *The Atomic Nucleus.* McGraw-Hill, 1955.
78. H. Fahimi and A. Macovski. Reducing the effects of scattered photons in x-ray projection imaging. *IEEE T. Med. Imag.*, 8:56–63, 1989.
79. A. Faridani, R. Hass, and D.C. Solmon. Numerical and theoretical explorations in helical and fan-beam tomography. *J. Phys. Conf. Ser.*, 124:012024, 2008.
80. J.-J. Fernandez, D. Gordon, and R. Gordon. Efficient parallel implementation of iterative reconstruction algorithms for electron tomography. *J. Par. Dist. Comput.*, 68:626–640, 2008.
81. S. Fourey and R. Malgouyres. Normals estimation for digital surfaces based on convolutions. *Comput. & Graph.*, 33:2–10, 2009.
82. K. Fourmont. Non-equispaced fast Fourier transform with applications to tomography. *J. Fourier Anal. Appl.*, 9:431–450, 2003.
83. J. Frank. *Electron Tomography: Methods for Three-Dimensional Visualization of Structures in the Cell.* Springer, 2nd edition, 2006.
84. J. Frank. *Three-Dimensional Electron Microscopy of Macromolecular Assemblies: Visualization of Biological Molecules in their Native State.* Oxford University Press, 2006.
85. R.A. Frazin. Tomography of the solar corona. I. A robust regularized, positive estimation method. *Astrophys. J.*, 530:1026–1035, 2000.
86. H. Fuchs, Z.M. Kedem, and S.P. Uselton. Optimal surface reconstruction from planar contours. *Commun. ACM*, 20:693–702, 1977.
87. M.J. Gallagher and G.L. Raff. Use of multislice CT for the evaluation of emergency room patients with chest pain: the so-called "Triple Rule-Out". *Catheter. Cardio. Inte.*, 71:92–99, 2008.
88. H.W. Gao, L. Zhang, Y.X. Xing, Z.Q. Chen, and J.P. Cheng. An improved form of linogram algorithm for image reconstruction. *IEEE T. Nucl. Sci.*, 55:552–559, 2008.
89. E. Garduño and G.T. Herman. Implicit surface visualization of reconstructed biological molecules. *Theor. Comput. Sci.*, 346:281–299, 2005.
90. E. Garduño and G.T. Herman. Parallel fuzzy segmentation of multiple objects. *Internat. J. Imag. Syst. Tech.*, 18:336–344, 2008.

91. A.P. Gibson, J.C. Hebden, and S.R. Arridge. Recent advances in diffuse optical tomography. *Phys. Med. Biol.*, 50:R1–R43, 2005.
92. B.K. Gilbert, A. Chu, D.E. Atkins, E.E. Schwartzlander, and E.L. Ritman. Ultra high speed transaxial image reconstruction of the heart, lung and circulation via numerical approximation methods and optimized processor architecture. *Comput. Biomed. Res.*, 12:17–38, 1979.
93. P. Gilbert. Iterative methods for the three-dimensional reconstruction of an object from projections. *J. Theor. Biol.*, 36:105–117, 1972.
94. W.V. Glenn, R.J. Johnston, P.E. Morton, and S.J. Dwyer. Image generation and display techniques for CT scan data. *Invest. Radiol.*, 10:403–416, 1975.
95. G. Glover and N. Pelc. The nonlinear partial volume artifact. *J. Comput. Assist. Tomo.*, 3:573–574, 1979.
96. W.C. Godoi, K. de Geus, V. Swinka-Filho, and R.R. de Silva. Volumetric and surface measurements of flows in polymeric insulators using X-ray computed tomography. *Insight*, 50:554–559, 2008.
97. T.A. Gooley and H.H. Barrett. Evaluation of statistical methods for image reconstruction through ROC analysis. *IEEE T. Med. Imag.*, 11:276–282, 1992.
98. R. Gordon. A tutorial on ART (Algebraic Reconstruction Techniques). *IEEE T. Nucl. Sci.*, 21:78–93, 1974.
99. R. Gordon, R. Bender, and G.T. Herman. Algebraic Reconstruction Techniques (ART) for three-dimensional electron microscopy and x-ray photography. *J. Theor. Biol.*, 29:471–481, 1970.
100. R. Gordon and G.T. Herman. Three-dimensional reconstruction from projections: a review of algorithms. In G.H. Bourne and J.F. Danielli, editors, *International Review of Cytology*, pages 111–151. Academic Press, 1974.
101. J.F. Greenleaf, S.A. Johnson, S. Lee, E.H. Wood, and G.T. Herman. Algebraic reconstruction of spatial distributions of acoustic absorption within tissue from their two-dimensional acoustic projections. In P. Green, editor, *Acoustical Holography*, pages 591–603. Springer-Verlag, 1974.
102. J.F. Greenleaf, J.S. Tu, and E.H. Wood. Computer generated three-dimensional oscilloscopic images and associated techniques for display and study of the spatial distribution of pulmonary blood flow. *IEEE T. Nucl. Sci.*, 17:353–359, 1970.
103. L.G. Gubin, B.T. Polyak, and E.V. Raik. The method of projections for finding a common point of convex sets. *USSR Comput. Math. Math. Phys.*, 7:1–24, 1967.
104. G.T. Gullberg. The reconstruction of fan-beam data by filtering back-projection. *Comput. Graph. Image Proc.*, 10:30–47, 1979.
105. P.R. Halmos. *Finite-Dimensional Vector Spaces.* Van Nostrand-Reinhold, 2nd edition, 1958.
106. C. Hamaker and D.C. Solomon. The angles between the null spaces of x-rays. *J. Math. Anal. Appl.*, 62:1–23, 1978.
107. K.M. Hanson. Method of evaluating image-recovery algorithms based on task performance. *J. Opt. Soc. Am. A*, 7:1294–1304, 1990.
108. G.T. Herman. Two direct methods for reconstruction pictures from their projections: a comparative study. *Comput. Graph. Image Proc.*, 1:123–144, 1972.
109. G.T. Herman. Reconstruction of binary patterns from a few projections. In A. Gunther, B. Levrat, and H. Lipps, editors, *International Computing Symposium*, pages 371–379. North-Holland Publ., 1973.

110. G.T. Herman. A relaxation method for reconstructing objects from noisy x-rays. *Math. Program.*, 8:1–19, 1975.
111. G.T. Herman. Correction for beam hardening in computed tomography. *Phys. Med. Biol.*, 24:81–106, 1979.
112. G.T. Herman. Demonstration of beam hardening correction in computerized reconstruction of the head. *J. Comput. Assist. Tomo.*, 3:373–378, 1979.
113. G.T. Herman. *Image Reconstruction from Projections: Implementation and Applications.* Springer-Verlag, 1979.
114. G.T. Herman. On modifications to the algebraic reconstruction techniques. *Comput. Biol. Med.*, 9:271–276, 1979.
115. G.T. Herman. Advanced principles of reconstructing algorithms. In T.H. Newton and D.G. Potts, editors, *Radiology of Skull and Brain*, volume 5: Technical Aspects of Computed Tomography, pages 3888–3903. C.V. Mosby Company, 1981.
116. G.T. Herman. Image reconstruction from projections. *Real-Time Imag.*, 1:3–18, 1995.
117. G.T. Herman. Algebraic reconstruction techniques in medical imaging. In C.T. Leondes, editor, *Medical Imaging Systems Techniques and Applications: Computational Techniques*, pages 1–42. Gordon and Breach, 1998.
118. G.T. Herman. *Geometry of Digital Spaces.* Birkhäuser, 1998.
119. G.T. Herman. Boundaries in digital spaces. *Appl. Gen. Topol.*, 8:93–149, 2007.
120. G.T. Herman and W. Chen. A fast algorithm for solving a linear feasibility problem with application to intensity-modulated radiation therapy. *Lin. Alg. Appl.*, 428:1207–1217, 2008.
121. G.T. Herman and R. Davidi. On image reconstruction from a small number of projections. *Inverse Problems*, 24:045011, 2008.
122. G.T. Herman, A.R. De Pierro, and N. Gai. On methods for maximum a posteriori image reconstruction with a normal prior. *J. Vis. Com. Imag. Rep.*, 3:316–324, 1992.
123. G.T. Herman, H. Hurwitz, and A. Lent. A storage efficient algorithm for finding the regularized solution of a large inconsistent system of equations. *IMA J. Appl. Math.*, 25:361–366, 1980.
124. G.T. Herman, H. Hurwitz, A. Lent, and H.P. Lung. On the Bayesian approach to image reconstruction. *Inform. Control.*, 42:60–71, 1979.
125. G.T. Herman and A. Kuba. *Advances in Discrete Tomography and Its Applications.* Birkhäuser, 2007.
126. G.T. Herman, A.V. Lakshminarayanan, and S.W. Rowland. The reconstruction of objects from shadowgraphs with high contrast. *Pattern Recognition*, 7:157–165, 1975.
127. G.T. Herman and A. Lent. Iterative reconstruction algorithms. *Comput. Biol. Med.*, 6:273–294, 1976.
128. G.T. Herman and A. Lent. Quadratic optimization for image reconstruction I. *Comput. Graph. Image Proc.*, 5:319–332, 1976.
129. G.T. Herman and A. Lent. A family of iterative quadratic optimization algorithms for pairs of inequalities with application in diagnostic radiology. *Math. Program. Stud.*, 9:15–29, 1978.
130. G.T. Herman, A. Lent, and P.H. Lutz. Relaxation methods for image reconstruction. *Commun. ACM.*, 21:152–158, 1978.
131. G.T. Herman and R.M. Lewitt. Evaluation of a preprocessing algorithm for truncated CT projections. *J. Comput. Assist. Tomo.*, 5:127–135, 1981.

132. G.T. Herman and H.K. Liu. Display of three-dimensional information in computed tomography. *J. Comput. Assist. Tomo.*, 1:155–160, 1977.
133. G.T. Herman and H.K. Liu. Three-dimensional display of human organs from computed tomograms. *Comput. Graph. Image Proc.*, 9:1–21, 1979.
134. G.T. Herman and H.P. Lung. Reconstruction from divergent beams: a comparison of algorithms with and without rebinning. *Comput. Biol. Med.*, 10:131–139, 1980.
135. G.T. Herman and L.B. Meyer. Algebraic reconstruction techniques can be made computationally efficient. *IEEE T. Med. Imag.*, 12:600–609, 1993.
136. G.T. Herman and A. Naparstek. Fast image reconstruction based on a Radon inversion formula appropriate for rapidly collected data. *SIAM J. Appl. Math.*, 33:511–533, 1977.
137. G.T. Herman and D. Odhner. Performance evaluation of iterative image reconstruction algorithms for positron emission tomography. *IEEE T. Med. Imag.*, 10:336–346, 1991.
138. G.T. Herman and S.W. Rowland. Three methods for reconstructing objects from x-rays: a comparative study. *Comput. Graph. Image Proc.*, 2:151–178, 1973.
139. G.T. Herman, S.W. Rowland, and M.M. Yau. A comparative study of the use of linear and modified cubic spline interpolation for image reconstruction. *IEEE T. Nucl. Sci.*, 26:2879–2894, 1979.
140. G.T. Herman and R.G. Simmons. Illustration of a beam hardening correction method in computerized tomography. *Proc. SPIE*, 173:264–270, 1979.
141. G.T. Herman and S.S. Trivedi. A comparative study of two postreconstuction beam hardening correction methods. *IEEE T. Med. Imag.*, 2:128–135, 1983.
142. G.T. Herman and H.K. Tuy. Image reconstruction from projections: An approach from mathematical analysis. In P.C. Sabatier, editor, *Basic Methods of Tomography and Inverse Problems*, pages 1–124. Institute of Physics Publishing, 1988.
143. G.T. Herman, H.K. Tuy, K.J. Langenberg, and P.C. Sabatier. *Basic Methods of Tomography and Inverse Problems.* Institute of Physics Publishing, 1988.
144. G.T. Herman and K.T.D. Yeung. Evaluators of image reconstruction algorithms. *Internat. J. Imag. Syst. Tech*, 1:187–195, 1989.
145. G.N. Hounsfield. A method and apparatus for examination of a body by radiation such as x or gamma radiation. Patent Specification 1283915, The Patent Office, London, England, 1972.
146. G.N. Hounsfield. Computerized transverse axial scanning tomography: Part I, description of the system. *Brit. J. Radiol.*, 46:1016–1022, 1973.
147. H.M. Hudson and R.S. Larkin. Accelerated image reconstruction using ordered subsets of projection data. *IEEE T. Med. Imag.*, 13:601–609, 1994.
148. A.A. Isola, A. Ziegler, T. Koehler, W.J. Niessen, and M. Grass. Motion-compensated iterative cone-beam CT image reconstruction with adapted blobs as basis functions. *Phys. Med. Biol.*, 53:6777–6797, 2008.
149. S. Jin, O.F. Luo, and P. Park. GPS observations of the ionospheric F2-layer behavior during the 20th November 2003 geomagnetic storm over South Korea. *J. Geod.*, 82:883–892, 2008.
150. G. Johnson, A. King, M.G. Honnicke, J. Marrow, and W. Ludwig. X-ray diffraction contrast tomography: a novel technique for three-dimensional grain mapping of polycrystals. II. The combined case. *J. Appl. Cryst.*, 41:310–318, 2008.

151. S.A. Johnson, T. Abbott, R. Bell, M. Berggren, D. Borup, D. Robinson, J. Wiskin, S. Olsen, and B. Hanover. Non-invasive breast tissue characterization using ultrasound speed and attenuation. In M.P. André, editor, *Acoustical Imaging*, volume 28, pages 147–154. Springer, 2007.
152. P.M. Joseph. Sampling errors in projection reconstruction MRI. *Magn. Reson. Med.*, 40:460–466, 1998.
153. P.M. Joseph and R.D. Spital. A method for correcting bone induced artifacts in computed tomography scanners. *J. Comput. Assist. Tomo.*, 2:100–108, 1978.
154. S. Kaczmarz. Angenäherte Auflösung von Systemen linearer Gleichungen. *Bull. Internat. Acad. Polo. Sci. Lettres. A.*, 35:355–357, 1937.
155. W.A. Kalender. *Computed Tomography: Fundamentals, System Technology, Image Quality, Applications.* Wiley-VCH, 2nd edition, 2006.
156. W.A. Kalender, W. Seissler, E. Klotz, and P. Vock. Spiral volumetric CT with single-breath-hold technique, continuous transport, and continuous scanner rotation. *Radiology*, 176:181–183, 1990.
157. A. Katsevich. Theoretically exact filtered backprojection-type inversion algorithm for spiral CT. *SIAM J. Appl. Math.*, 62:2012–2026, 2002.
158. M.B. Katz. *Questions of Uniqueness and Resolution in Reconstruction from Projections.* Springer-Verlag, 1978.
159. S. Kawata and J. Sklansky. Elimination of nonpivotal plane images from x-ray motion tomograms. *IEEE T. Med. Imag.*, 4:153–159, 1985.
160. P.E. Kinahan, S. Matej, J.P. Karp, G.T. Herman, and R.M. Lewitt. A comparison of transform and iterative reconstruction techniques for a volume-imaging PET scanner with a large axial acceptance angle. *IEEE T. Nucl. Sci.*, 42:2181–2287, 1995.
161. A.N. Kolmogorov and S.V. Fomin. *Elements of the Theory of Functions and Functional Analysis.* Dover Publications, 1999.
162. A.B. Konovalov, V.V. Vlasov, D.V. Mogilenskikh, O.V. Kravtsenyuk, and V.V. Lyubimov. Algebraic reconstruction and postprocessing in one-step diffuse optical tomography. *Quant. Electr.*, 38:588–596, 2008.
163. M. Krumm, S. Kasperl, and M. Franz. Reducing non-linear artifacts of multi-material objects in industrial 3D computed tomography. *NDT&E Internat.*, 41:242–251, 2008.
164. D.E. Kuhl and R.Q. Edwards. Image separation radioisotope scanning. *Radiology*, 80:653–662, 1963.
165. J.-O. Lachaud and A. Montevert. Continuous analogs of digital boundaries: A topological approach to isosurfaces. *Graph. Models*, 62:129–164, 2000.
166. A.V. Lakshminarayanan and A. Lent. Methods of least squares and SIRT in reconstruction. *J. Theor. Biol.*, 76:267–295, 1979.
167. L. Landweber. An iterative formula for Fredholm integral equations of the first kind. *Amer. J. Math.*, 73:615–624, 1951.
168. K.J. Langenberg. Applied inverse problems for accoustic, electromagnetic and elastic wave scattering. In P.C. Sabatier, editor, *Basic Methods of Tomography and Inverse Problems*, pages 125–467. Institute of Physics Publishing, 1988.
169. D.J. Larkman and R.G. Nunes. Parallel magnetic resonance imaging. *Phys. Med. Biol.*, 52:R15–R55, 2007.
170. P.C. Lauterbur. Medical imaging by nuclear magnetic resonance zeugmatography. *IEEE T. Nucl. Sci.*, 26:2808–2811, 1979.
171. R.S. Ledley, G. Di Chiro, A.J. Luessenhop, and H.L. Twigg. Computerized transaxial X-ray tomography of the human body. *Science*, 186:207–212, 1974.

172. J.M. Lees. Seismic tomography of magmatic systems. *J. Volcanol. Geotherm. Res.*, 167:37–56, 2007.
173. E. Lehmann and N. Kardjilov. Neutron absorption tomography. In J. Banhart, editor, *Advanced Tomographic Methods in Materials Research*, pages 375–408. Oxford University Press, 2007.
174. S. Leng, J. Tang, J. Zambelli, B. Nett, R. Tolakanahalli, and G.H. Chen. High temporal resolution and streak-free four-dimensional cone-beam computed tomography. *Phys. Med. Biol.*, 53:5653–5673, 2008.
175. S. Leng, J. Zambelli, R. Tolakanahalli, B. Nett, P. Munro, J. Star-Lack, B. Paliwal, and G.H. Chen. Streaking artifacts reduction in four-dimensional cone-beam computed tomography. *Med. Phys.*, 35:4649–4659, 2008.
176. A. Lent. A convergent algorithm for maximum entropy image restoration, with a medical x-ray application. In R. Shaw, editor, *Image Analysis and Evaluation*, pages 249–257. Society of Photographic Scientists and Engineers, 1977.
177. A. Lent and Y. Censor. Extensions of Hildreth's row generation method for quadratic programming. *SIAM J. Control Optim.*, 18:444–454, 1980.
178. A. Lent and Y. Censor. The primal-dual algorithm constraint-set-manipulation device. *Math. Program.*, 50:343–357, 1991.
179. A. Lent and H. Tuy. An iterative method for the extrapolation of band-limited functions. *J. Math. Anal. Appl.*, 83:554–565, 1981.
180. R.D. Levine and M. Tribus, editors. *The Maximum Entropy Formalism*. MIT Press, 1979.
181. E. Levitan and G.T. Herman. A maximum a posteriori probability expectation maximization algorithm for image reconstruction in emission tomography. *IEEE T. Med. Imag.*, 6:185–192, 1987.
182. R.M. Lewitt. Processing of incomplete measurement data in computed tomography. *Med. Phys.*, 6:412–417, 1979.
183. R.M. Lewitt. Multidimensional digital image representation using generalized Kaiser-Bessel window functions. *J. Opt. Soc. Am. A*, 7:1834–1846, 1990.
184. R.M. Lewitt. Alternatives to voxels for image representation in iterative reconstruction algorithms. *Phys. Med. Biol.*, 37:705–716, 1992.
185. H.Y. Liao and G.T. Herman. A method for reconstructing label images from a few projections, as motivated by electron microscopy. *Ann. Oper. Res.*, 148:117–132, 2006.
186. H.K. Liu. Two- and three-dimensional boundary detection. *Comput. Graph. Image Proc.*, 6:123–134, 1977.
187. W. Lorensen and H. Cline. Marching cubes: A high-resolution 3D surface reconstruction algorithm. *Comput. Graph.*, 21(4):163–169, 1987.
188. D. Ludwig. The Radon transform on Euclidean space. *Commun. Pur. Appl. Math.*, 19:49–81, 1966.
189. W. Ludwig, P. Reischig, A. King, M. Herbig, E.M. Lauridsen, G. Johnson, T.J. Marrow, and J.Y. Buffière. Three-dimensional grain mapping by x-ray diffraction contrast tomography and the use of Friedel pairs in diffraction data analysis. *Rev. Sci. Instrum.*, 80:033905, 2009.
190. D.G. Luenberger. *Optimization by Vector Space Methods*. Wiley, 1969.
191. A. Macovski, R.E. Alvarez, J.L.-H. Chan, J.P. Stonestrom, and L.M. Zatz. Energy dependent reconstruction in x-ray computerized tomography. *Comput. Biol. Med.*, 6:325–336, 1976.

192. D.D. Maki, B.A. Birnbaum, D.P. Chakraborty, J.E. Jacobs, B.M. Carvalho, and G.T. Herman. Renal cyst pseudo-enhancement: Beam hardening effects on CT numbers. *Radiology*, 213:468–472, 1999.
193. S.H. Manglos, D.A. Bassano, F.D. Thomas, and Z.D. Grossman. Imaging of the human torso using cone-beam transmission CT implemented on a rotating gamma camera. *J. Nucl. Med.*, 33:150–156, 1992.
194. R. Marabini, G.T. Herman, and J.-M. Carazo. 3D reconstruction in electron microscopy using ART with smooth spherically symmetric volume elements (blobs). *Ultramicroscopy*, 72:53–65, 1998.
195. R. Marabini, E. Rietzel, R. Schroeder, G.T. Herman, and J.M. Carazo. Three-dimensional reconstruction from reduced sets of very noisy images acquired following a single-axis tilt schema: Application of a new three-dimensional reconstruction algorithm and objective comparison with weighted backprojection. *J. Struct. Biol.*, 120:363–371, 1997.
196. R. Marabini, C.O.S. Sorzano, S. Matej, J.J. Fernández, and G.T. Herman. 3D reconstruction of 2D crystals in real space. *IEEE T. Image Proc.*, 13:549–561, 2004.
197. S. Matej, S.S. Furuie, and G.T. Herman. Relevance of statistically significant differences between reconstruction algorithms. *IEEE T. Image Proc.*, 5:554–556, 2006.
198. S. Matej, G.T. Herman, T.K. Narayan, S.S. Furuie, R.M. Lewitt, and P.E. Kinahan. Evaluation of task-oriented performance of several fully 3D PET reconstruction algorithms. *Phys. Med. Biol.*, 39:355–367, 1994.
199. S. Matej and R.M. Lewitt. Efficient 3-D grids for image reconstruction using spherically symmetrical volume elements. *IEEE T. Nucl. Sci.*, 42:1361–1370, 1995.
200. S. Matej and R.M. Lewitt. Practical consideration for 3D image-reconstruction using spherically-symmetrical volume elements. *IEEE T. Med. Imag.*, 15:68–78, 1996.
201. R.M. Mersereau. Direct Fourier transform techniques in 3-D image reconstruction. *Comput. Biol. Med.*, 6:247–258, 1976.
202. C.E. Metz. Some practical isues of experimental design and data analysis in radiological ROC studies. *Invest. Radiol.*, 24:234–243, 1989.
203. G. Minerbo. MENT: A maximum entropy algorithm for reconstructing a source from projection data. *Comput. Graph. Image Proc.*, 10:48–68, 1979.
204. W.E. Moore and G.P. Garmire. The X-ray structure of the Vela supernova remnant. *Astrophys. J.*, 199:680–690, 1975.
205. R.F. Mould. *Introductory Medical Statistics.* Taylor & Francis, 3rd edition, 1998.
206. K. Mueller and R. Yagel. Rapid 3-D cone-beam reconstruction with the Simultaneous Algebraic Reconstruction Technique (SART) using 2-D texture mapping hardware. *IEEE T. Med. Imag.*, 19:1227–1237, 2000.
207. G.R. Myers, T.E. Guryev, D.M. Paganin, and S.C. Mayo. The binary dissector: phase contrast tomography of two- and three-material objects from few projections. *Opt. Express*, 16:10736–10749, 2008.
208. O. Nalcioglu, Z.H. Cho, and R.Y. Lou. Limited field of view reconstruction in computerized tomography. *IEEE T. Nucl. Sci.*, 26:546–551, 1979.
209. J. Näppi and H. Yoshida. Adaptive correction of pseudo-enhancement of CT attenuation for fecal-tagging CT colonography. *Med. Image Anal.*, 12:413–426, 2008.

210. T.K. Narayan and G.T. Herman. Prediction of human observer performance by numerical observers: an experimental study. *J. Opt. Soc. Am. A*, 16:679–693, 1999.
211. F. Natterer and F. Wübbeling. *Mathematical Methods in Image Reconstruction.* SIAM, 2001.
212. F. Noo, J. Pack, and D. Heuscher. Exact helical reconstruction using native cone-beam geometries. *Phys. Med. Biol.*, 48:3787–3818, 2003.
213. W.H. Oldendorf. Isolated flying-spot detection of radiodensity discontinuities; displaying the internal structural pattern of a complex object. *IRE T. Biomed. Electr.*, BME-8:68–72, 1961.
214. N. Oliveira, N. Matela, R. Bugalho, N. Ferreira, and P. Almeida. Optimization of 2D image reconstruction for positron emission mammography using IDL. *Comput. Biol. Med.*, 39:119–129, 2009.
215. J.R. Palta and T.R. Mackie. *Intensity-Modulated Radiation Therapy: The State of the Art.* Medical Physics Publishing, 2003.
216. D.Y. Parkison, G. McDermott, L.D. Etkin, M.A. Le Gros, and C.A. Larabell. Quantitative 3-D imaging of eukaryotic cells using soft X-ray tomography. *J. Struct. Biol.*, 162:380–386, 2008.
217. E. Parzen. *Modern Probability Theory and Its Applications.* Wiley, 1960.
218. J. Pavkovich. Apparatus and method for reconstructing data. U.S. Patent Office, Washington DC, 1979. U.S. Patent 4,149,248.
219. M.E. Phelps, E.J. Hoffman, and M.M. Ter-Pogossian. Attenuation coefficients of various body tissues, fluids, and lesions at photon energies of 18 to 136 keV. *Radiology*, 117:573–583, 1975.
220. C. Popa. Constrained Kaczmarz extended algorithm for image reconstruction. *Lin. Alg. Appl.*, 429:2247–2267, 2008.
221. H.F. Poulsen. *Three-Dimensional X-Ray Diffraction Microscopy: Mapping Polycrystals and Their Dynamics.* Springer-Verlag, 2004.
222. F. Prino, C. Ceballos, A. Cabal, A. Samelli, M. Gambaccini, and L. Ramello. Effect of x-ray energy dispersion in digital subtraction imaging of the iodine K-edge – A Monte Carlo study. *Med. Phys.*, 35:13–24, 2008.
223. L.R. Rabiner and B. Gold. *Theory and Application of Digital Signal Processing.* Prentice-Hall, 1975.
224. M. Radermacher. Weighted back-projection methods. In J. Frank, editor, *Electron Tomography: Methods for Three-Dimensional Visualization of Structures in the Cell*, pages 245–274. Springer, 2nd edition, 2006.
225. J. Radon. Über die Bestimmung von Funktionen durch ihre Integralwerte längs gewisser Mannigfaltigkeiten. *Ber. Verh. Sächs. Akad. Wiss., Leipzig, Math. Phys. Kl.*, 69:262–277, 1917.
226. A. Ralston, E.D. Reilly, and D. Hemmendinger, editors. *Encyclopedia of Computer Science.* Wiley, 4th edition, 2000.
227. G.N. Ramachandran and A.V. Lakshminarayanan. Three-dimensional reconstruction from radiographs and electron micrographs: application of convolutions instead of Fourier transforms. *P. Natl. Acad. Sci. USA.*, 68:2236–2240, 1971.
228. V.R. Ravindran, C. Sreelakshmi, and S. Vibinkumar. Digital radiography-based 3D-CT imaging for the NDE of solid rocket propellant systems. *Insight*, 50:564–568, 2008.
229. J. Raviv, J.F. Greenleaf, and G.T. Herman. *Computer Aided Tomography and Ultrasonics in Medicine.* North-Holland, 1979.

230. A.J. Reader. The promise of new PET image reconstruction. *Physica Medica*, 24:49–56, 2008.
231. E.L. Ritman, R.A. Robb, and L.D. Harris. *Imaging Physiological Functions: Experience with the Dynamic Spatial Reconstructor*. Praeger, 1985.
232. E.L. Ritman, R.A. Robb, S.A. Johnson, P.A. Chevalier, B.K. Gilbert, J.F. Greenleaf, R.E. Strum, and E.H. Wood. Quantitative imaging of the structure and function of the heart, lungs and circulation. *Mayo Clin. Proc.*, 53:3–11, 1978.
233. L. Rodek, H.F. Poulsen, E. Knudsen, and G.T. Herman. A stochastic algorithm for the reconstruction of grain maps of moderately deformed specimens based on X-ray diffraction. *J. Appl. Cryst.*, 40:313–321, 2007.
234. S.W. Rowland. Computer implementation of image reconstruction formulas. In G.T. Herman, editor, *Image Reconstruction from Projections: Implementation and Applications*, pages 9–80. Springer-Verlag, 1979.
235. A.P. Sage and J.L. Melsa. *Estimation Theory with Application to Communications and Control*. McGraw-Hill, 1971.
236. C. San Martín, J.N. Glasgow, A. Borovjagin, M.S. Beatty, E.A. Kashentseva, D.T. Curiel, R. Marabini, and I.P. Dimitriev. Localization of the N-terminus of minor coat protein IIIa in the adenovirus capsid. *J. Mol. Biol.*, 383:923–934, 2008.
237. S.H.W. Scheres, H. Gao, M. Valle, G.T. Herman, P.P.B. Eggermont, J. Frank, and J.-M. Carazo. Disentangling conformational states of macromolecules in 3D-EM through likelihood optimization. *Nat. Methods*, 4:27–29, 2007.
238. S.H.W. Scheres, R. Marabini, S. Lanzavechia, F. Cantele, T. Rutten, S.D. Fuller, J.M. Carazo, R.M. Burnett, and C. San Martín. Classification of single-projection reconstructions for cryo-electron microscopy data of icosahedral viruses. *J. Struct. Biol.*, 151:79–91, 2005.
239. S.H.W. Scheres, R. Nuñez-Ramirez, C.O.S. Sorzano, J.M. Carazo, and R. Marabini. Image processing for electron microscopy single-particle analysis using XMIPP. *Nat. Protocols*, 3:977–990, 2008.
240. R. Schulte, V. Bashkirov, T. Li, J.Z. Liang, K. Mueller, J. Heimann, L.R. Johnson, B. Keeney, H.F.-W. Sadrozinski, A. Seiden, D.C. Williams, L. Zhang, Z. Li, S. Peggs, T. Satogata, and C. Woody. Conceptual design of a proton computed tomography system for applications in proton radiation therapy. *IEEE T. Nucl. Sci.*, 51:866–872, 2004.
241. L.A. Shepp and B.F. Logan. The Fourier reconstruction of a head section. *IEEE T. Nucl. Sci.*, 21:21–43, 1974.
242. L.A. Shepp and Y. Vardi. Maximum likelihood reconstruction for emission tomography. *IEEE T. Med. Imag.*, 1:113–122, 1982.
243. A.R. Smith. Vision 20/20: Proton therapy. *Med. Phys.*, 36:556–568, 2009.
244. K.T. Smith, D.C. Solmon, and S.L. Wagner. Practical and mathematical aspects of the problem of reconstructing objects from radiographs. *B. Am. Math. Soc.*, 83:1227–1270, 1977.
245. K.T. Smith, D.C. Solmon, S.L. Wagner, and C. Hamaker. Mathematical aspects of divergent beam radiography. *P. Natl. Acad. Sci. USA.*, 75:2055–2058, 1978.
246. P.R. Smith, U. Aebi, R. Josephs, and M. Kessel. Studies of the structure of the T4 bacteriophage tail sheath. I. The recovery of three-dimensional information from the extended sheath. *J. Mol. Biol.*, 106:243–275, 1976.

247. P.R. Smith, T.M. Peters, and R.H.T. Bates. Image reconstruction from a finite number of projections. *J. Phys. A*, 6:361–382, 1973.
248. R. Smith and B. Carragher. Software tools for molecular biology. *J. Struct. Biol.*, 163:224–228, 2008.
249. C.O.S. Sorzano, R. Marabini, N. Boisset, E. Rietzel, R. Schröder, G.T. Herman, and J.M. Carazo. The effect of overabundant projection directions on 3D reconstruction algorithms. *J. Struct. Biol.*, 133:108–118, 2001.
250. C.O.S. Sorzano, R. Marabini, G.T. Herman, Y. Censor, and J.M. Carazo. Transfer function restoration in 3D electron microscopy via iterative data refinement. *Phys. Med. Biol.*, 49:509–522, 2004.
251. A. Srivastava, D. Singh, and K. Muralidhar. Reconstruction of time-dependent concentration gradients around a KDP crystal growing from its aqueous solution. *J. Cryst. Growth*, 311:1166–1177, 2009.
252. J.P. Stonestrom and A. Macovski. Scatter considerations in fan beam computerized tomographic systems. *IEEE T. Nucl. Sci.*, 23:1453–1458, 1976.
253. J.W. Strohbehn, H.Y. Carter, B.H. Curren, and E.S. Sternick. Image enhancement of conventional transverse-axial tomograms. *IEEE T. Bio-Med Eng.*, 26:253–262, 1979.
254. J.A. Swets. ROC analysis applied to the evaluation of medical imaging techniques. *Invest. Radiol.*, 14:109–112, 1979.
255. E. Tanaka and T.A. Iinuma. Correction functions for optimizing the reconstructed image in transverse section scan. *Phys. Med. Biol.*, 20:789–798, 1975.
256. M. Tanaka, M. Honda, M. Mitsuhara, S. Hata, K. Kaneko, and K. Higashida. Three-dimensional observation of dislocations by electron tomography in a silicon crystal. *Materials T.*, 49:1953–1956, 2008.
257. J.H. Taylor. Two-dimensional brightness distribution of radio sources from lunar occultation observations. *Astrophys. J.*, 150:421–426, 1967.
258. D. Thomas, P. Bron, T. Weimann, A. Dautant, M.-F. Giraud, P. Paumard, B. Salin, A. Cavalier, J. Velours, and D. Bréthes. Supramolecular organization of the yeast F_1F_0-ATP synthase. *Biol. Cell*, 100:591–601, 2008.
259. M. Tseitlin, T. Czechowski, S.S. Eaton, and G.R. Eaton. Regularized optimization (RO) reconstruction for oximetric EPR imaging. *J. Magn. Reson.*, 194:212–221, 2008.
260. J.K. Udupa and G.T. Herman. *3D Imaging in Medicine*. CRC Press, 2nd edition, 1999.
261. J.K. Udupa, G.T. Herman, L.S. Chen, P.S. Margasayaham, and C.R. Meyer. 3D98: A turnkey system for the 3D display and analysis of medical objects in CT data. *Proc. SPIE*, 671:154–168, 1986.
262. J.K. Udupa and S. Samarasekera. Fuzzy connectedness and object definition: Theory, algorithms, and applications in image segmentation. *Graph. Models Image Proc.*, 58:246–261, 1996.
263. P.E. Valk, D. Delbeke, D.L. Bailey, D.W. Townsend, and M.N. Maisey. *Positron Emission Tomography: Clinical Practice*. Springer-Verlag, 2006.
264. V.S.V.M. Vedula and P. Munshi. An improved algorithm for beam-hardening corrections in experimental X-ray tomography. *NDT&E Internat.*, 41:25–31, 2008.
265. S. Walrand, A. van Dulmen, H. van Rossem, and S. Pauwels. Acquisition of linograms in SPET: implementation and benefits. *Euro. J. Nucl.. Med. Mol. Imag.*, 29:1188–1197, 2002.

266. G. Wang, Y. Yangbo, and H. Yu. Approximate and exact cone-beam reconstruction with standard and non-standard spiral scanning. *Phys. Med. Biol.*, 52:R1–R13, 2007.
267. J. Wang, H. Lu, Z. Liang, D. Eremina, G. Zhang, S. Wang, J. Chen, and J. Manzione. An experimental study on the noise properties of x-ray CT sinogram data in Radon space. *Phys. Med. Biol.*, 53:3327–3341, 2008.
268. S. Webb. *Contemporary IMRT: Developing Physics and Clinical Implementation.* Institute of Physics Publishing, 2005.
269. J. Wiskin, D.T. Borup, S.A. Johnson, M. Berggren, T. Abbott, and R. Hanover. Full-wave, nonlinear, inverse scattering. In M.P. André, editor, *Acoustical Imaging*, volume 28, pages 183–193. Springer, 2007.
270. W. Withayachumnankul, G. M. Png, X. Yin, S. Atakaramians, I. Jones, H. Lin, B.S.Y. Ung, J. Balakrishnan, B.W.-H. Ng, B. Ferguson, S.P. Mickan, B.M. Fischer, and D. Abbott. T-ray sensing and imaging. *Proc. IEEE*, 95:1528–1558, 2007.
271. E.H. Wood. New vistas for the study of structural and functional dynamics of the heart, lungs and circulation by noninvasive numerical tomographic vivisection. *Circulation*, 56:506–520, 1977.
272. E.H. Wood, J.H. Kinsey, R.A. Robb, B.K. Gilbert, L.D. Harris, and E.L. Ritman. Applications of high temporal resolution computerized tomography to physiology and medicine. In G.T. Herman, editor, *Image Reconstruction from Projections: Implementation and Applications*, pages 247–279. Springer-Verlag, 1979.
273. N.A. Worth and T.B. Nickels. Acceleration of Tomo-PIV by estimating the initial volume distribution. *Exp. Fluids*, 45:847–856, 2008.
274. F. Xu and K. Mueller. Accelerating popular tomographic reconstruction algorithms on commodity PC graphics hardware. *IEEE T. Nucl. Sci.*, 52:654–663, 2005.
275. T. Yoshinaga, Y. Imakura, K. Fujimoto, and T. Ueta. Bifurcation analysis of iterative image reconstuction method for computed tomography. *Int. J. Bifurc. Chaos*, 18:1219–1225, 2008.
276. D.M. Young. *Iterative Solution of Large Linear Systems.* Academic Press, 1971.
277. H. Yu, S. Zhao, E.A Hoffman, and G. Wang. Ultra-low dose lung CT perfusion regularized by a previous scan. *Acad. Radiol.*, 16:363–373, 2009.
278. R. Zdunek. On image reconstruction algorithms for binary electromagnetic geotomography. *Theor. Comput. Sci.*, 406:160–170, 2008.
279. J. Zhao, Y. Lu, Y. Jin, E. Bai, and G. Wang. Feldkamp-type reconstruction algorithms for spiral cone-beam CT with variable pitch. *J. X-Ray Sci. Tech.*, 15:177–196, 2007.
280. L. Zhu, L. Lee, Y. Ma, Y. Ye, R. Mazzeo, and L. Xing. Using total-variation regularization for intensity modulated radiation therapy inverse planning with field-specific numbers of segments. *Phys. Med. Biol.*, 53:6653–6672, 2008.

Index